DIAGNOSTIC
ATLAS
of the
HEART

DIAGNOSTIC ATLAS of the HEART

EDITORS

Robert C. Schlant, M.D.
Professor of Medicine (Cardiology)
Emory University School of Medicine
Chief of Cardiology
Grady Memorial Hospital
Atlanta, Georgia

R. Wayne Alexander, M.D., Ph.D.
R. Bruce Logue Professor of Medicine
Director, Division of Cardiology
Emory University School of Medicine
Chief of Cardiology
Emory Hospital and Emory Clinic
Atlanta, Georgia

Martin J. Lipton, M.D.
Professor of Radiology and Medicine
Chairman, Department of Radiology
The University of Chicago
Chicago, Illinois

McGraw-Hill
Health Professions Division

New York   St. Louis   San Francisco   Auckland   Bogotá   Caracas   Lisbon   London   Madrid
Mexico City   Milan   Montreal   New Delhi   San Juan   Singapore   Sydney   Tokyo   Toronto

McGraw-Hill
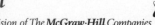
A Division of The **McGraw·Hill** Companies

Diagnostic Atlas of the Heart

1234567890 KGPKGP 9876

ISBN 0-07-055029-8

This book was set in Times Roman by V&M Graphics, Inc.
The editors were Martin J. Wonsiewicz and Muza Navrozov.
The production supervisor was Clare B. Stanley.
The text was designed by José Fonfrias.
The cover and color insert were designed by Marsha Cohen/Parallelogram.
The index was prepared by Geraldine Beckford.
Quebecor Printing/Kingsport was printer and binder.

Library of Congress Cataloging-in-Publication Data

Diagnostic atlas of the heart / editors, Robert C. Schlant, R. Wayne
    Alexander, Martin K. Lipton.
            p. cm.
     Includes bibliographical references and index.
     ISBN 0-07-055029-8 (hardcover : alk. paper)
      1. Heart—Diseases—Diagnosis—Atlases. I. Schlant, Robert C.,
    date. II. Alexander, R. Wayne. III. Lipton, Martin J.
      [DNLM: 1. Heart—Physiopathology—atlases, 2. Heart Diseases—
    diagnosis—atlases. 3. Diagnostic Imaging—atlases. WG 17 D5361
    1996]
    RC683.D462 1996
    616. 1'2075—dc20
    DNLM/DLC
    for Library of Congress

To our families, our patients, and our students

CONTENTS

CONTRIBUTORS*

W. Banks Anderson, Jr., M.D.   [2]
Professor of Ophthalmology
Vice Chairman, The Department of Opthalmology
Duke University Medical Center
Durham, North Carolina

Gerald G. Blackwell, M.D.   [6]
Assistant Professor of Medicine
Clinical Director, Cardiovascular MMR
Department of Medicine, Division of Cardiovascular Disease
University of Alabama
Birmingham, Alabama

Bruce H. Brundage, M.D.   [7]
Professor of Medicine and Radiological Sciences
UCLA School of Medicine
Scientific Director
Saint John's Cardiovascular Research Center
Torrance, California

Roxana Campisi, M.D.   [8]
Postgraduate Researcher
UCLA School of Medicine
Los Angeles, California

John D. Carroll, M.D.   [12]
Associate Professor of Medicine
Director, Hans Hecht Cardiac Catheterization Laboratory
The University of Chicago
Chicago, Illinois

Agustin Castellanos, M.D.   [1]
Professor of Medicine
Director, Clinical Electrophysiology
University of Miami School of Medicine
Miami, Florida

James T. T. Chen, M.D.   [3]
Professor of Radiology
Department of Radiology
Duke University Medical Center
Durham, North Carolina

Shiuh-Yung Chen, Ph.D.   [12]
Assistant Professor of Medicine, Research Associate
The University of Chicago
Chicago, Illinois

Anthony De Franco, M.D.   [9]
Assistant Professor of Medicine
Ohio State University
Cleveland, Ohio

Bart L. Dolmatch, M.D.   [10]
Section Head, Vascular and Interventional Radiology
Cleveland Clinic Foundation
Cleveland, Ohio

Neal L. Eigler, M.D.   [13]
Associate Professor of Medicine
UCLA School of Medicine
Co-Director, Cardiovascular Intervention Center
Cedars-Sinai Medical Center
Los Angeles, California

Joel M. Felner, M.D.   [4]
Associate Dean (Clinical Education)
Professor of Medicine (Cardiology)
Emory University School of Medicine
Atlanta, Georgia

James S. Forrester, M.D.   [13]
Professor of Medicine, Burns and Allen Chair in Cardiology
UCLA School of Medicine
Director, Cardiovascular Research
Cedars-Sinai Medical Center
Los Angeles, California

Steven A. Goldstein, M.D.   [10]
Clinical Professor of Medicine, George Washington University
Director, Noninvasive Cardiology
Washington Hospital Center
Washington, DC

Kenneth R. Hoffmann, Ph.D.   [12]
Assistant Professor of Radiology
The University of Chicago
Chicago, Illinois

* The numbers in brackets following the contributor name refer to chapter(s) written or co-written by the contributor.

Lynne L. Johnson, M.D. [5]
Professor of Medicine, Brown University
Director, Nuclear Cardiology
Rhode Island Hospital
Providence, Rhode Island

Jeffrey A. Leef, M.D. [11]
Assistant Professor of Radiology
Section Chief/Angiography/Interventional
The University of Chicago
Chicago, Illinois

Joseph Lindsay, Jr., M.D. [10]
Director, Section of Cardiology
Washington Hospital Center
Washington, DC

Martin J. Lipton, M.D. [11,12]
Professor of Radiology and Medicine
Chairman, Department of Radiology
The University of Chicago
Chicago, Illinois

Frank Litvack, M.D. [13]
Associate Professor of Medicine
UCLA School of Medicine
Co-Director, Cardiovascular Intervention Center
Cedars-Sinai Medical Center
Los Angeles, California

Song Shou Mao, M.D. [7]
Research Associate
Saint John's Cardiovascular Research Center
Torrance, California

Randolph P. Martin, M.D. [4]
Professor of Medicine (Cardiology)
Associate Dean for Clinical Development
Director of Noninvasive Cardiology
Associate Director of Emory Clinic
Emory University School of Medicine
Atlanta, Georgia

Robert J. Myerburg, M.D. [1]
Professor of Medicine and Physiology
Director, Division of Cardiology
University of Miami School of Medicine
Miami, Florida

Steven E. Nissen, M.D. [9]
Professor of Medicine (Cardiology)
Vice Chairman, Department of Cardiology
Director, Clinical Cardiology
Cleveland Clinic
Cleveland, Ohio

Gerald M. Pohost, M.D. [6]
Mary Gertrude Waters Professor of Cardiovascular Medicine
Director, Division of Cardiovascular Disease
University of Alabama at Birmingham
Birmingham, Alabama

Heinrich R. Schelbert, M.D., Ph.D. [8]
Professor of Pharmacology and Radiological Sciences
Vice Chairman, Department of Pharmacology
Medical Director, Division of Nuclear Medicine
UCLA School of Medicine
Los Angeles, California

Vipul B. Shah, M.D. [4]
Assistant Professor of Medicine
Director of Echocardiography Laboratory
Medical College of Georgia
Augusta, Georgia

Robert J. Siegel, M.D. [13]
Professor of Medicine in Residence
UCLA School of Medicine
Director, Cardiac Noninvasive Laboratory
Division of Cardiology
Cedars-Sinai Medical Center
Los Angeles, California

E. Murat Tuzcu, M.D. [9]
Associate Professor of Medicine
Ohio State University
Staff Cardiologist
Cleveland Clinic
Cleveland, Ohio

Susanne Weismüller, M.D. [8]
Postgraduate Researcher
UCLA School of Medicine
Los Angeles, California

PREFACE

In the last few decades there has been a dramatic increase in the development of our understanding and application of established diagnostic techniques for displaying the function and the anatomic changes of the heart and peripheral circulation. These advances have occurred concurrently with the rapid development of many new techniques for imaging and studying the heart and blood vessels.

The present volume was created in response to these developments. Its goal is to present a relatively concise atlas with illustrations of many of these techniques, including characteristic findings. We hope that this volume will be an extension of the presentations in a general textbook on cardiology. We have purposely omitted a detailed discussion of how a particular procedure is performed, its advantages or disadvantages, its cost-effectiveness, etc. These topics are well discussed in larger cardiology texts or in books devoted either to cardiac imaging or to the individual technique.

Because advances have occurred so fast in so many technologies, it is increasingly difficult to keep abreast of all the exciting diagnostic methods now available. It is our hope that practicing physicians as well as physicians in training will benefit from the open architectural design of this atlas, which provides a rapid guide and reference to the broad spectrum of diagnostic cardiac imaging techniques in the nineties.

We wish to acknowledge with grateful appreciation the efforts of Muza Navrozov and Martin Wonsiewicz of McGraw-Hill in helping to bring this book to publication. In particular, we wish to thank our authors, each of whom is an established authority in his or her field. Each has worked diligently to produce a chapter of significant clinical value. It is our hope that this volume will help those responsible for the care of patients to become more familiar with modern cardiovascular imaging so that they may apply these remarkable techniques optimally.

ROBERT C. SCHLANT, M.D.
R. WAYNE ALEXANDER, M.D., PH.D.
MARTIN J. LIPTON, M.D.

ABBREVIATIONS

AIDS = acquired immunodeficiency syndrome
ASD = atrial septal defect
AV = atrioventricular
BP = blood pressure
BPM = beats per minute
CABG = coronary artery bypass graft
CAD = coronary artery disease
CCU = coronary care unit
CSP = carotid sinus pressure
CT = computed tomography
DSA = digital subtraction arteriography
      (or angiography)
EBCT = electron beam computed tomography
ECG = electrocardiogram
ED = end-diastolic
ES = end-systolic
FWHM = full width at half maximum
HBE = His bundle electrocardiographic lead
HIV = human immunodeficiency virus
HLA = horizontal long axis
HR = heart rate
HRA = high right atrium
HTN = hypertension
IVC = inferior vena cava
IVCD = inferior vena cava defect;
      intraventricular conduction delay
LAD = left anterior descending (coronary artery)
LAO = left anterior oblique
LCF = left circumflex artery
LCX = left coronary circumflex artery
LPO = left posterior oblique
LRA = low right atrium

LV = left ventricle
LVEF = left ventricular ejection fraction
LVH = left ventricular hypertrophy
MAA = macroaggregated albumin
METS = metabolic equivalents
MI = myocardial infarction
MRI = magnetic resonance imaging
NURD = nonuniform rotational distortion
OM1 = obtuse marginal (coronary artery), first
PA = posteroanterior
PBF = pulmonary blood flow
PDA = patent ductus arteriosus;
      posterior descending artery
PE = pulmonary embolism
PET = positron emission tomography
PTCA = percutaneous transluminal coronary
      angioplasty
RAGE = rapid acquisition gradient echo
RAO = right anterior oblique
RCA = right coronary artery
RPO = right posterior oblique
SA = short axis
SPAMM = spatial modulation of magnetization
SPECT = single photon emission tomography
SNR = signal-to-noise ratio
SVC = superior vena cava
TEE = transesophageal echocardiography
TOF = tetralogy of Fallot
TR = repetition time
VLA = vertical long axis
VPD = ventricular premature depolarization
VSD = ventricular septal defect

DIAGNOSTIC
ATLAS
of the
HEART

CHAPTER 1

ELECTROCARDIOGRAPHY

Agustin Castellanos, M.D.
Robert J. Myerburg, M.D.

THE material presented in this chapter complements and extends the static illustrations shown in "The Resting Electrocardiogram," which is the title of our chapter in the eighth edition of *Hurst's The Heart*.[1] Historically, there was a time when the electrocardiographic leads were recorded sequentially.[2] At present, most electrocardiographic printouts consist of four sets of three simultaneously recorded leads complemented by one or more rhythm strips on the bottom, also aligned with those on top.[3] This facilitates the interpretation of the 12-lead electrocardiogram (ECG), especially in those frequent cases where the rhythm is not perfectly regular or totally irregular. When it is recorded with simultaneous rhythm strips, the ECG becomes more dynamic than the conventional, static, 12-lead ECG, but obviously less so than "long rhythm strips" or Holter recordings. At times, other displays are used. Thus, the classic 12 leads can be recorded simultaneously. An additional 13th lead (usually V_{4R}) is helpful for the diagnosis of right ventricular infarction and of certain congenital cardiac abnormalities.[4] At present, few authors still use the three orthogonal (X, Y, Z) leads of the Frank system, which can be analyzed for rhythm disturbances as well as for vectorial representations of the forces moving in a left-to-right, inferior-superior, posterior-anterior direction.[5] In our institution, the "semiorthogonal" leads I, II, and V_1 are used. Although didactically, certain ECG patterns can best be observed in illustrations showing only one cycle of each lead, sometimes the rich dynamic structure of certain abnormalities is lost. Besides, that is not the type of display encountered in everyday electrocardiographic practice. Therefore, according to circumstances, our illustrations show different features.[3] In addition, other types of recordings (e.g., intracavitary) that expand our understanding of electrocardiographic changes are presented. As the twentieth century is drawing to a close, the written and oral teaching of the earlier resting but currently more dynamic ECG is or will be performed in different ways, requiring the various modes of presentation shown in this chapter. Currently, we depend on the classroom interactive method; conceivably in the future, however, we may have interactive computerized textbooks.[3] That development remains for a future edition of this atlas.

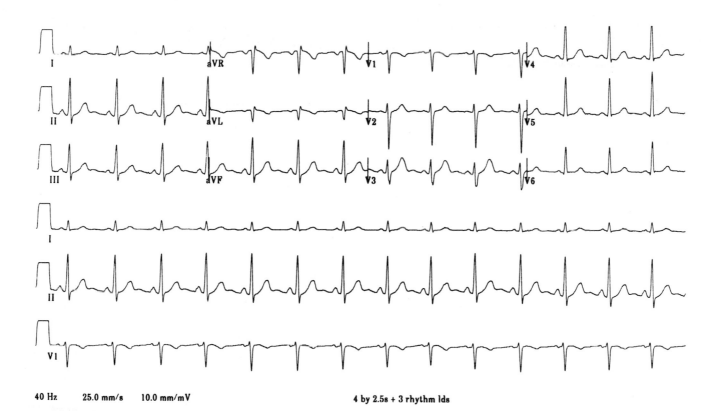

40 Hz   25.0 mm/s   10.0 mm/mV   4 by 2.5s + 3 rhythm lds

FIGURE 1-1   Normal ECG in a patient with the so-called electrocardio-graphically vertical heart. Note negative P and T waves in lead aV_L. In this display, four groups of three vertically aligned leads, separated by switching artifacts (*top*), were recorded simultaneously with three (also aligned) semiorthogonal leads (*bottom*). The latter are not interrupted by switching artifacts.

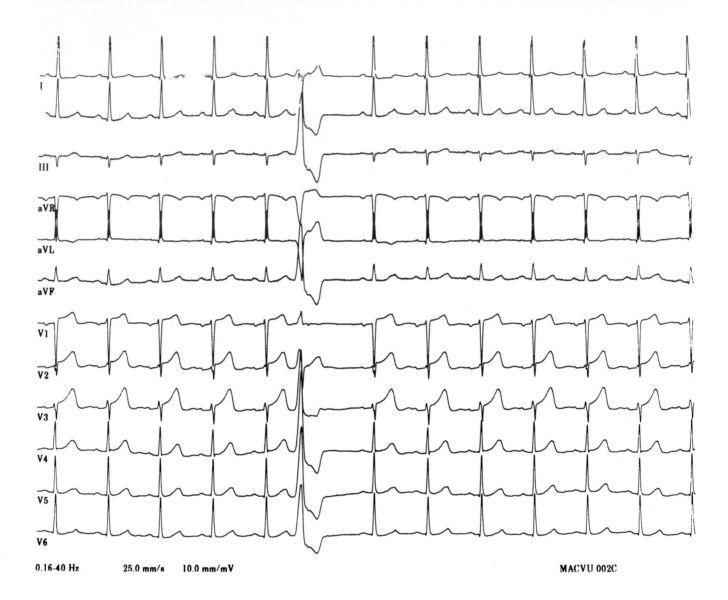

0.16–40 Hz   25.0 mm/s   10.0 mm/mV   MACVU 002C

FIGURE 1-2 Simultaneously recorded 12-lead ECG showing sinus rhythm with one ventricular premature beat. The three leads on top were recorded in the part of the page which, in the conventional format, would have included patient information, computer-measured intervals, etc. This type of display is useful for analysis of both rhythm and QRS-T morphology.

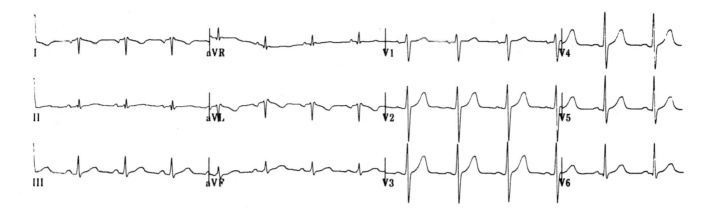

FIGURE 1-3   Electrocardiogram obtained from a normal patient with reversal of right and left arm electrodes, resulting in inversion of lead I (note negative P wave) and reversal of leads II and III as well as of aV_R and aV_F.

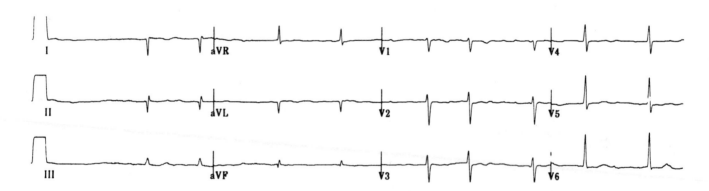

FIGURE 1-4   Electrocardiogram obtained with reversal of right and left arm electrodes in a patient with atrial fibrillation. Because negative P waves in lead I were not present and the patient had nonspecific ST-T-wave changes (see Figs. 1-10 and 1-11), the ECG could have been interpreted as showing a high lateral (or anterosuperior) myocardial infarction.

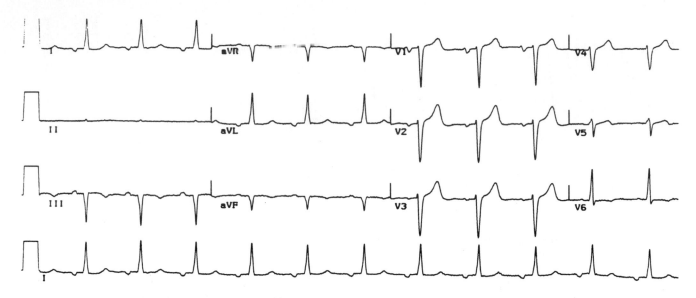

FIGURE 1-5 Electrocardiogram obtained with reversal of right arm and right leg (ground) electrode. In this case, lead II records the difference in potential between both legs (almost a straight line). Lead I = reversed lead III; lead III = lead III. The patient had an old inferior wall myocardial infarction. This figure shows that a negative P wave in lead I can be seen with switching of electrodes other than right and left arm.

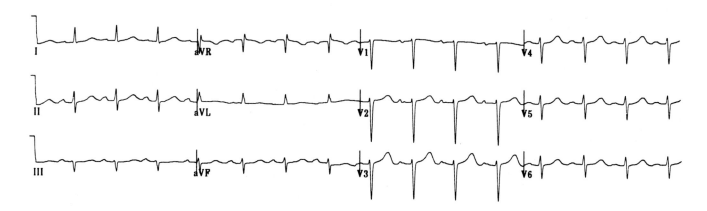

FIGURE 1-6 Improper (low) placement of leads V_5 and V_6, a common technical problem. When this occurs, the latter resemble lead aV_F.

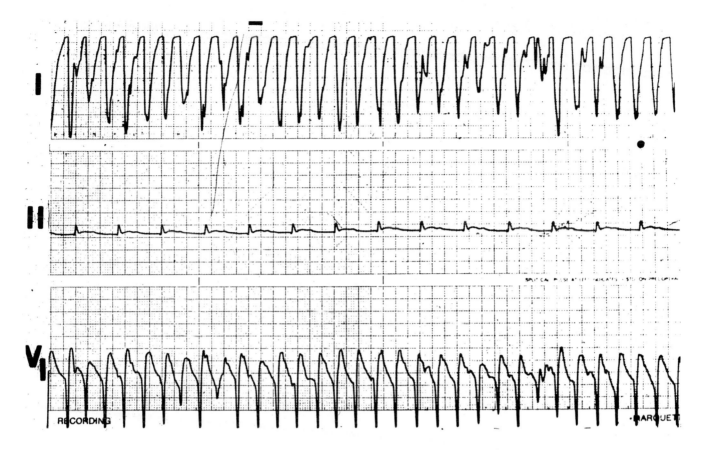

FIGURE 1-7   **Rhythm strip of simultaneously recorded leads I, II, and V₁ showing artifacts resembling ventricular tachycardia (in this case in all leads except standard lead II). The artifacts were due to a loose attachment of the left arm cable to the corresponding electrode. With the particular electrocardiographic machine used, these artifacts affected the chest leads.**

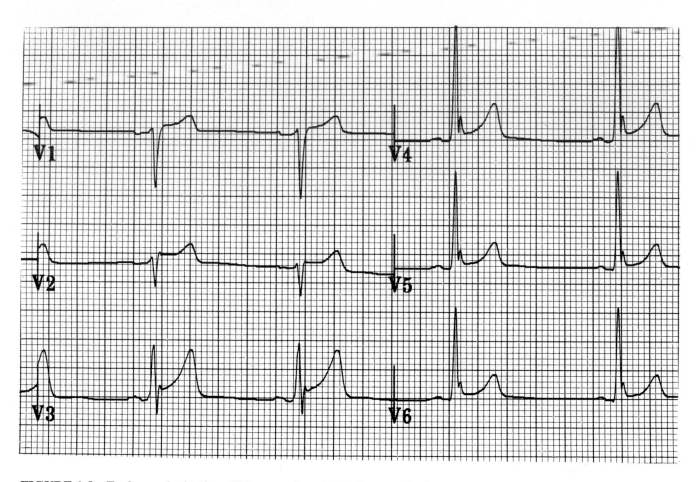

FIGURE 1-8 Early repolarization. This normal variant, characterized by an upwardly concave ST segment that is elevated beginning at the take-off at the J-point, is frequently associated with a tall R wave having a distinct notch or slur on its downstroke.

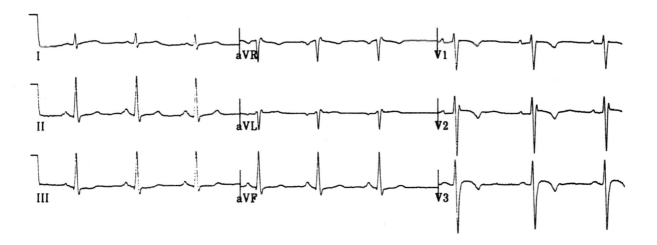

FIGURE 1-9 Electrocardiogram obtained from a normal 19-year-old female showing "juvenile" T-wave inversion in leads V_1, V_2, and V_3.

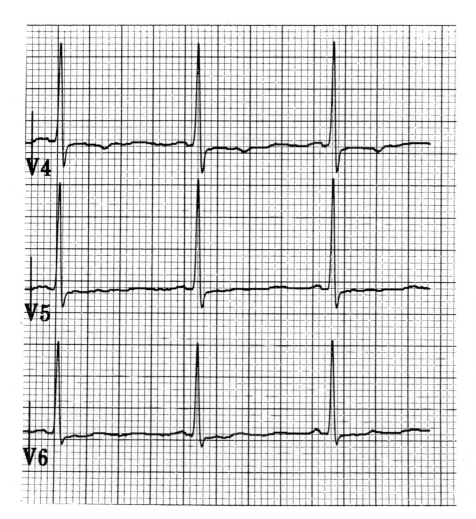

FIGURE 1-10 Nonspecific ST-segment and T-wave changes in left chest leads. This, the most common abnormality diagnosed in routine ECG interpretation, accounts for approximately 50 percent of abnormal tracings recorded in a general hospital. Such a relatively high number can be reduced (to about 10 percent) when appropriate clinical information is made available to the interpreter.

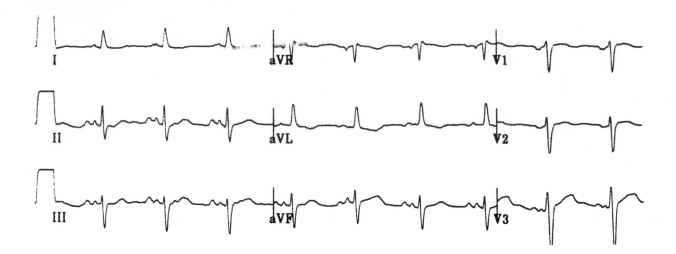

FIGURE 1-11 Nonspecific ST-segment T-wave changes in leads I and aV$_L$. From a patient with tachycardia-bradycardia syndrome who had intraatrial block with no echocardiographic evidence of left atrial enlargement.

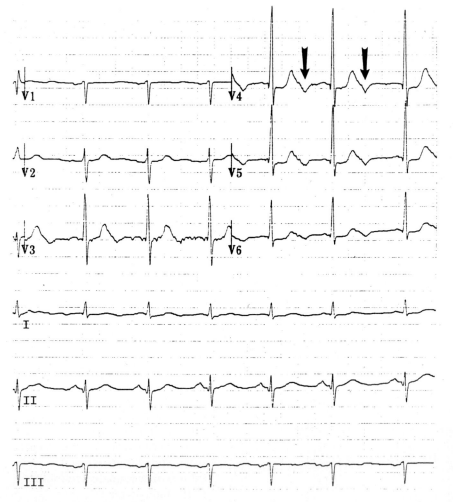

FIGURE 1-12 Negative U wave in left chest leads (*arrows*). The patient had an old (small high lateral wall) myocardial infarction and a recent ischemic episode. The U waves were positive in leads V$_1$ and V$_2$ and almost invisible in leads I and II.

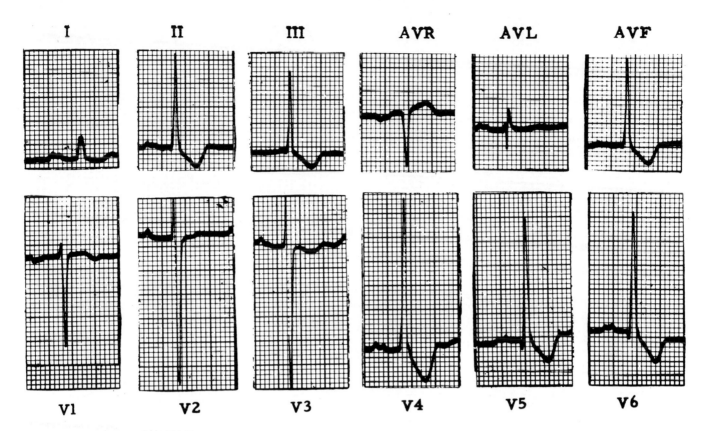

FIGURE 1-13   Left atrial hypertrophy associated with left ventricular hypertrophy and secondary ST-segment T-wave changes. The patient was receiving digoxin. Small q waves were not present in leads I and AVL because of the electrical position of the heart ("semivertical"). (From Lemberg L, Castellanos A Jr: *Vectorcardiography*, 2d ed. New York, Appleton-Century-Crofts, 1975. Reproduced with permission from the publisher and authors.)

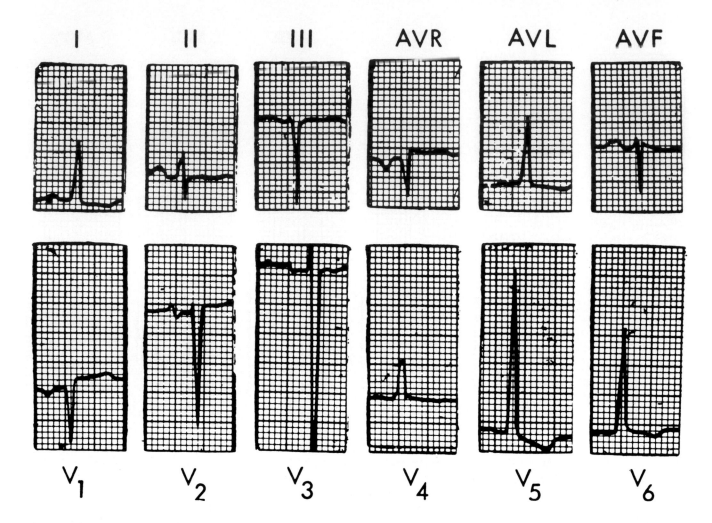

FIGURE 1-14 Left ventricular hypertrophy and secondary ST-segment T-wave changes. Absent q waves in leads I, AVL, V_5, and V_6 are probably due to an associated incomplete left bundle branch block. (From Lemberg L, Castellanos A Jr: *Vectorcardiography*, 2d ed. New York, Appleton-Century-Crofts, 1975. Reproduced with permission from the publisher and authors.)

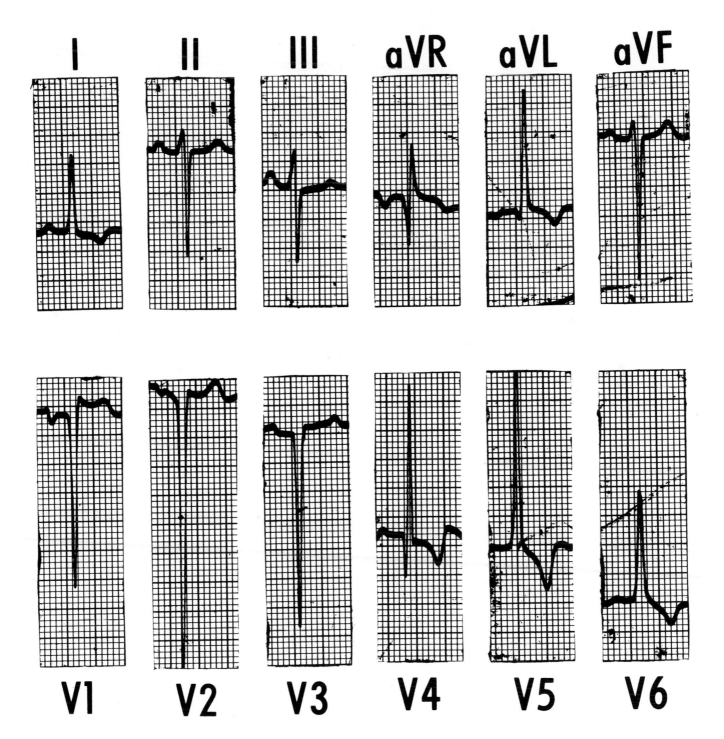

FIGURE 1-15 Left ventricular hypertrophy and secondary ST-segment T-wave changes in a patient with an old anteroseptal wall myocardial infarction and left anterior fascicular block. (From Castellanos A, Myerburg RJ: *The Hemiblocks in Myocardial Infarction*. New York, Appleton-Century-Crofts, 1976. Reproduced with permission from the publisher and authors.)

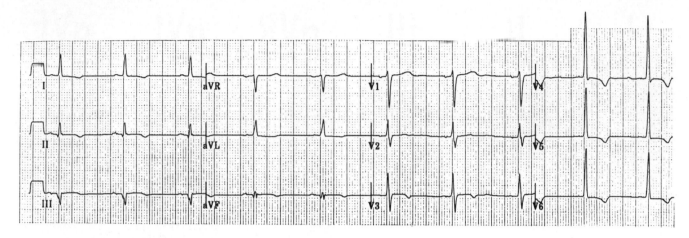

FIGURE 1-16   Left ventricular hypertrophy and secondary ST-segment
T-wave changes in a patient with an inferior wall myocardial infarction.
Absent q waves in left ventricular leads may be due to septal extension of
the infarction or to an associated incomplete left bundle branch block.

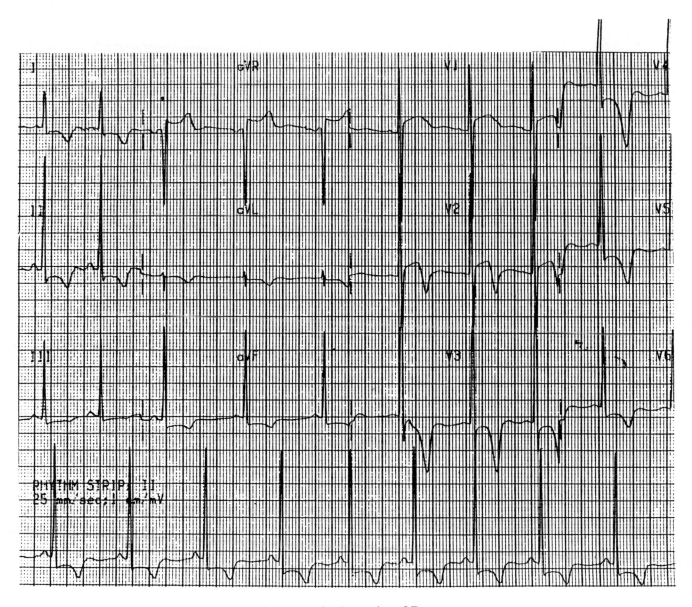

FIGURE 1-17 Left and right ventricular hypertrophy (note size of R wave in lead V_1) in a 23-year-old Asian male with apical hypertrophic cardiomyopathy. Note ischemic T waves in anterior chest leads. In this patient, a conventional M-mode echocardiogram had shown no evidence of hypertrophy.

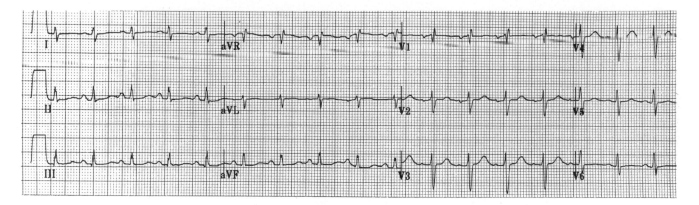

FIGURE 1-18   Right ventricular enlargement in a patient with atrial septal defect (secundum type). There is an incomplete right bundle branch block pattern associated with only a slight deviation of the electrical axis to the right.

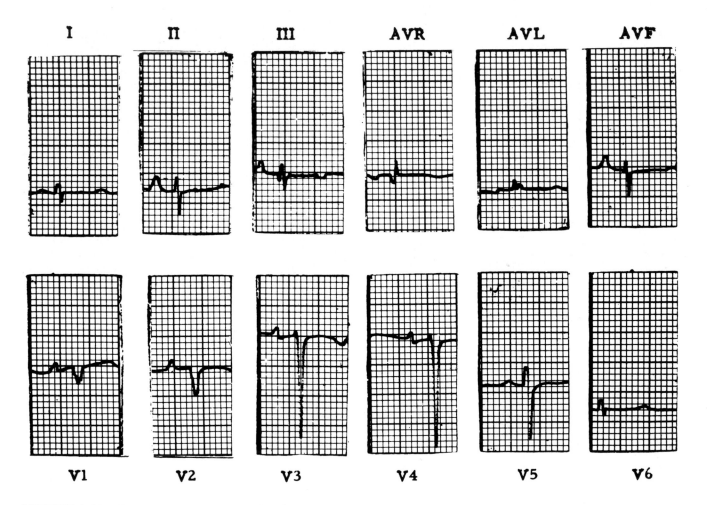

FIGURE 1-19   Pulmonary emphysema showing low voltage, an S_1-S_2-S_3 pattern, and QS complexes in V_1 and V_2. The latter can be interpreted as suggestive of anteroseptal wall myocardial infarction. (From Lemberg L, Castellanos A Jr: *Vectorcardiography*, 2d ed. New York, Appleton-Century-Crofts, 1975. Reproduced with permission from the publisher and authors.)

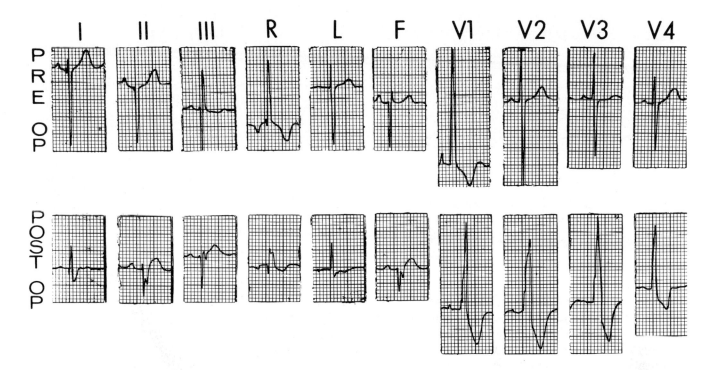

FIGURE 1-20 Right ventricular hypertrophy due to tetralogy of Fallot. The preoperative (PRE OP) ECG shows extreme right axis deviation. The latter is substituted by the surgically induced left anterior hemiblock, which deviates the axis to the left in spite of persistent right ventricular hypertrophy (POST OP). (From Rosenbaum MB, Corrado G, Oliveri R, et al: Right bundle branch block with left anterior hemiblock surgically induced in tetralogy of Fallot. *Am J Cardiol* 1970; 26:12–19. Reproduced with permission from the publisher and authors.)

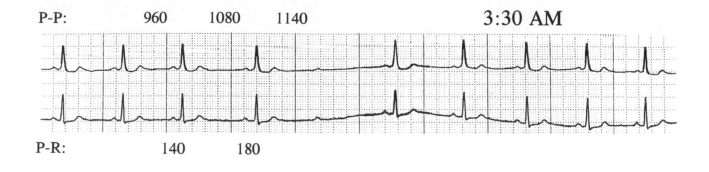

P-P: 960   1080   1140   3:30 AM

P-R: 140   180

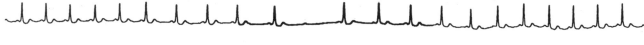

P-P: 760   1040

FIGURE 1-21   Atypical type I (Wenckebach) vagally induced second-degree atrioventricular (AV) block. There is only a minimal increase in the PR interval before the blocked P wave. In contrast, the PP intervals show a more detectable gradual increase. The QRS complexes are narrow. In this figure, values were expressed in milliseconds. The bottom strip was recorded at half normal paper speed (12.5 mm/s) to provide a greater number of cycles for analysis.

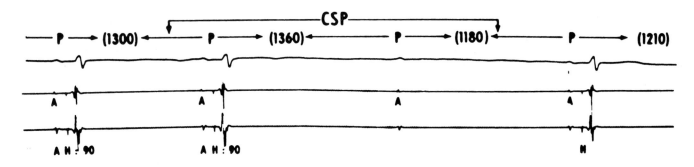

FIGURE 1-22   His bundle recording from another patient with vagally induced second-degree AV block. This tracing was recorded at four times normal paper speed (100 mm/s) to make measurements more accurately. Carotid sinus pressure (CSP) was applied at a moment of the cycle that did not cause prolongation of the PR, or AH, interval prior to the blocked P wave but resulted in an increase in the corresponding PP interval. The QRS complexes are narrow. A and H refer to the atrial and His bundle deflections recorded in the His bundle electrographic lead. Block occurred at the AV node, since the A was not followed by an H. Values are expressed in milliseconds. (From Zaman L, Moleiro F, Rozanski JJ, et al: Multiple electrophysiologic manifestations and clinical implications of vagally mediated AV block. *Am Heart J* 1983; 106:92–99. Reproduced with permission from the publisher and authors.)

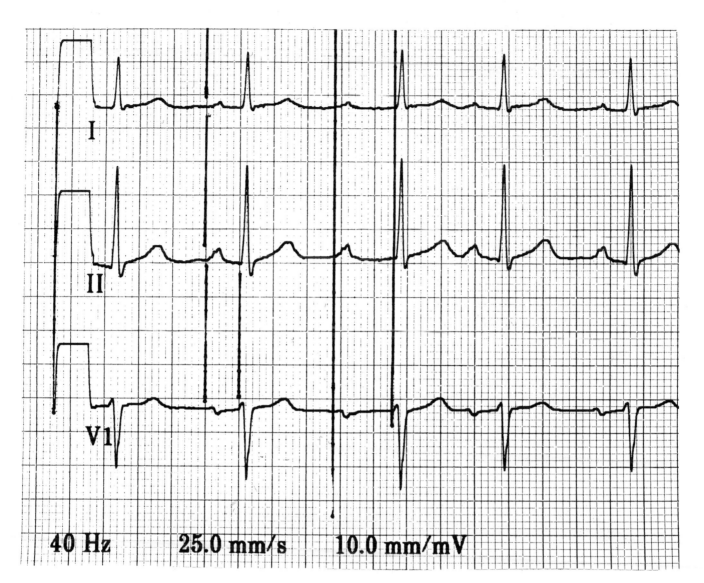

40 Hz   25.0 mm/s   10.0 mm/mV

FIGURE 1-23   Carotid sinus pressure (vagal) induced changes in PR
intervals without occurrence of second-degree AV block. This ECG also
shows one way of measuring the PR intervals using three semiorthogonal
leads (I, II, and V₁). This interval is measured from the earliest onset
of the P wave to the earliest beginning of the QRS complex on any of the
simultaneously recorded leads. Also, the proper alignment of the leads can
be assessed by determining whether the onsets of the standardization
signals coincide.

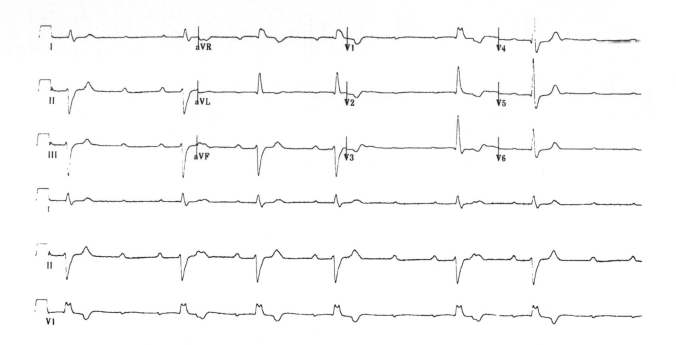

FIGURE 1-24   Twelve-lead ECG and simultaneously recorded rhythm strips in a patient with left anterior fascicular block and complete right bundle branch block. There is also a type II (Mobitz) AV block during which runs of 2:1 alternated with 3:1 block. An episode with a 7:3 AV ratio (2:1+2:1+3:1) is seen toward the middle of the tracing. This ECG was obtained at half standardization.

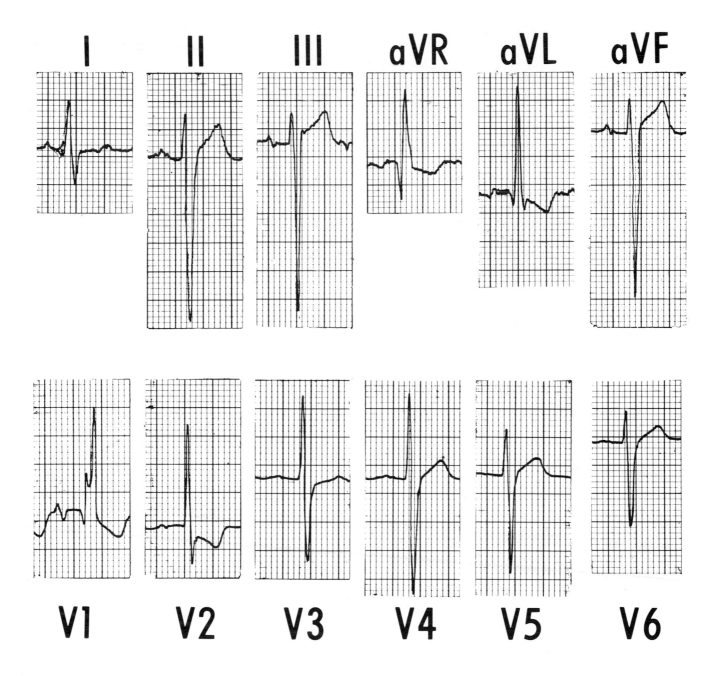

FIGURE 1-25 **Left anterior fascicular block and complete right bundle branch block with normal PR interval. (From Castellanos A, Myerburg RJ:** *The Hemiblocks in Myocardial Infarction.* **New York, Appleton-Century-Crofts, 1976. Reproduced with permission from the publisher and authors.)**

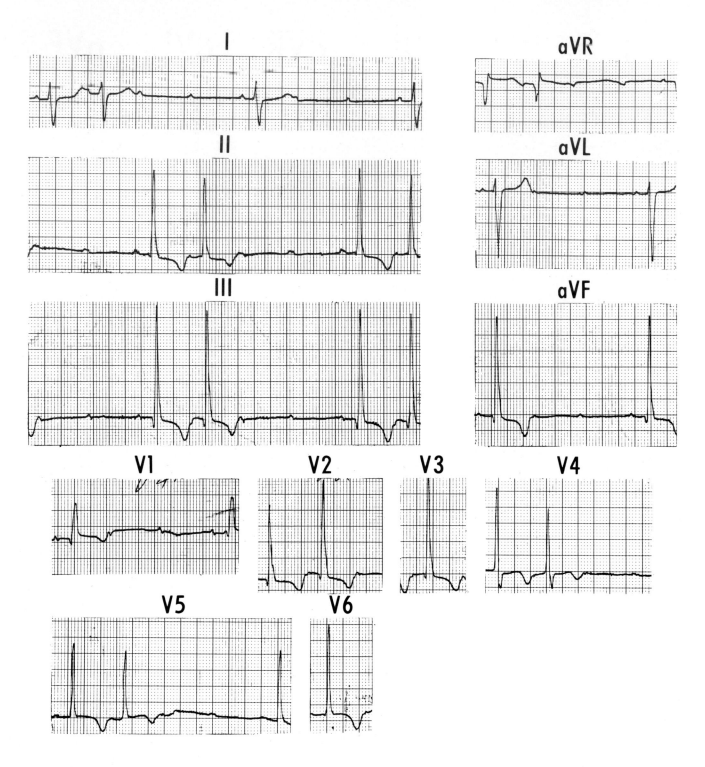

FIGURE 1-26 (Same patient as in previous figure.) There is now type II second-degree (Mobitz) AV block with a 4:2 ratio. The previously present left anterior fascicular block has now been replaced by a left posterior fascicular block. Complete right bundle branch block persists. (From Castellanos A, Myerburg RJ, *The Hemiblocks in Myocardial Infarction*. New York, Appleton-Century-Crofts, 1976. Reproduced with permission from the publisher and authors.)

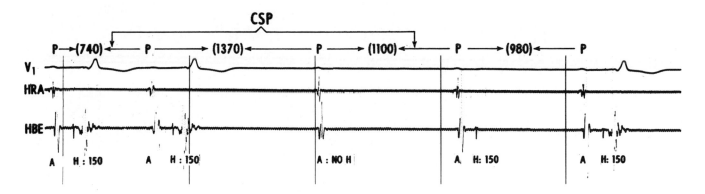

FIGURE 1-27 His bundle recordings depicting block above and below the bundle of His. Whereas the first A was blocked at the AV node (since it was not followed by an H), the second was blocked below the His bundle recording site because the corresponding H was not followed by a ventricular electrogram. Note wide QRS complexes. HRA = high right atrium; HBE = His bundle electrocardiographic lead. Other abbreviations and paper speed as in Fig. 1-22. (From Zaman L, Moleiro F, Rozanski JJ, et al: Multiple electrophysiologic manifestations and clinical implications of vagally mediated AV block. *Am Heart J* 1983; 106:92–99. Reproduced with permission from the publisher and authors.)

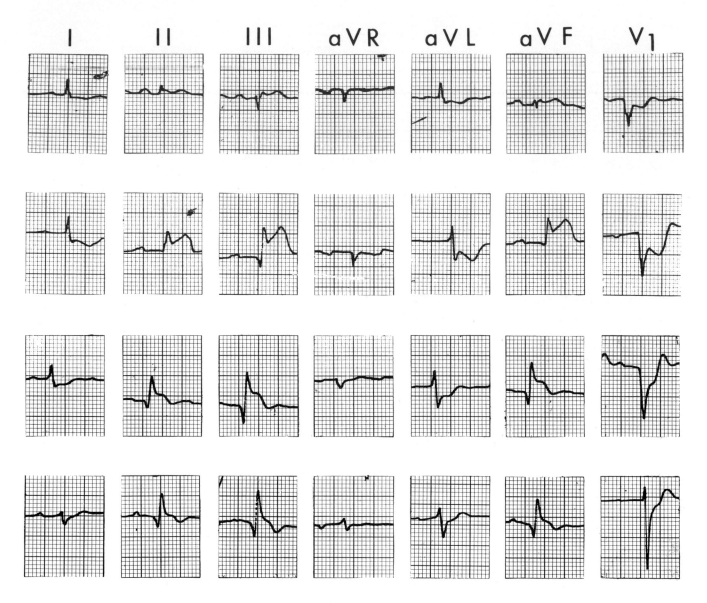

FIGURE 1-28 Evolution of inferior wall myocardial infarction prior to the thrombolytic era. The top strip was recorded on arrival at the emergency room, the second strip 6 h later, and the third strip 24 h later. The bottom strip, obtained after transfer from the coronary care unit, shows right-axis deviation (without right bundle branch block), which could be due to pure left posterior fascicular block.

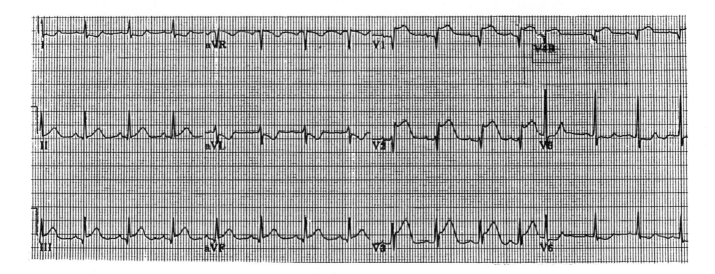

FIGURE 1-29 Acute inferior wall myocardial infarction with right ventricular myocardial infarction (diagnosed by V_{4R}, which, in this ECG, was recorded in the usual position of V_4). ST-segment elevation is more marked in the anteroseptal than the inferior leads.

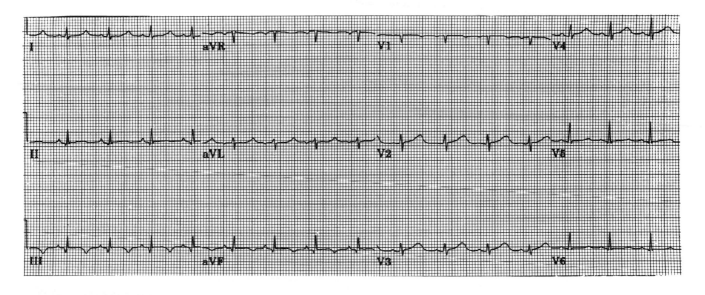

FIGURE 1-30 (Same patient as in previous figure.) Evolutionary changes of inferior wall myocardial infarction without evidence of anteroseptal wall myocardial infarction. This tracing was obtained 1 day after thrombolytic therapy.

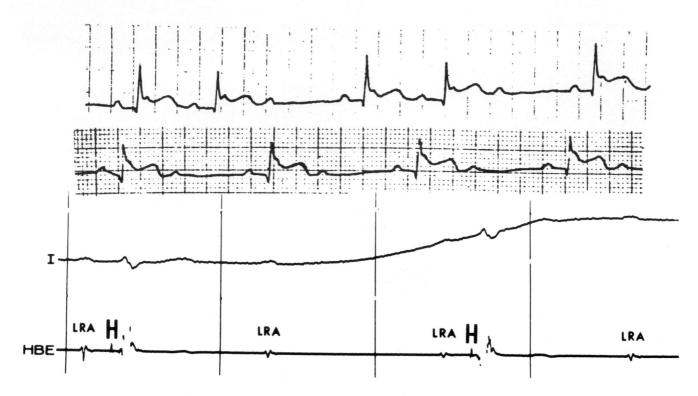

FIGURE 1-31 Type I (Wenckebach) second-degree (3:2) AV block in acute inferior wall myocardial infarction (*top strip in upper panel*) and 2:1 AV block (*bottom strip in upper panel*). The His bundle recording in the bottom panel shows that block occurred at the AV node, since nonconducted atrial (LRA) deflections were not followed by H deflections. (From Castellanos A, Myerburg RJ: *The Hemiblocks in Myocardial Infarction*. New York, Appleton-Century-Crofts, 1976. Reproduced with permission from the publisher and authors.)

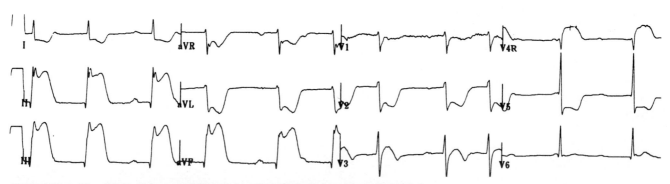

FIGURE 1-32 High-degree AV block in acute inferior wall myocardial infarction. V_{4R} is diagnostic of right ventricular infarction.

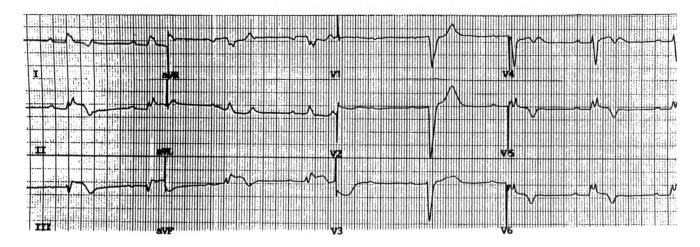

FIGURE 1-33   Two-to-one AV block (best seen in right chest leads) in
acute inferior wall myocardial infarction with left bundle branch block.
The latter, rare in infarctions with this location, may obscure the abnormal
Q waves characteristic of transmural infarction.

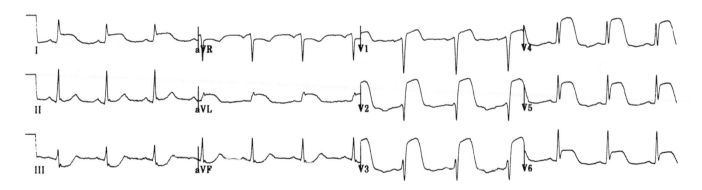

FIGURE 1-34   Acute, extensive anterior wall myocardial infarction.
The ECG was recorded prior to the occurrence of abnormal Q waves.

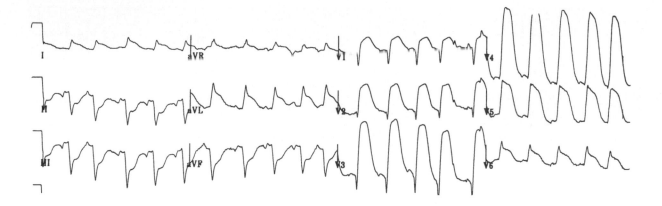

FIGURE 1-35   Ectopic atrial rhythm and premature atrial contractions in a patient with an acute, extensive anterior wall myocardial infarction. Left anterior fascicular block and q waves in anteroseptal leads were due to a previous anteroseptal wall myocardial infarction.

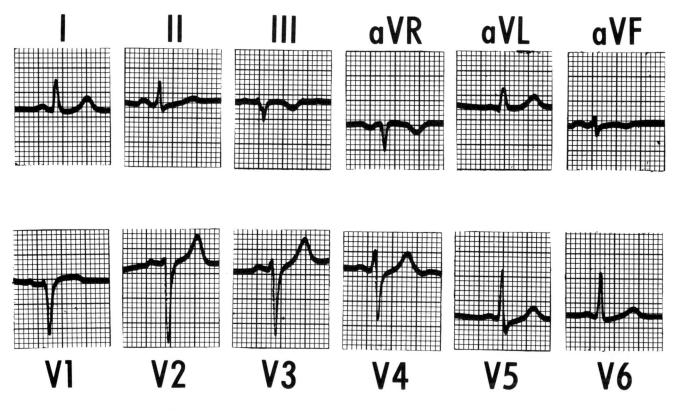

FIGURE 1-36   Control tracing recorded on arrival at the emergency room. Figures 1-36 to 1-41 were obtained before the thrombolytic era. (From Castellanos A, Myerburg RJ: *The Hemiblocks in Myocardial Infarction.* New York, Appleton-Century-Crofts, 1976. Reproduced with permission from the publisher and authors.)

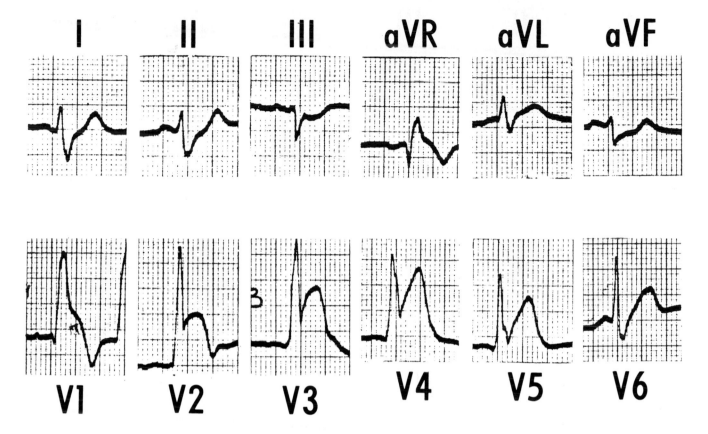

FIGURE 1-37   (Same patient as in previous tracing on arrival at the coronary care unit.) Acute anterior wall myocardial infarction, complete right bundle branch block, and left anterior fascicular block. (From Castellanos A, Myerburg RJ: *The Hemiblocks in Myocardial Infarction.* New York, Appleton-Century-Crofts, 1976. Reproduced with permission from the publisher and authors.)

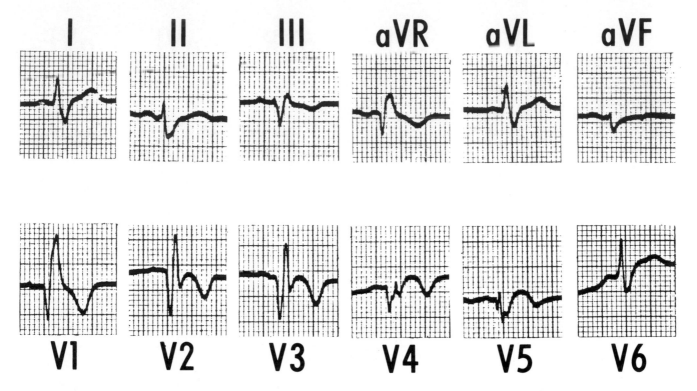

FIGURE 1-38   (Same patient, 5 days later.) Evolving anterior wall myocardial infarction with similar conduction disturbances after appearance of abnormal Q waves. (From Castellanos A, Myerburg RJ: *The Hemiblocks in Myocardial Infarction*. New York, Appleton-Century-Crofts, 1976. Reproduced with permission from the publisher and authors.)

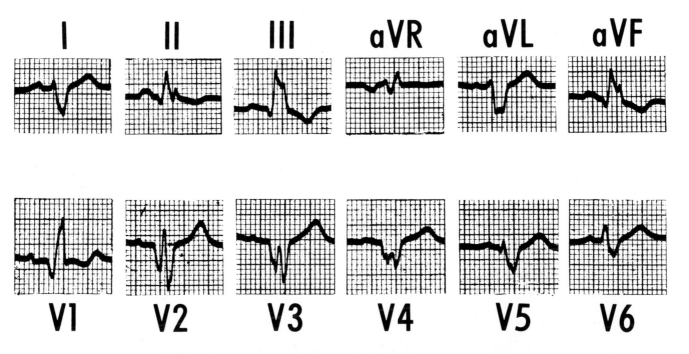

FIGURE 1-39   (Same patient, 1 h later.) Left anterior fascicular block is no longer present. The ECG now shows left posterior fascicular block. Right bundle branch block persists. (From Castellanos A, Myerburg RJ: *The Hemiblocks in Myocardial Infarction*. New York, Appleton-Century-Crofts, 1976. Reproduced with permission from the publisher and authors.)

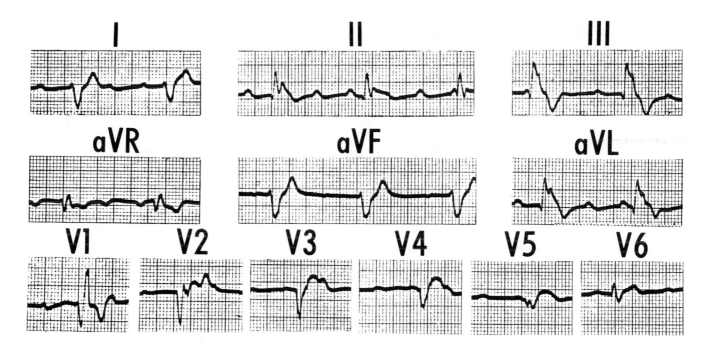

FIGURE 1-40   (Same patient, 5 days later.) Complete AV block is now present.

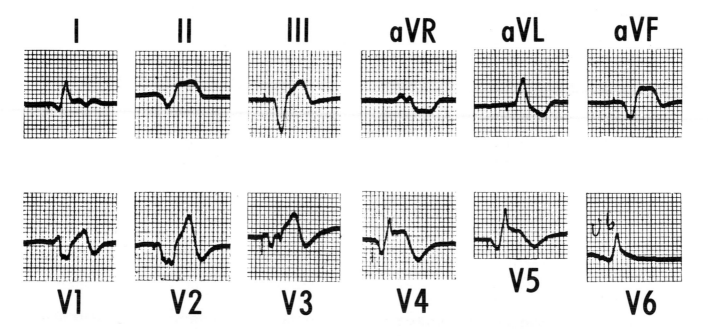

FIGURE 1-41   (Same patient after insertion of a temporary pacemaker.) Electrocardiogram obtained during ventricular pacing. In leads I, V_4, V_5, and V_6, the small bipolar spikes are followed by small q waves. This "stimulus-qR pattern" is frequently seen with bipolar right ventricular stimulation in patients with anterior wall myocardial infarction, as when, during sinus rhythm, the latter coexists with left bundle branch block. (From Castellanos A, Myerburg RJ: *The Hemiblocks in Myocardial Infarction*. New York, Appleton-Century-Crofts, 1976. Reproduced with permission from the publisher and authors.)

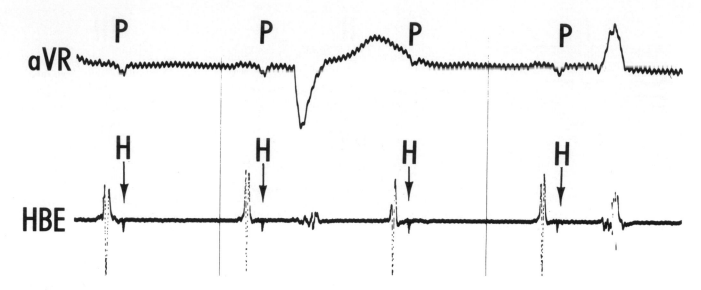

FIGURE 1-42   His bundle readings from a patient with acute myocardial infarction showing that block occurs below the His bundle (in contrast to what happens in inferior wall myocardial infarction, as shown in Fig. 1-31).

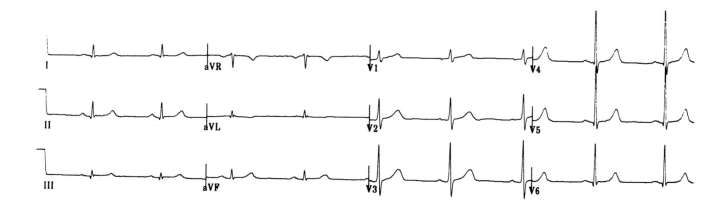

FIGURE 1-43   True posterior (basal) myocardial infarction without concomitant inferior wall myocardial infarction. Note prominent R waves and upright T waves in leads V_1, V_2, and V_3.

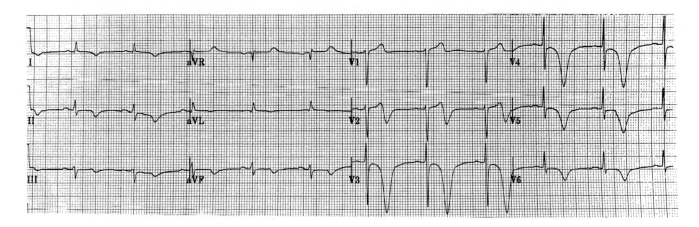

FIGURE 1-44 Acute non-Q-wave myocardial infarction. Note diffuse T-wave inversion in almost all leads.

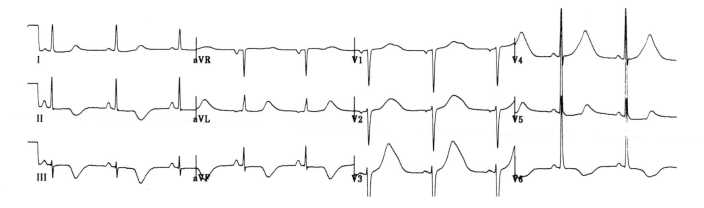

FIGURE 1-45 Acute intracerebral bleeding simulating acute non-Q-wave myocardial infarction. This process is also one of the many that can cause marked prolongation of the QT interval.

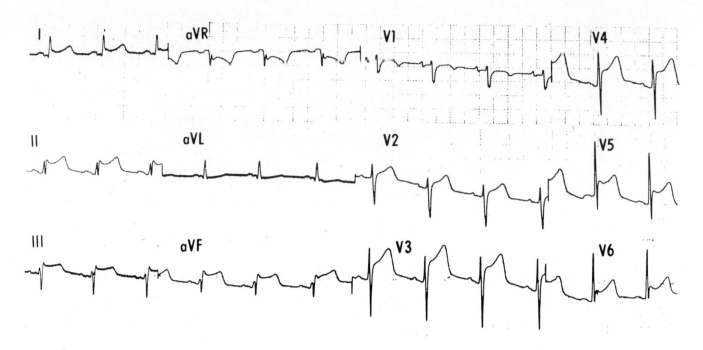

FIGURE 1-46 Acute nonspecific pericarditis simulating acute myocardial infarction.

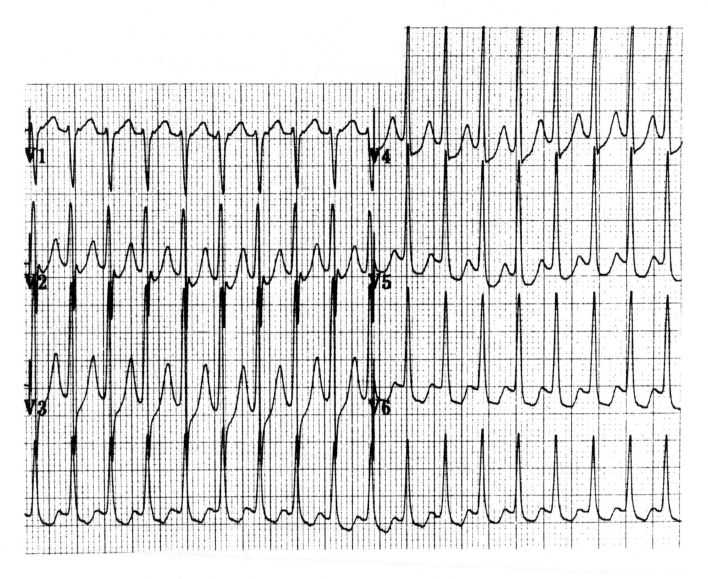

FIGURE 1-47 Chest leads from a young patient with recurrent sustained AV-nodal reciprocating tachycardia showing rate-related pseudoischemic ST-segment changes. The latter are not necessarily followed by the better-known posttachycardia T-wave syndrome.

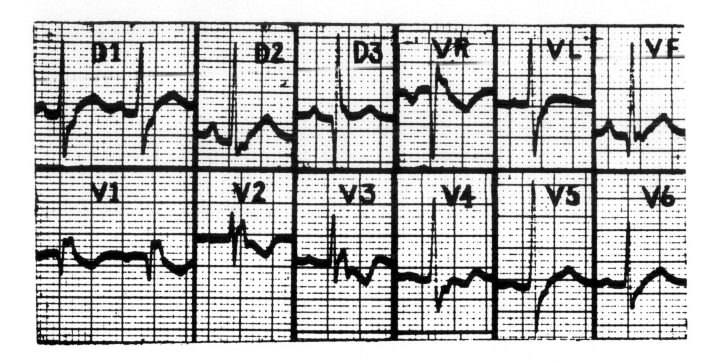

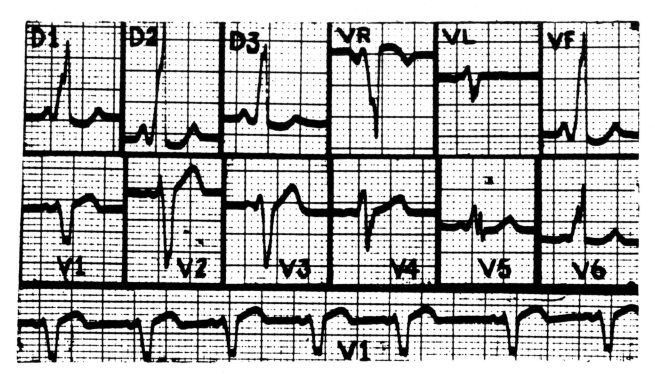

FIGURE 1-48 **Wolff-Parkinson-White syndrome in a 19-year-old male with Ebstein's anomaly. The top panel shows sinus rhythm, normal PR interval, and complete right bundle branch block. When AV conduction occurred through an accessory pathway, the right ventricular preexcitation obscured the right bundle branch block (*bottom panel*).**

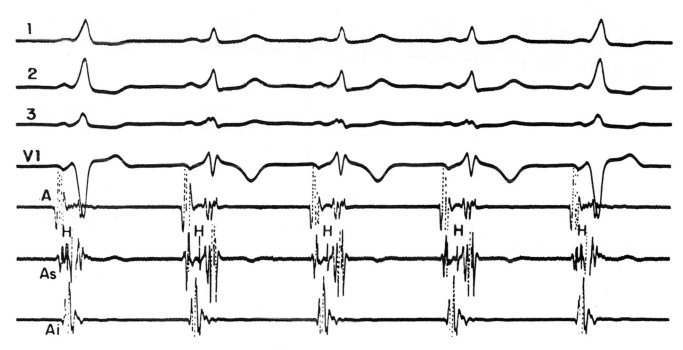

FIGURE 1-49   His bundle recordings in a patient with Wolff-Parkinson-White syndrome. The PR interval is 120 ms. Delta waves are best seen in leads 2 and V$_1$ when beats show a right bundle branch block morphology and in leads 3 and V$_1$ when they display a left bundle branch block pattern. The HV interval is shorter than normal or has a negative (H after V) value. Surface leads show sinus rhythm with two distinct QRS morphologies due to AV conduction through two separate accessory pathways. A = high right atrium; As = A in His bundle lead; Ai = proximal coronary sinus. Paper speed was 100 mm/s.

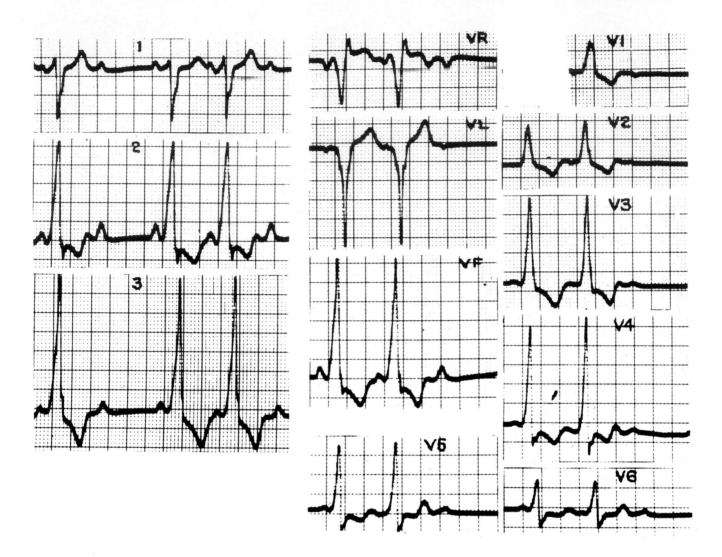

FIGURE 1-50 Electrocardiogram from a 68-year-old female with Wolff-Parkinson-White syndrome, complete block (see Fig. 1-51) in the normal pathway, exclusive AV conduction through the accessory pathway, and type II (Mobitz) block in the latter.

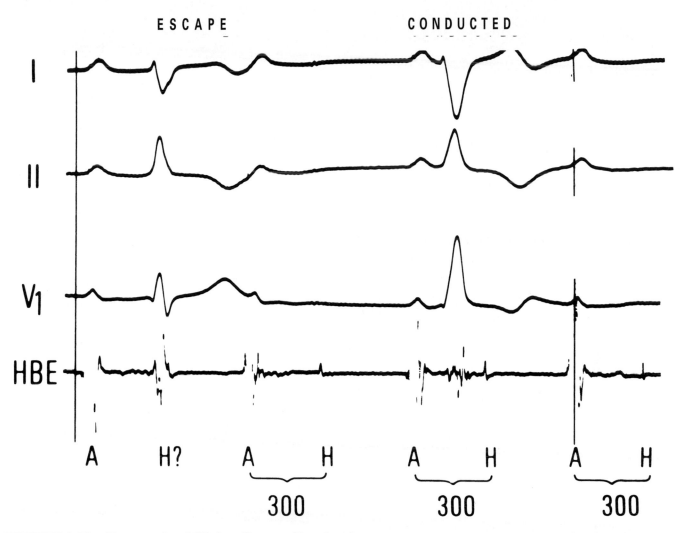

FIGURE 1-51 (Same patient.) His bundle recording showing an escape beat followed by a beat conducted to the ventricles through the accessory pathway. There is complete infra-Hisian block in the normal pathway, since H deflections are not followed by ventricular deflections.

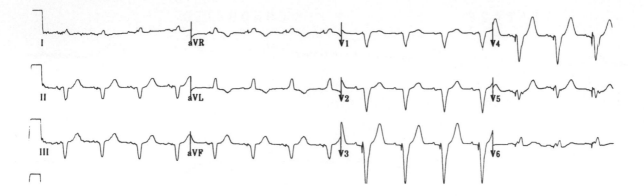

FIGURE 1-52 Right ventricular apical pacing showing the corresponding left bundle branch block–left axis deviation pattern. Special care has to be taken not to miss small spikes (usually best seen in chest leads) when bipolar stimulation is performed.

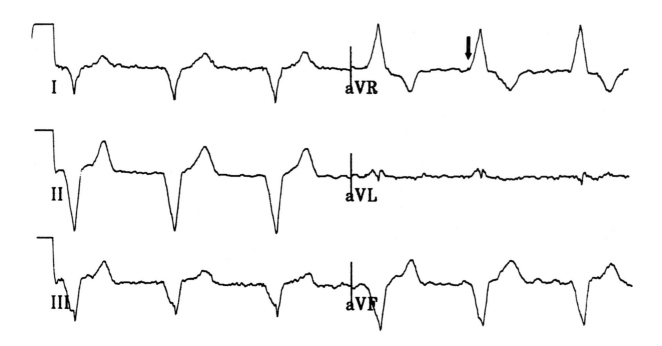

FIGURE 1-53 Ventricular pacing. The small bipolar spikes (*arrow*) are hardly detected in the standard and unipolar leads.

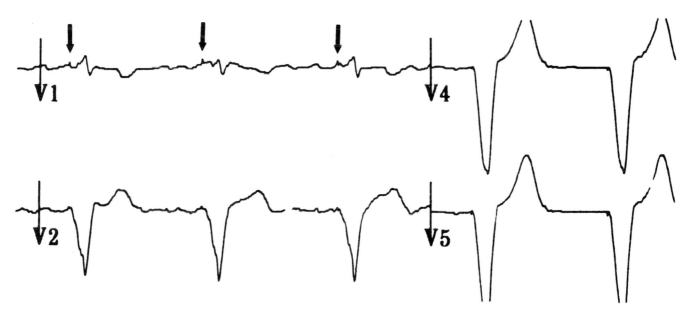

FIGURE 1-54 (Same patient.) Small bipolar spikes are best seen in lead V₁ (*arrows*) and, with great difficulty, in lead V₅.

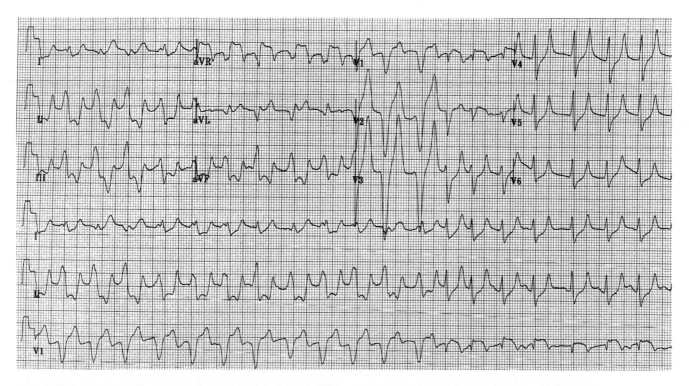

FIGURE 1-55 "Dialyzable current of injury" in a patient with hyperkalemia (8.2 meq/L) simulating acute anteroseptal myocardial infarction. The wide QRS complexes became narrower toward the end of the tracing. The rhythm was most likely sinus tachycardia with premature atrial beats throughout the entire recording time. Hyperkalemia is more easily diagnosed when the ventricular complexes are narrower.

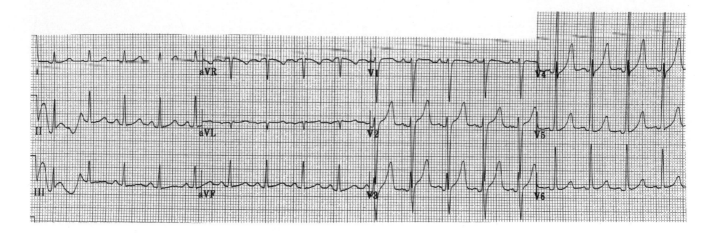

FIGURE 1-56 (Same patient as in previous figure.) Electrocardiogram obtained after dialysis showing sinus tachycardia, narrow QRS complexes, and slightly peaked T waves (mainly in lead V$_4$).

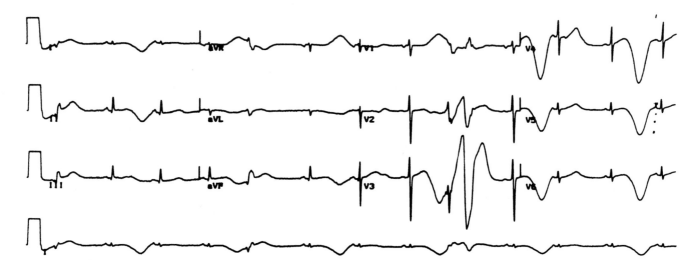

FIGURE 1-57 Prolonged QT interval with ST-T alternans in a patient with torsades de pointes (not shown) due to pentamidine.

REFERENCES

1. Castellanos A, Kessler KM, Myerburg RJ: The resting electrocardiogram. In: Schlant RC, Alexander RW, O'Rourke RA, et al (eds): *Hurst's the Heart*, 8th ed. New York, McGraw-Hill, 1994; 321–356.
2. Burch GE, DePasquale NP: *A History of Electrocardiography*. Chicago, Year Book Medical Publishers, Inc., 1964.
3. Wagner GS: *Marriotts's Practical Electrocardiography*, 9th ed. Boston, Williams & Wilkins, 1994.
4. Task Force Report of the American College of Cardiology and the American Heart Association: ACC/AHA Guidelines for Electrocardiography. *Circulation* 1992; 19:473–481.
5. Castellanos A, Sung RJ, Richter S, Myerburg RJ: XYZ Electrocardiography: Correlation with conventional 12-lead electrocardiogram. *Cardiovasc Clin* 1977; 8/3:285–299.

CHAPTER 2

EXAMINATION OF THE RETINA

W. Banks Anderson, Jr., M.D.

THE microcirculation participates in the pathophysiology of most cardiovascular disease. Clinicians may easily observe a human capillary bed by examining the retina with an ophthalmoscope. Here in a two-dimensional array are displayed the afferent arterioles, tributary venules, and interposed capillary net. No other human capillary bed is as accessible to direct observation. With the light and magnification of the ophthalmoscope, the astute physician may detect emboli and observe the microcirculatory effects of diabetes, hypertension, and arteriolarsclerosis.[1]

The calibre of the retinal vessels may be directly observed and vascular wall thickness assessed at arteriovenous crossings. In hypoxic patients, as in those with left to right shunts, the retinal veins may be dark and dilated. Dark and dilated veins are more frequently seen distal to a retinal venous outflow obstruction at an arteriovenous crossing. At the crossing, a hard, thick, sclerotic arterial wall may obstruct the vein within their confining common adventitial sheath. The consequent breakdown in vascular endothelial integrity is made manifest by leakage of serum with retinal edema and agglomeration of large molecules into hard retinal exudates. Larger endothelial openings permit the passage of red blood cells, and these hemorrhages can be observed in the retina or in front of the retina. Such leakage marks the capillary watershed area behind the venous obstruction. Hemorrhages and exudates are also very characteristic of the retinal capillary disease occurring in diabetes of ten or twenty years duration.[2,3]

Microischemic infarcts of the retinal capillary bed produce swelling of the adjacent nerve fiber layer of the retina, which can be observed as cotton wool spots. These white fluffy appearing lesions are not exudates but indices of microinfarction. In years past usually associated with untreated severe hypertension, they now are most commonly seen, particularly in younger individuals, as a result of HIV infection. At times cotton wool spots may be found downstream from an obstructing arterial embolus. Bits of cholesterol from carotid plaques and calcium from aortic valvular lesions remain as visible evidence of embolic disease for months to years. In patients with amaurosis fugax, however, platelet emboli may be visible only during the symptomatic phase. Bits of atrial myxoma may end up in the retinal arterial tree with ominous prognosis. Septic emboli to the retina from subacute bacterial endocarditis are now rare. They usually manifest themselves as hemorrhagic blots and may have a white center as described by Roth. Such hemorrhages may also be seen in the other visible micro-circulation, that of the nail beds.

Embolic retinopathy occurs following intracardiac instrumentation and surgery. Although these emboli are usually asymptomatic, blot retinal hemorrhages are not rare in the period immediately following cardiac interventions. They may serve as markers for similar embolic occurrences in other areas of the central nervous system.

The retina and eye participate in multisystem congenital and inherited diseases, affecting the cardiovascular system. The retinitis of rubella and the retinitis pigmentosa of Kearn-Sayre syndrome are examples. Marfan syndrome patients commonly have visual complaints, but these are usually related to their subluxed lenses and not to retinopathy.

Familiarity with the use of the ophthalmoscope and with the ocular signs of cardiovascular disease may assist the clinician in assessing prognosis and severity as well as in making a diagnosis. Below are representative photographs of some of the more common conditions of cardiovascular significance affecting the retina.

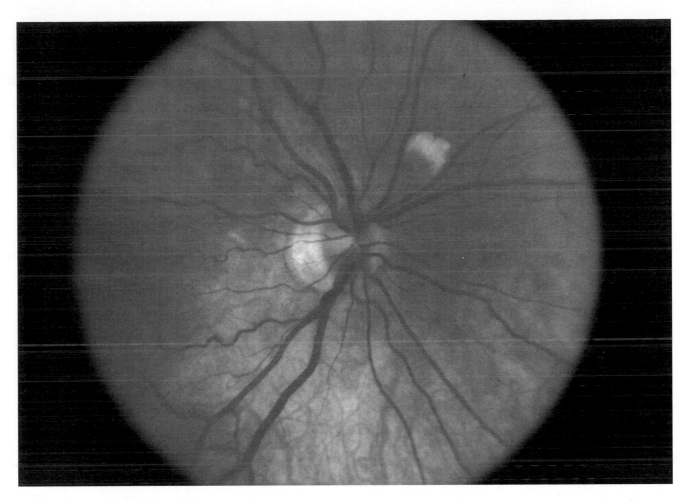

FIGURE 2-1   Retinal cotton-wool spot. Cotton-wool spots are most frequently found close to the optic disk. Although they occur in acute uncontrolled systemic hypertension, the more common cause now, in younger patients, is infection with the human immunodeficiency virus. This normotensive 37-year-old man had no visual symptoms and no other retinopathy. There is a myopic crescent at the temporal disk edge, which is not abnormal. He died of complications related to the acquired immunodeficiency syndrome (AIDS) two years later. (*See color Plate 1.*)

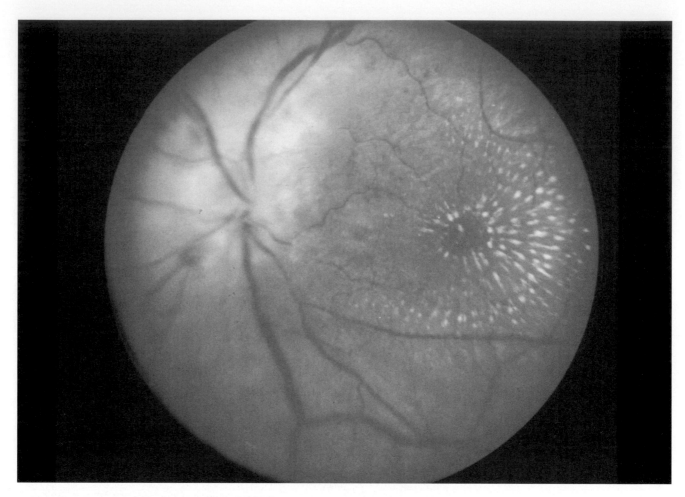

FIGURE 2-2 **Disk swelling and hard exudate in a macular "star" pattern. In this hypertensive patient with periarteritis nodosa, vascular leakage has led to the deposit of hard exudates around the fovea. Radial perifoveal connective tissue results in the star pattern of the exudate. Note also that the optic disk is edematous, with blurred margins, secondary to hypertension.** (*See color Plate 2.*)

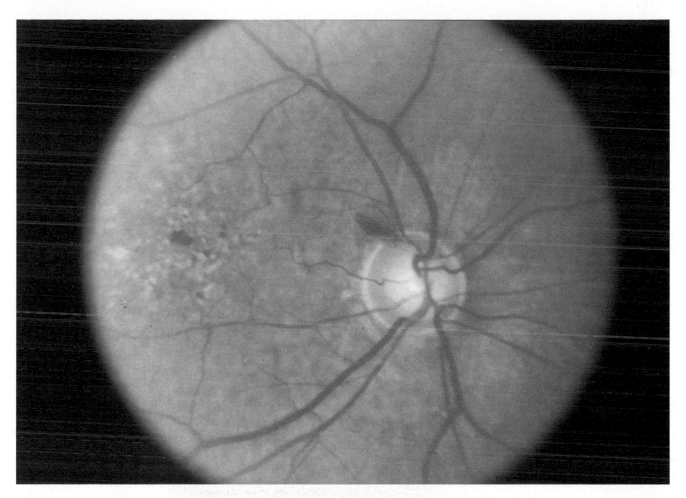

FIGURE 2-3   Splinter or flame hemorrhage at the optic disk. Superficial hemorrhages such as this may be seen in hypertensive patients. Such hemorrhages may also be associated with glaucoma. In glaucoma, the hemorrhages usually overlie a portion of the disk as in this 61-year-old normotensive man. Note the temporal cupping of the disk, which is also a sign of glaucoma. Macular degeneration, another very common condition of the elderly, is also evident in this photograph. At the temporal edge of the field, pigment clumps can be seen in the macular area. Such retinal pigment disorganization is typical of the dry form of macular degeneration. (*See color Plate 3.*)

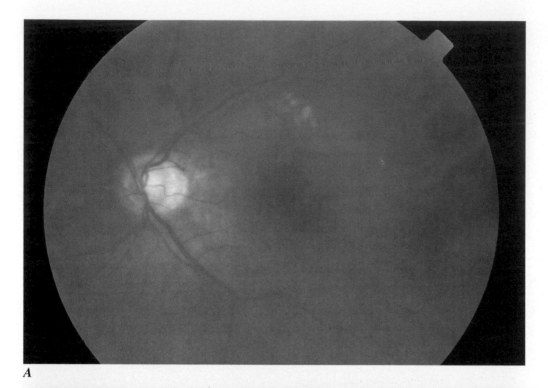

A

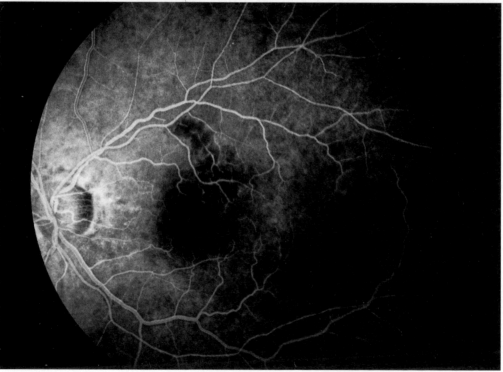

B

FIGURE 2-4   Hypertensive retinal vaso-occlusion. *A*. Noting a spot in her vision, this previously healthy 63-year-old physician was found to have a small retinal venous occlusion with a patch of edematous retina superior to the left fovea. Hypertension and diabetes are associated with retinal vascular obstructions. After this lesion was discovered, brachial blood pressure was found to be 220/120. (*See color Plate 4.*) On the fluorescein angiogram (*B*), note the dark, ischemic, edematous area just below the superior arcade of vessels which corresponds to the pale area on the color photograph.

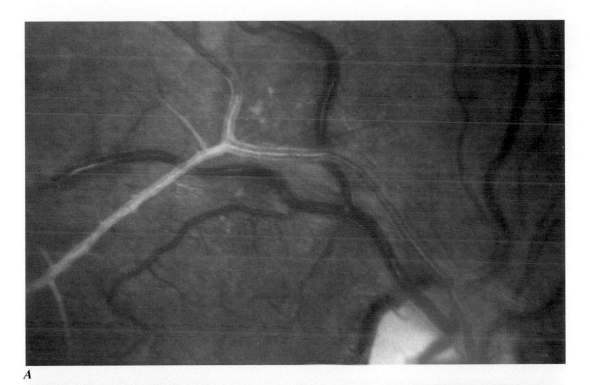

A

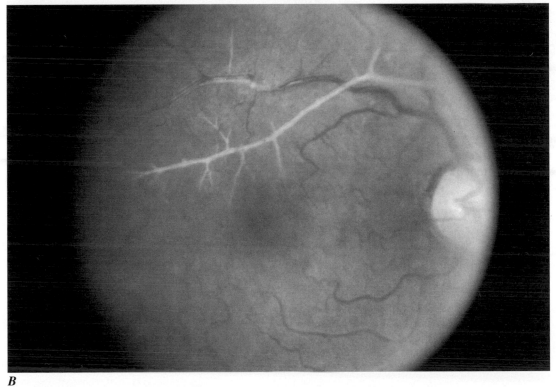

B

FIGURE 2-5   *A.* **Retinal arteriosclerosis. This 75-year-old hypertensive woman has marked arteriosclerosis of the upper temporal retinal arteriole and its branches. When the narrowed blood column can no longer be seen, the thickened wall produces the "silver-wire" appearance seen here. Where the arteriole crosses its associated vein, the course of the vein is altered, and its blood column cannot be seen. This venous "nicking" and "banking" is associated with impairment of outflow, and the affected veins become darker, larger, and more tortuous.** *B.* **Low-power view showing the silver-wire arteriole.** (*See color Plate 5A and B.*)

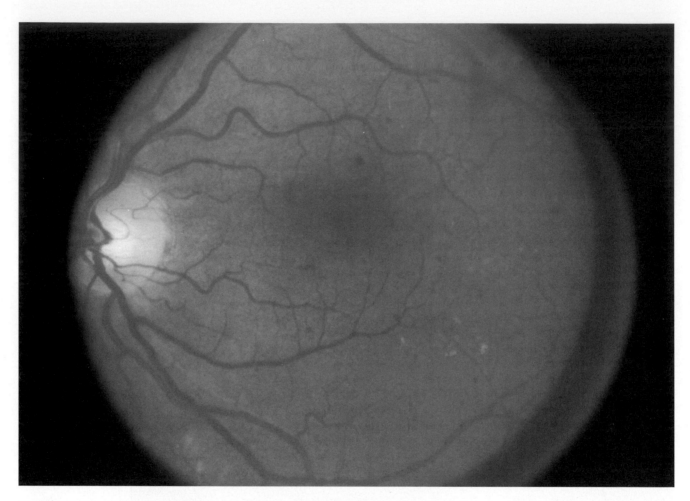

FIGURE 2-6   **Background diabetic retinopathy. Retinal microaneurysms, dot-and-blot hemorrhages, and a few fine upper temporal hard exudates are diagnostic of early diabetic retinopathy. The patient had no visual symptoms, but retinopathy of this magnitude can often be seen in patients with insulin-requiring diabetes of 15 or more years duration.** (*See color Plate 6.*)

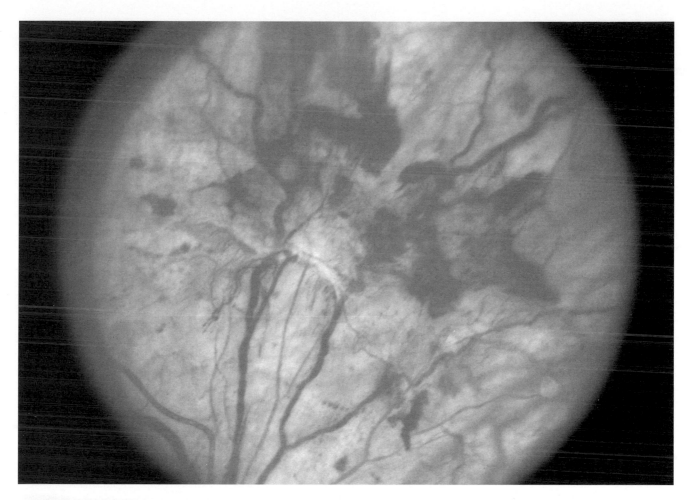

FIGURE 2-7   **Proliferative diabetic retinopathy with preretinal hemorrhage. When neovascularization develops, preretinal and vitreous hemorrhages are much more likely to occur. Easily visible neovascularization either in the periphery of the retina, as in this diabetic patient, or at the disk is an indication for immediate panretinal laser photocoagulation.** (*See color Plate 7.*)

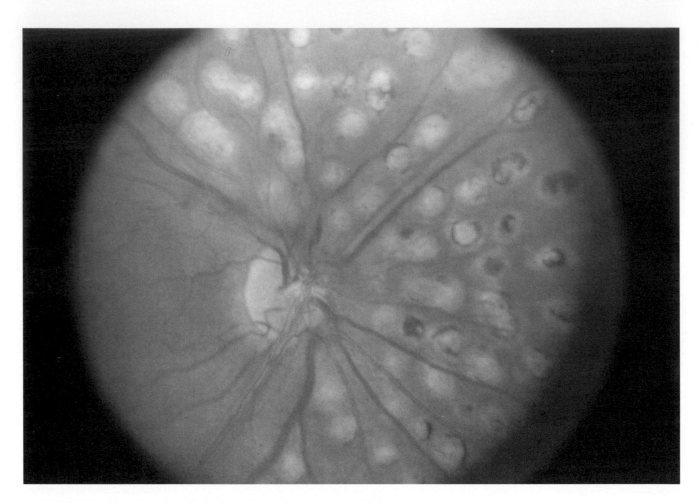

FIGURE 2-8 **Proliferative diabetic retinopathy treated with laser photocoagulation. The retina nasal to the optic disk has been treated with a panretinal pattern. Note the neovascularization at the disk, which is evidence of proliferative retinopathy and an indication for panretinal laser photocoagulation. Untreated, there is a high risk of blinding hemorrhage when neovascularization is present at the disk or in the periphery.** (*See color Plate 8.*)

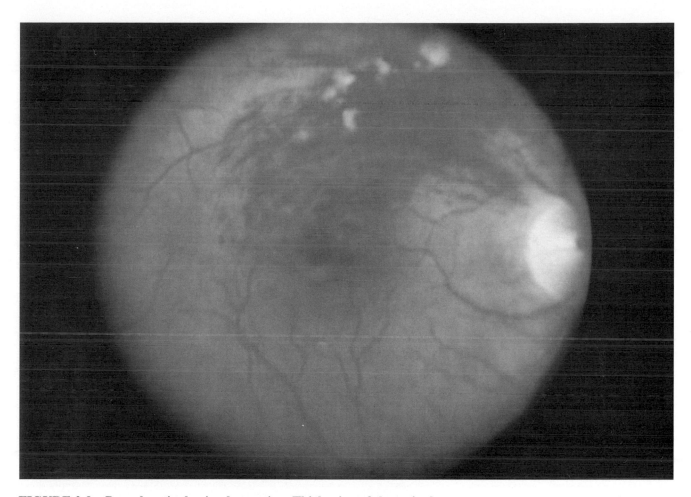

FIGURE 2-9   Branch retinal vein obstruction. Thickening of the retinal arterial wall in diabetes and hypertension may compromise the lumen of the vein where they share a common adventitial sheath at an arteriovenous crossing. The resulting obstruction produces hemorrhagic retinopathy in the drainage area of the affected vein. Note here how the flame-shaped pattern of blood outlines the arcuate pattern of the nerve fibers as they run toward the optic disk. (*See color Plate 9.*)

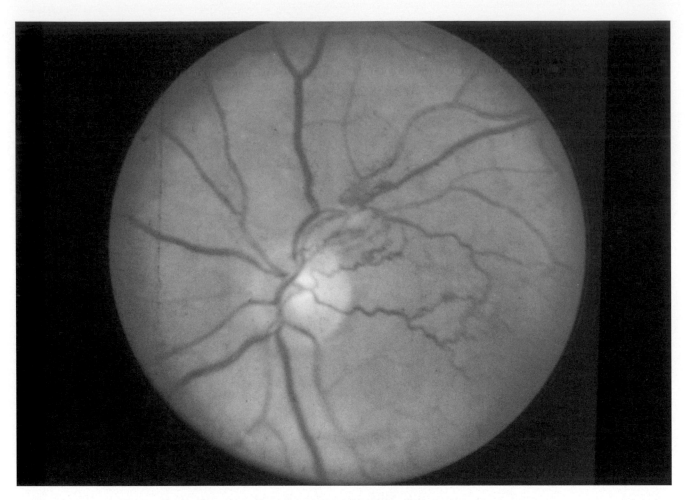

FIGURE 2-10 Neovascularization after branch retinal vein obstruction. New vessels may develop late after obstruction of a branch of the central retinal vein. These most often serve to shunt flow around the obstructed vessel site and are thus not as exuberantly proliferative as those seen in diabetic retinopathy. (*See color Plate 10.*)

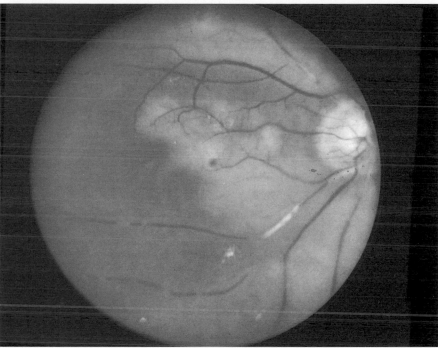

A

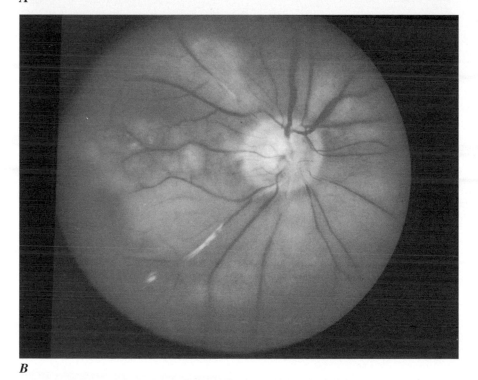

B

FIGURE 2-11 Embolic retinal arterial obstruction (*A* and *B*). Cholesterol crystals may dislodge from the walls of the heart, aortic arch, or carotids. Carried into the retinal circulation as Hollenhorst plaques, they seldom completely obstruct the arterioles. Although amaurosis fugax is more common, the embolic burden may occasionally be so large as to produce retinal infarction. Note in the photograph of the macular area (*A*) that this patient's fovea remains red, while there is a pale, cloudy swelling nasal to it. This has produced a half "cherry-red" spot. With complete central retinal artery occlusion, the red foveal area is completely surrounded by pale swollen retina. Hollenhorst cholesterol plaques can be seen in both the upper and lower temporal retinal arteries. In *A*, the inferior temporal arteriole demonstrates "boxcar" segmentation of the blood column, indicative of very slow flow. (*See color Plate 11A and B.*)

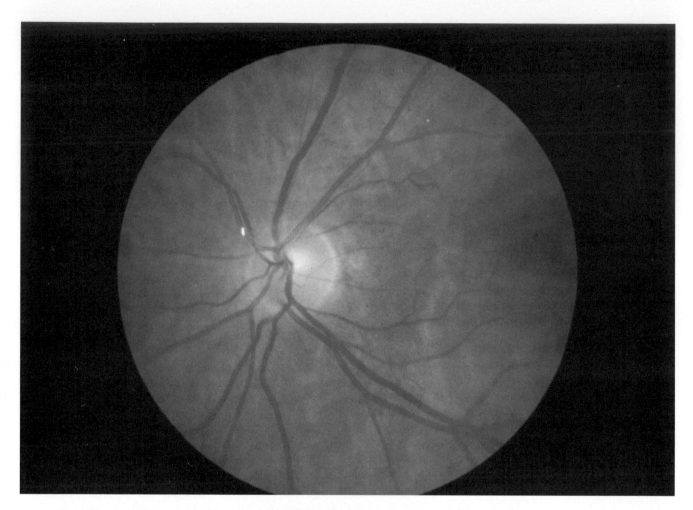

FIGURE 2-12   Calcific retinal embolus associated with aortic valvular disease. Calcific aortic valvular disease and valve replacement surgery may result in retinal emboli. Like cholesterol emboli, these calcific flecks lodge at arterial bifurcations but seldom completely obstruct flow. They are white and glitter in the ophthalmoscope beam. Somewhat similar emboli may be seen after the intravenous injection of illicit drugs expanded with talc. (*See color Plate 12.*)

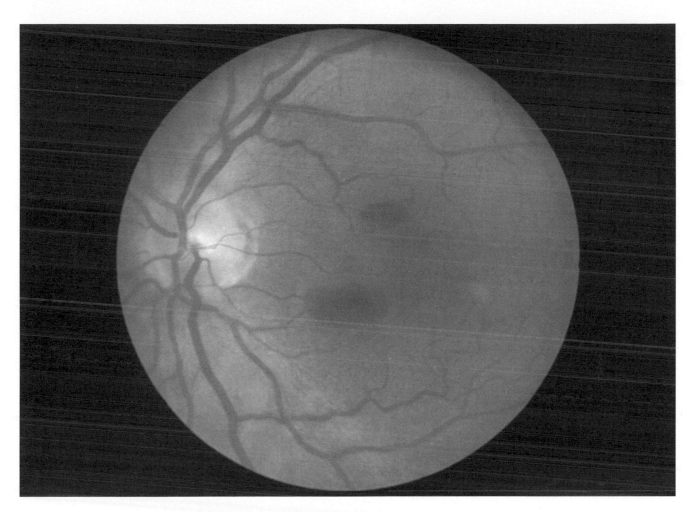

FIGURE 2-13   Retinal hemorrhages after cardiac catheterization.
Following cardiac catheterization, symptomatic and asymptomatic retinal
hemorrhages may occur. The latter are more common. Presumably, these
are the result of embolic events. Note, in this recently catheterized patient,
the two oval hemorrhages and a small area of cloudy swelling just inferior
and temporal to the fovea. (*See color Plate 13.*)

REFERENCES

1. Wise GN, Dollery CT, Henkind P: *The Retinal Circulation.* New York, Harper & Row, 1971.
2. The Diabetic Retinopathy Study Research Group: Photocoagulation treatment in proliferative diabetic retinopathy. The second report of diabetic retinopathy study findings. *Ophthalmology* 1978; 85:82–106.
3. Early Treatment Diabetic Retinopathy Study Research Group: Results from the early treatment diabetic retinopathy study. *Ophthalmology* 1991; 98:766–840.

CHAPTER 3

PLAIN FILM DIAGNOSIS OF HEART DISEASE: CONGENITAL AND ACQUIRED

James T. T. Chen, M.D.

T HIS chapter builds and expands upon the illustrations in the eighth edition of *Hurst's The Heart*.[1] The material falls into two parts: Figs. 3-2 through 3-23 deal with the roentgenographic interpretation of acquired heart disease[1–5] and Figs. 3-1 and 3-25 through 3-52 depict congenital heart defects, chosen mainly from the adult population.[2,6] The new materials provide anatomic or pathophysiologic details of certain important diseases. For example, a magnified view of notched ribs (Fig. 3-1) demonstrates not only the exquisite notches but also the earliest changes in the ribs, the wavy, sclerotic lower edge of which represents the reparative process of laying down new bone. Roentgenographic manifestations of volume overload versus pressure overload are best appreciated in side-by-side comparisons (e.g., Figs. 3-9 and 3-10). The same is true with regard to surgical benefits or complications (Fig. 3-7A and B). Some radiographic findings are virtually diagnostic (e.g., a calcified left ventricular aneurysm in its typical location, as in Figs. 3-13, 3-14, and 3-15).

Thanks to recent advances in medicine and surgery, an increasing number of pediatric patients with congenital heart disease now live into adulthood; therefore those physicians who have, in the past, dealt mainly with acquired cardiac diseases will certainly benefit from becoming familiar with the radiographic manifestations of adult congenital heart disease.

In the category of left-to-right shunts, the most common entity encountered among adult patients is secundum atrial septal defect (ASD; Fig. 3-25). Although patients with

ASD may remain asymptomatic throughout most of their adult lives, some may develop problems earlier; then their disease may be confused with mitral stenosis, because the auscultatory features of these two conditions are similar. One rarely sees a large ventricular septal defect (VSD; Fig. 3-26) in an adult, mainly because this will either have closed spontaneously or been treated by early surgery. A large patent ductus arteriosus (PDA; Fig. 3-27) is also a rarity in an adult. On the other hand, Eisenmenger syndrome (Figs. 3-30, 3-31, and 3-32) due to a large, long-standing left-to-right shunt is relatively more common in the young adult population.

Uncommonly, admixture lesions with increased pulmonary blood flow (Fig. 3-33) may be encountered in the adolescent or adult. Patients with D-loop transposition of the great arteries and VSD usually cannot survive into adulthood unless some natural protective mechanism is present, such as associated pulmonary stenosis (Fig. 3-35) or coexistent pulmonary arterial hypertension (Fig. 3-34).

Some patients with right-to-left shunts may first present with stroke or paradoxical embolism (Fig. 3-43). Others may appear with surgical complications (Fig. 3-47). Certain entities—such as a calcific bicuspid aortic valve (Fig. 3-38) or the scimitar syndrome (Fig. 3-52)—provide a radiographic diagnosis. Some anatomic features are extremely useful in suggesting a particular entity; for example, a mirror-image branching type of right aortic arch (Fig. 3-47) is associated with tetralogy of Fallot in over 90 percent of patients with this presentation.

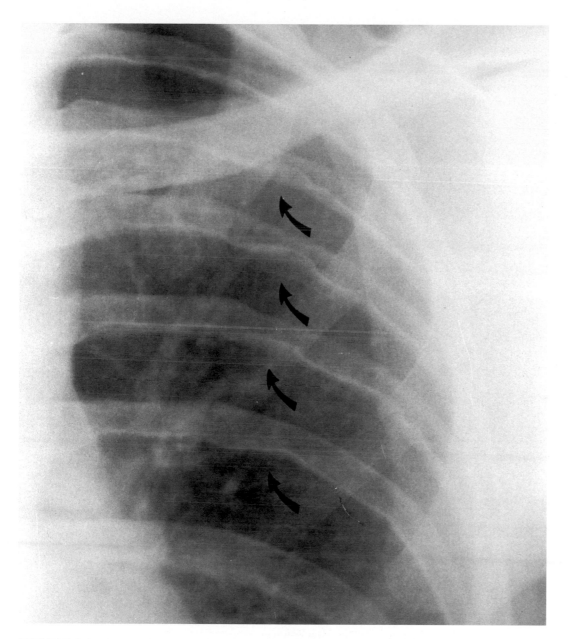

FIGURE 3-1   Magnified view of the left upper thorax showing multiple areas of rib notching (*arrows*) in a patient with severe coarctation of the aorta. The sclerotic margin of each notch represents a reparative process by which new bone is laid down in the defect.

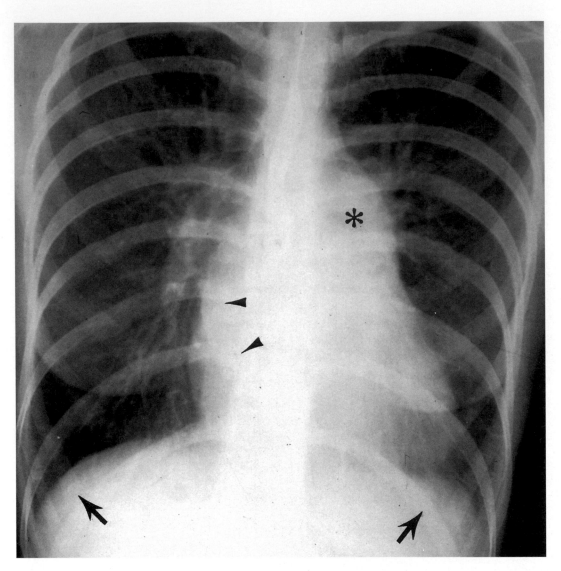

FIGURE 3-2   Striking cephalization of the pulmonary vasculature representing severe pulmonary venous hypertension in a patient with critical mitral stenosis. Note also the septal lines in both costophrenic sulci (*arrows*), double density of left atrial enlargement (*arrowheads*), and markedly dilated pulmonary trunk(*).

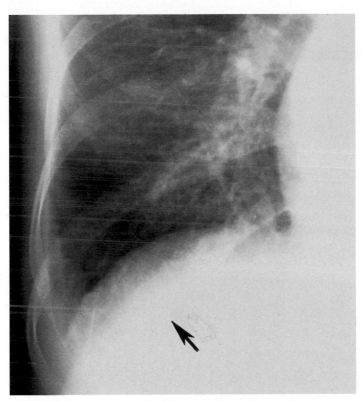

A

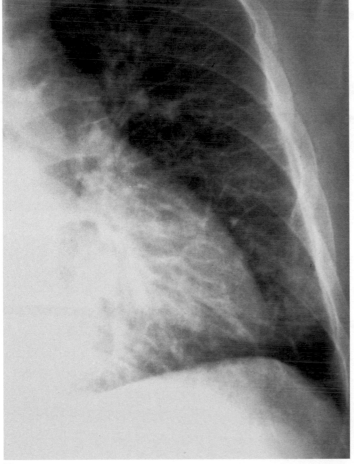

B

FIGURE 3-3   Magnified view of the right
costophrenic sulcus (A) of a patient with critical
mitral stenosis, showing multiple septal lines
(arrow). B. Patient with subacute left ventricular
failure. Note numerous septal lines. Kerley's "B"
lines are shorter and always perpendicular to the
pleural surface. "A" lines are longer, converging
to the hilum. Other signs of interstitial edema are
poor margination of vessels and peribronchial
cuffings.

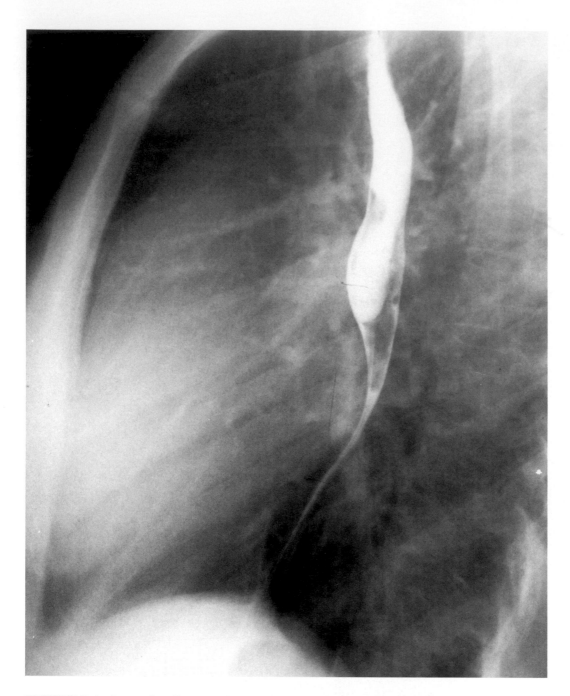

FIGURE 3-4   Lateral radiograph in a patient with pure mitral stenosis showing right ventricular–left atrial enlargement and abnormally small left ventricle. Note that the barium-filled esophagus is deviated posteriorly by the enlarged left atrium.

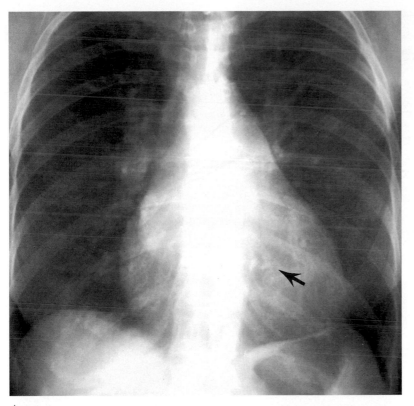

A

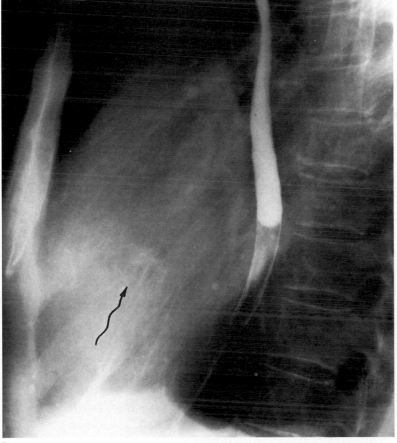

B

FIGURE 3-5 *A.* **Posteroanterior radiograph of an elderly woman with severe mitral stenosis and calcified mitral valve** (*arrow*)**. Lateral view** (*B*) **of a similar patient with calcified mitral valve** (*arrow*)**.**

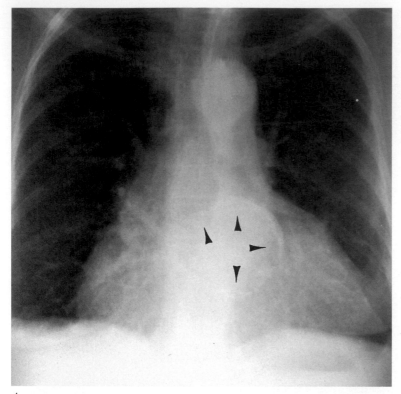

A

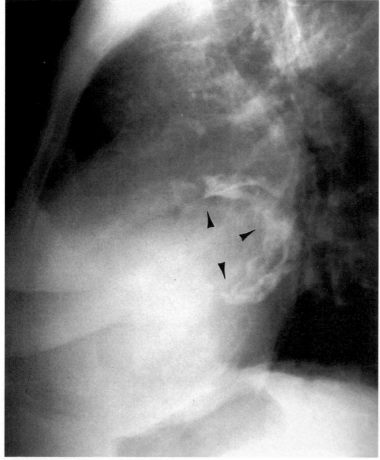

B

FIGURE 3-6   A 58-year-old woman
suffering from severe rheumatic mitral
stenosis, tricuspid regurgitation, atrial
fibrillation, and episodes of arterial
embolization. Note diffuse calcification
of the left atrial wall (*arrowheads*).
A. Posteroanterior view. *B.* Lateral view.

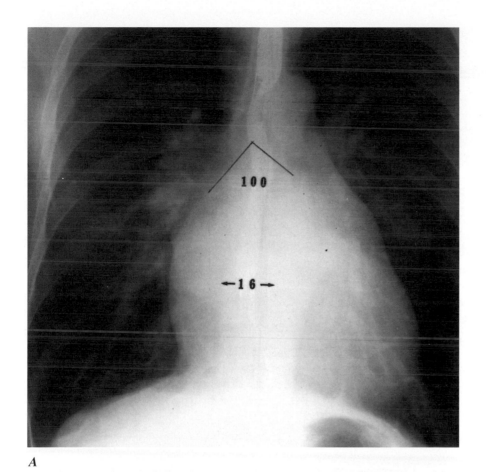

A

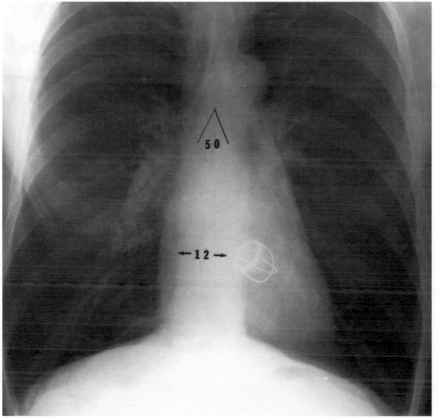

B

FIGURE 3-7   Patient with rheumatic mitral regurgitation and preserved left ventricular contractility. Radiograph prior to surgery (*A*) shows a huge left atrium, moderate biventricular enlargement, and widening of the subcarinal angle to 100°. Also note the cephalic pulmonary blood flow (PBF) pattern. The transverse diameter of the heart measures 16 cm. After mitral valve replacement (*B*), dramatic improvements are noted. The subcarinal angle now measures 50° and the heart 12 cm.

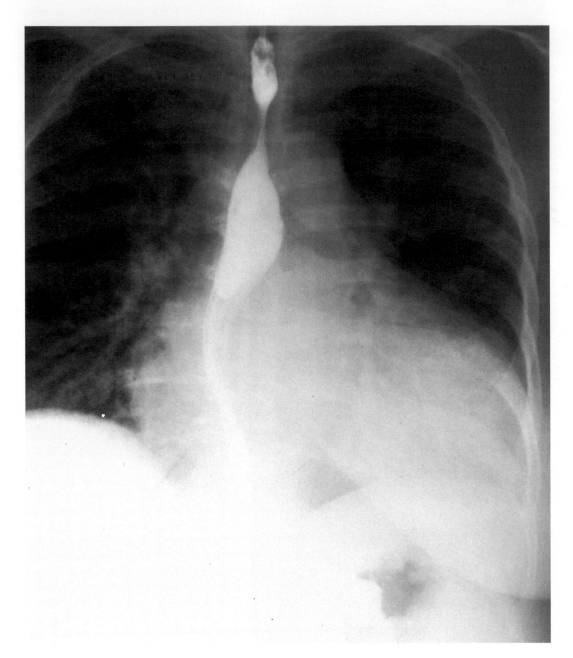

FIGURE 3-8 Posteroanterior radiograph of a patient with coronary heart disease, papillary muscle dysfunction, and mitral regurgitation. The left ventricle was markedly enlarged and contracting poorly. The regurgitant flow to the left atrium was small. Consequently, there is a huge left ventricle, a moderately enlarged left atrium, and a cephalic PBF pattern. Compare with Fig. 3-7.

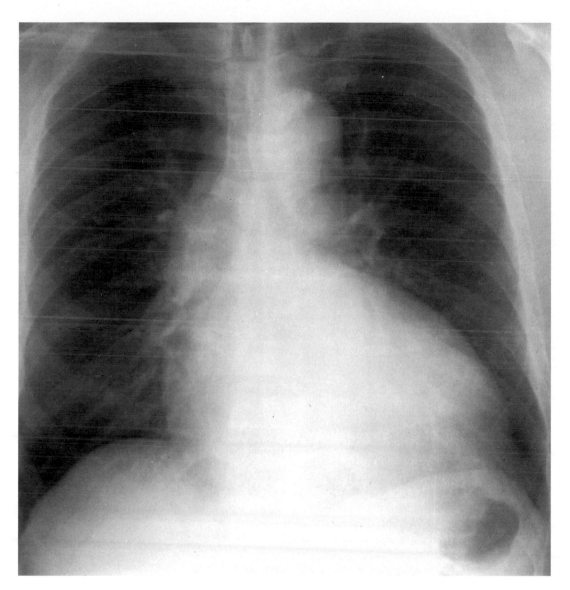

FIGURE 3-9   A 57-year-old man with severe aortic regurgitation prior
to left ventricular failure. Despite considerable volume overload to the left
ventricle and aorta, the lungs and their vasculature remain normal.

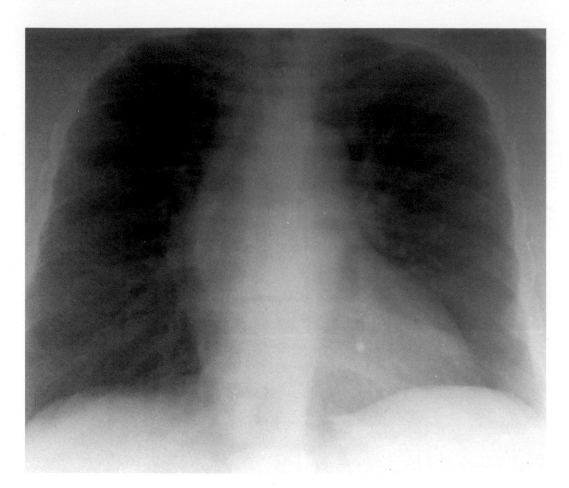

FIGURE 3-10   A 41-year-old man with systemic hypertension and pressure overload to the left ventricle and aorta. The aorta is too prominent for his relatively young age. The increased convexity of the left ventricle represents concentric hypertrophy. Compare with volume overload situation shown in Fig. 3-9.

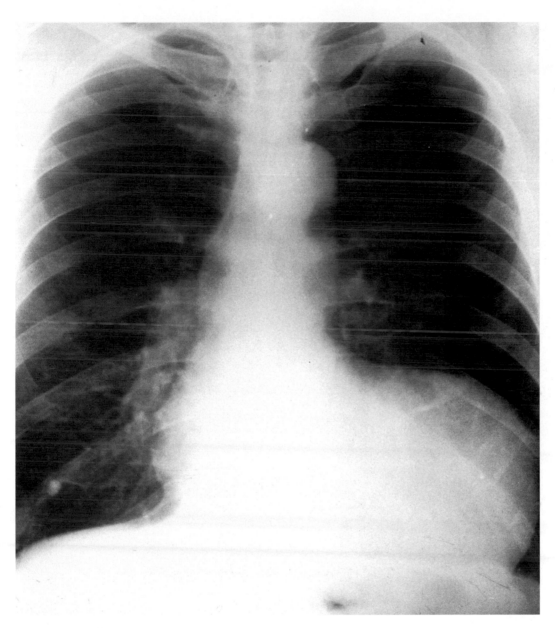

FIGURE 3-11   An elderly man with a huge anterolateral apical left ventricular aneurysm.

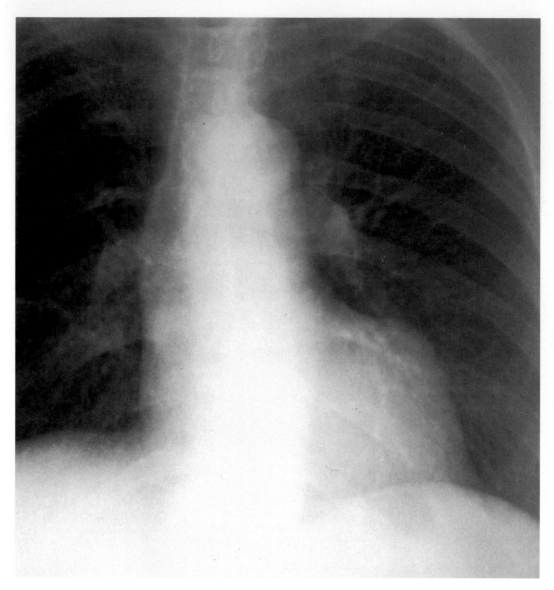

FIGURE 3-12   Posteroanterior radiograph of a 60-year-old man with a localized anterolateral left ventricular aneurysm.

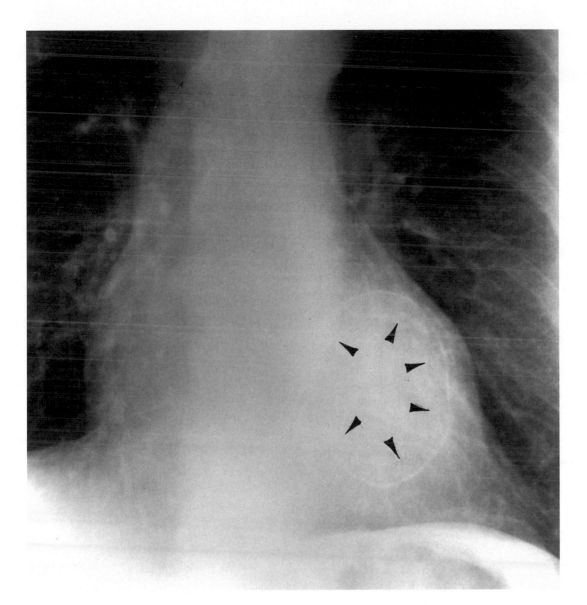

FIGURE 3-13 Posteroanterior radiograph of a 69-year-old man with a totally calcified anterolateral apical left ventricular aneurysm (*arrowheads*).

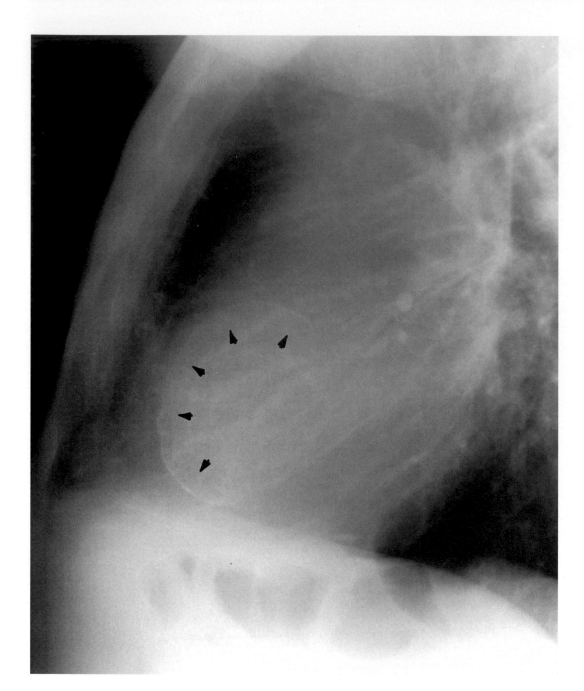

FIGURE 3-14   Lateral radiograph of same patient as in Fig. 3-13 showing the typical anterior location of such an aneurysm (*arrowheads*). (From Chen JTT: The significance of cardiac calcifications. *Appl Radiol* 1992, 2:11–19. Reproduced with permission from the publisher and author.)

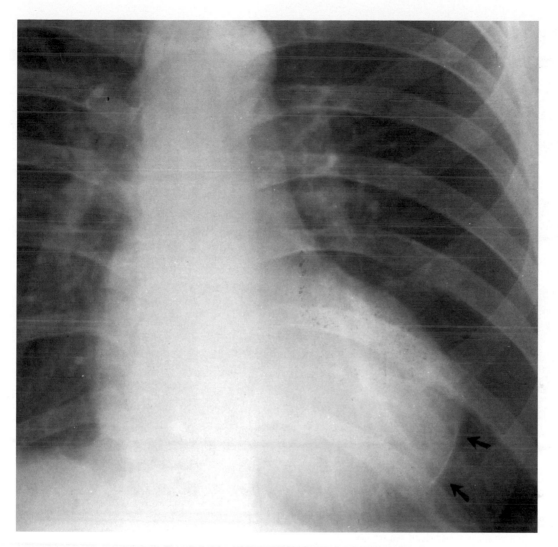

FIGURE 3-15   Patient with long-standing severe coronary heart disease showing a rather large anterolateral apical left ventricular aneurysm that was only partially calcified (*arrows*). Unfortunately, the patient expired, and we had postmortem proof of this diagnosis. (From Chen JTT: *Essentials of Cardiac Roentgenology*. Boston, Little, Brown, 1987. Reproduced with permission from the publisher and author.)

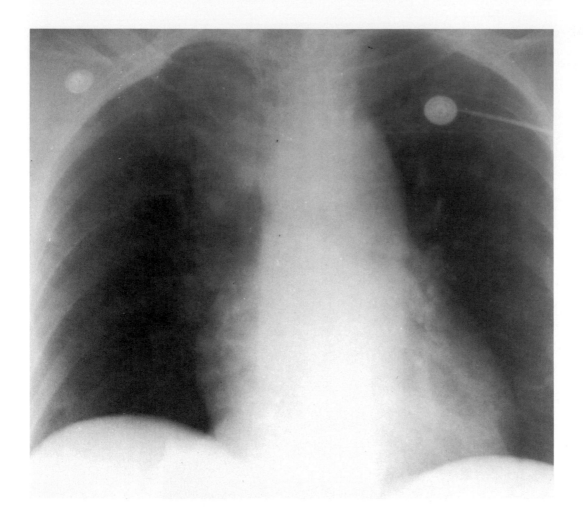

FIGURE 3-16 A 72-year-old woman suffering from acute chest pain and dyspnea. The chest radiograph shows marked dilatation of superior vena cava and azygous vein, moderate dilatation of the proximal right pulmonary artery, and oligemia of the right lower lung (Westermark sign). The patient expired shortly afterward. Autopsy showed massive embolism to right interlobar pulmonary artery from clots in right iliac vein. (See also Chap. 11.)

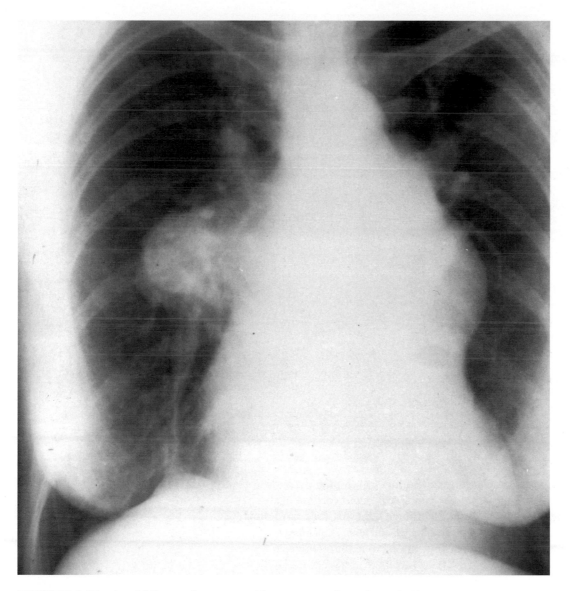

FIGURE 3-17 A middle-aged woman with recurrent thromboembolic disease showing a striking centralized PBF pattern indicating severe pulmonary arterial hypertension. Also note the calcified right pulmonary artery and a scar from previous pulmonary infarction in the right lower zone. The dilated right atrium and ventricle indicate right heart failure with tricuspid regurgitation. (See also Chap. 11.)

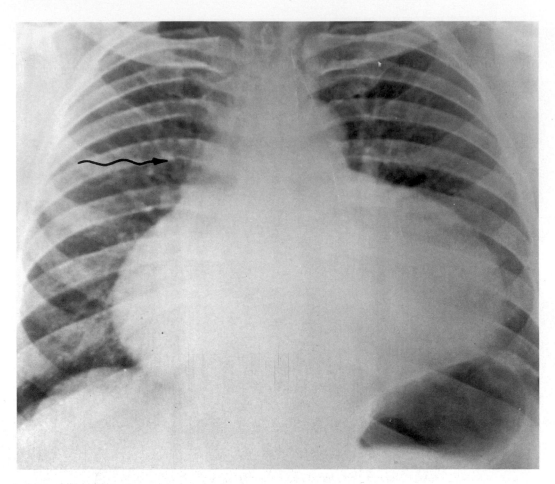

FIGURE 3-18   This patient suffered from rapidly developing dyspnea and became hypotensive. His roentgenogram shows gross cardiomegaly with a bulging border bilaterally. Note the dilated superior vena cava and azygous vein (*arrow*). Also note the cephalic PBF pattern. A prompt pericardiocentesis was performed to relieve his cardiac tamponade.

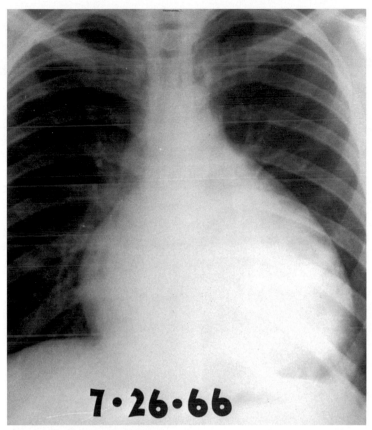

A

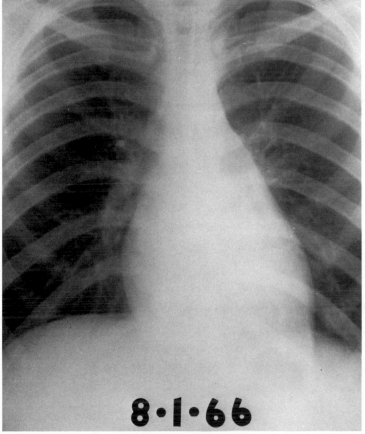

B

FIGURE 3-19   This young man suffered from acute pericarditis with effusion. The initial radiograph (*A*) shows a water-bottle-shaped cardiomegaly, clear lungs, and normal pulmonary vascularity. With appropriate therapy, the effusion resolved rapidly, as seen in (*B*), taken 5 days later.

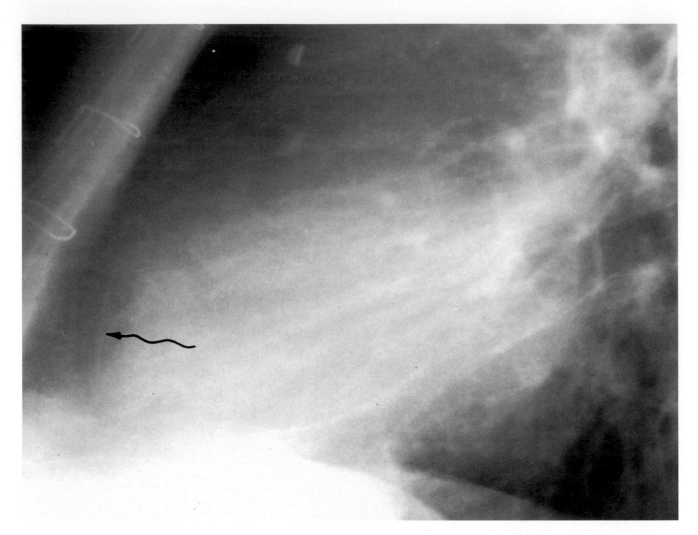

FIGURE 3-20   A magnified view of the retrosternal area showing the
hairlike normal pericardium (*arrow*) sandwiched between the subepicardial
fat stripe interiorly and mediastinal fat stripe exteriorly. The maximal
width of normal pericardium is 2 mm.

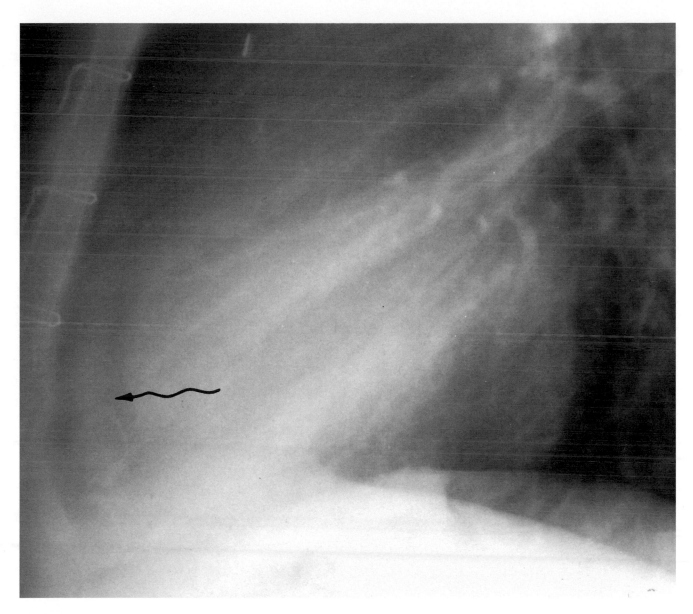

FIGURE 3-21   The same patient 2 weeks later, with moderate pericardial effusion. The pericardial cavity now measured >1 cm wide (*arrow*).

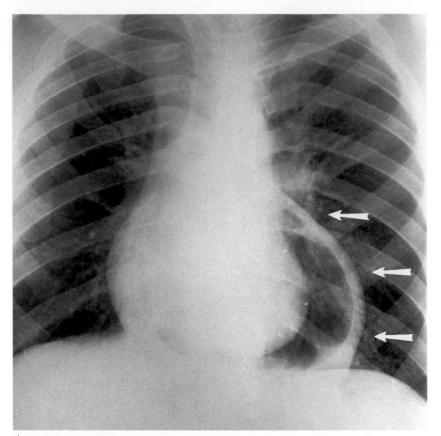

A

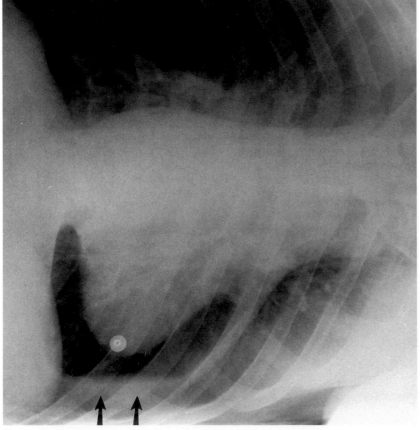

B

FIGURE 3-22   **This young man with traumatic constrictive-effusive pericarditis required emergent pericardiocentesis. The subsequent injection of air produced a hydropneumopericardium. In the supine position (*A*), air filled only the left side of the pericardium. Note the much thickened parietal layer (*arrows*). Even in a left lateral decubitus position (*B*), air could not rise to the right side of the pericardium because of adhesions. Note the horizontal air-fluid level (*arrows*).**

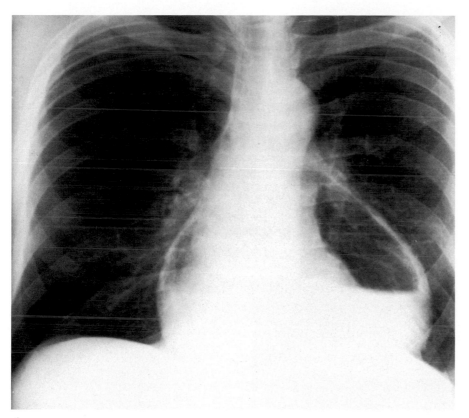

A

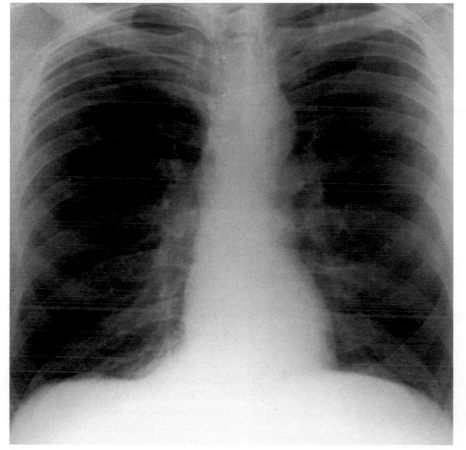

B

FIGURE 3-23   Patient with tuberculous effusive-constrictive pericarditis. The postpericardio-centesis erect film (*A*) shows thickening of the pericardium and partial obliteration of the pericardial cavity on the right side, owing to adhesions. Following pericardiectomy (*B*), the heart returned to normal.

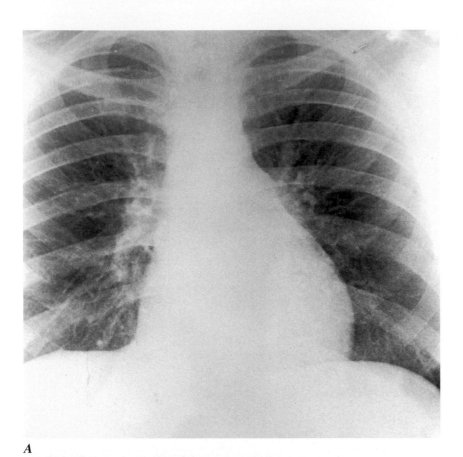

A

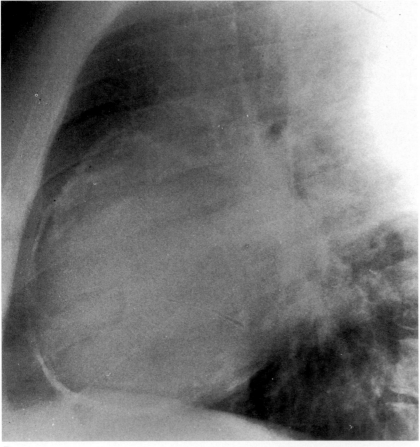

B

FIGURE 3-24   **Patient with constrictive calcific pericarditis. In PA view (*A*), one sees a cephalic PBF pattern and a peculiar cardiac contour due to thickening and adhesions of the pericardium. In the lateral view (*B*), heavy calcification of the pericardium is evident over the pulmonary trunk, the anterior border of the right ventricle, and the inferior border of both ventricles. Also note left atrial enlargement. (From Chen JTT:** *Essentials of Cardiac Roentgenology.* **Boston, Little, Brown, 1987. Reproduced with permission from the publisher and author.)**

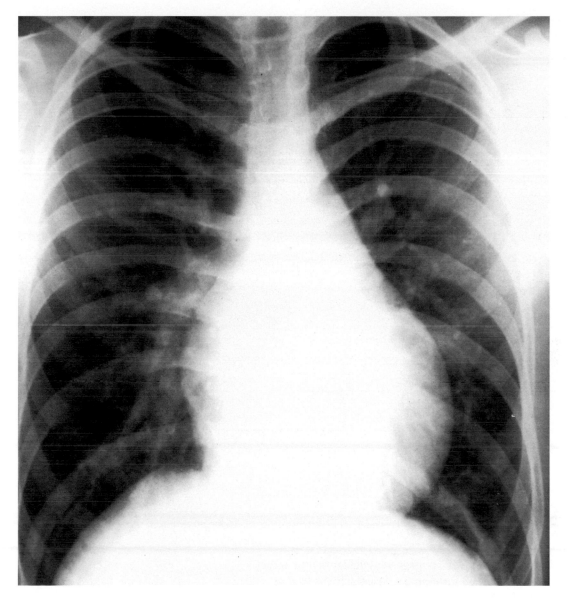

FIGURE 3-25   A 17-year-old man with a large secundum atrial septal defect. The radiograph shows increased pulmonary vascularity, right-sided cardiomegaly, a large pulmonary trunk, and small aortic arch.

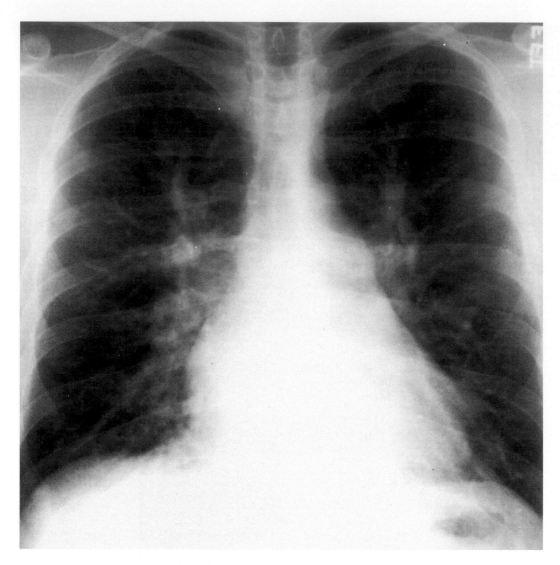

**FIGURE 3-26   A 28-year-old man with a large ventricular septal defect.
The PA radiograph shows increased pulmonary vascularity as well as
biventricular and left atrial enlargement. The aortic arch is normal in size.**

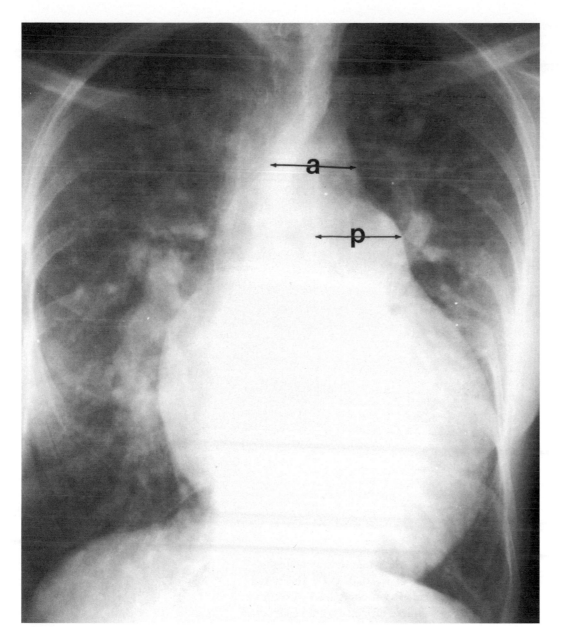

FIGURE 3-27   A 24-year-old woman with a very large patent ductus arteriosus. The radiograph shows increased pulmonary vascularity, left-sided cardiomegaly, and dilated aorta (a) and pulmonary trunk (p).

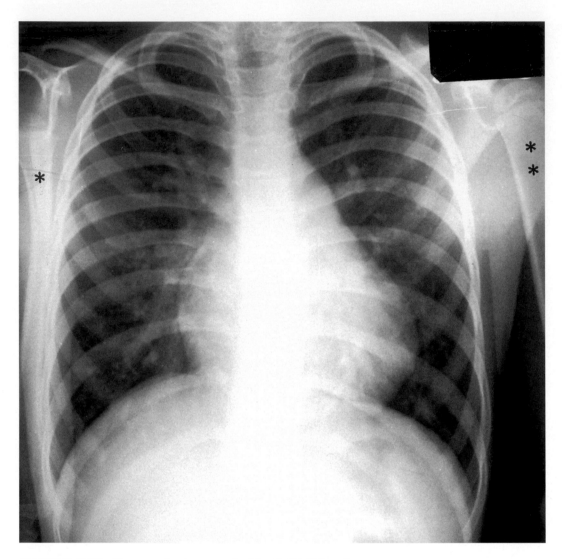

FIGURE 3-28 Same patient as seen in Fig. 3-25. When he was younger, the radiograph again showed a typical picture of isolated ASD. Also noted was a hypoplastic and subluxed right humerus (∗) as compared with the much better formed left humerus (*). An example of Holt-Oram syndrome.

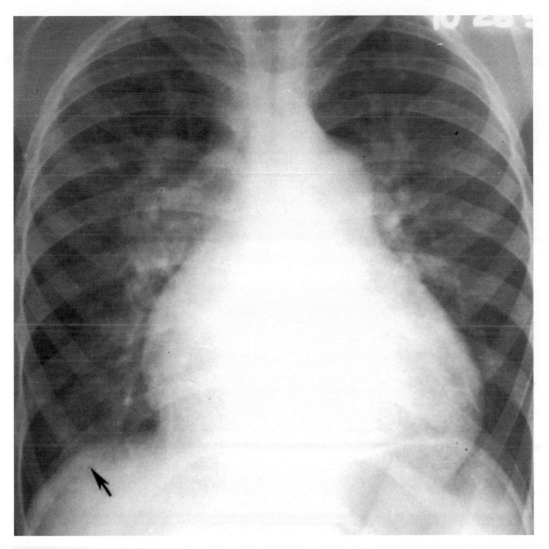

FIGURE 3-29   A child with a combination of secundum ASD and
rheumatic mitral stenosis (Lutembacher's syndrome). Note a cephalic
PBF pattern and Kerley's "B" lines (*arrow*). The upper vessels are much
bigger than those seen in a patient with isolated mitral stenosis due to the
presence of a large left-to-right shunt. Lateral view (not shown) depicts an
enlarged left atrium deviating the barium-filled esophagus posteriorly.

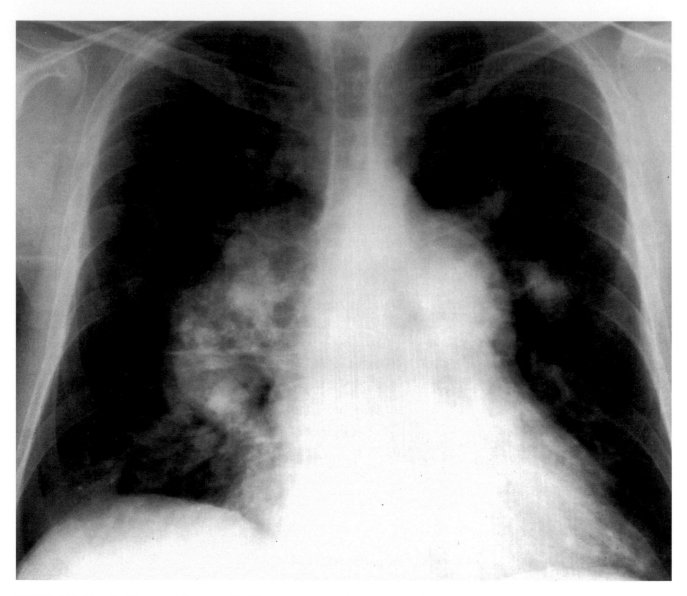

FIGURE 3-30   A 42-year-old man with Eisenmenger syndrome secondary to an ASD showing a striking centralized flow pattern and right-sided cardiomegaly. The aortic arch is quite small.

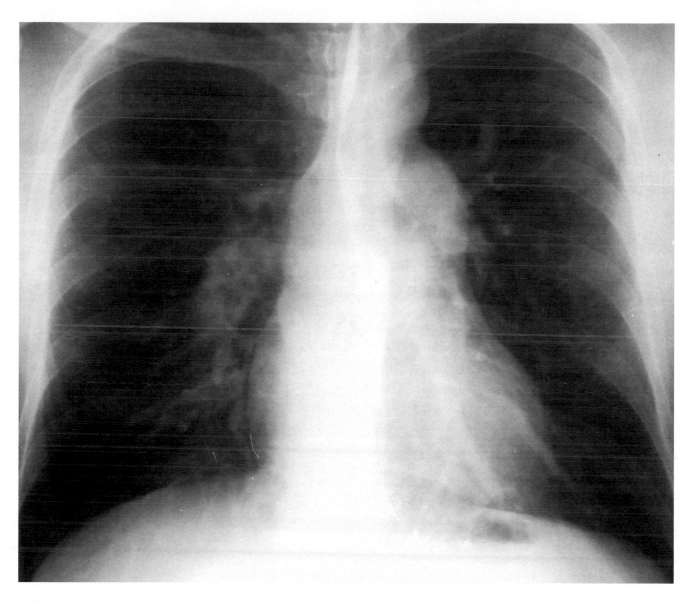

FIGURE 3-31   A 22-year-old man with Eisenmenger syndrome secondary to a VSD showing a centralized flow pattern and right-sided cardiomegaly. The aortic arch is normal.

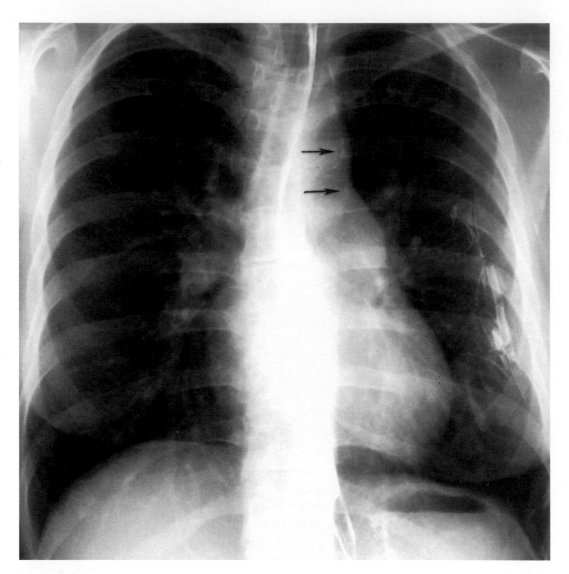

FIGURE 3-32   A 41-year-old woman with Eisenmenger syndrome secondary to a PDA showing a centralized flow pattern and right-sided cardiomegaly. Both the aortic arch and pulmonary trunk are dilated with curvilinear calcium deposits (*arrows*).

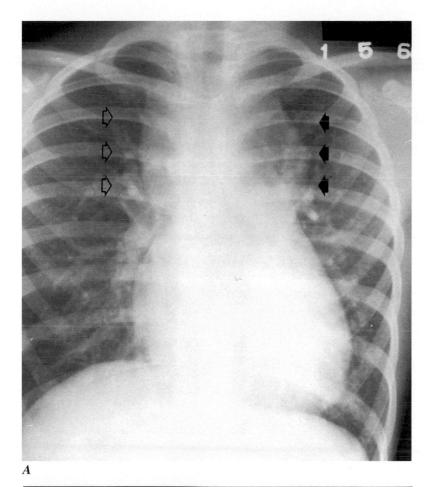

A

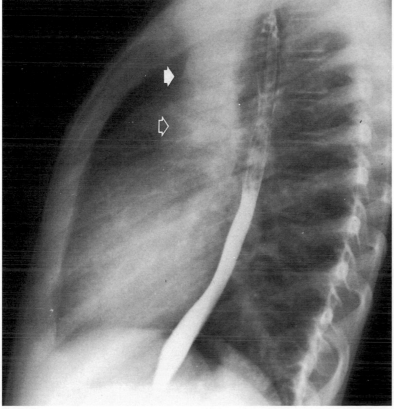

B

FIGURE 3-33 Patient with total anomalous pulmonary venous connection via the left vertical vein, forming a "snowman" cardiovascular configuration on PA view (*A*). The snowman's head is formed by the left vertical vein (*solid arrowheads*) on the left and the dilated superior vena cava (SVC; *open arrowheads*) on the right. The fat body of the snowman is formed by the right-sided cardiomegaly. Also note the increased pulmonary vascularity. On lateral view (*B*), in addition to right-sided cardiomegaly, there is a striking pretracheal double density (*solid and open arrowheads*) representing a superimposition of the large left vertical vein upon the dilated SVC.

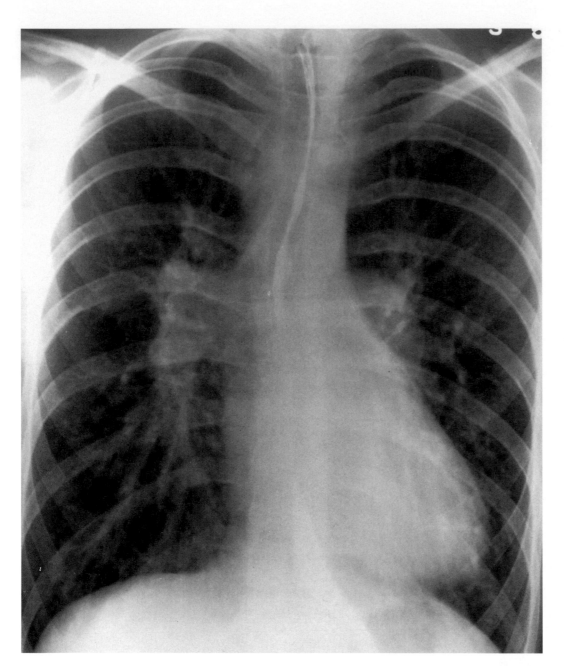

FIGURE 3-34   Young adult with D-loop transposition of the great
arteries, VSD, and pulmonary arterial hypertension. Note a centralized
PBF pattern, mild cardiomegaly with left ventricular preponderance, and
the narrow waist of the heart. (From Chen JTT: *Essentials of Cardiac
Roentgenology*. Boston, Little, Brown, 1987. Reproduced with permission
from the publisher and author.)

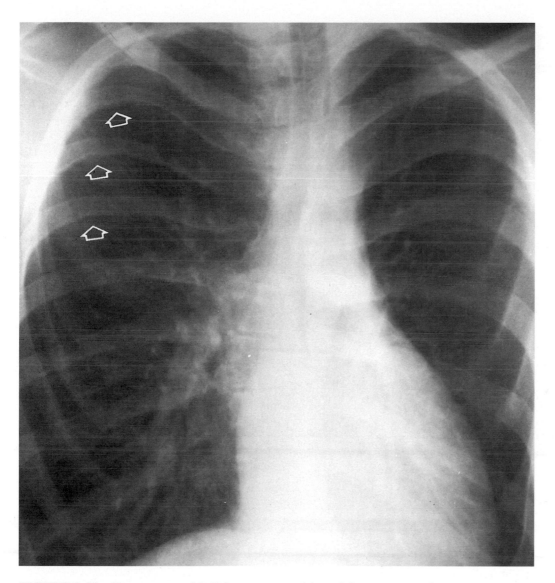

FIGURE 3-35   Young man with D-loop transposition of the great arteries and pulmonary stenosis following a right-sided Blalock-Taussig shunt. Note oligemia of the left lung, slight plethora of the right lung, notching of the right upper ribs (*arrowheads*), mild left ventricular enlargement, and narrowing of the cardiac waist.

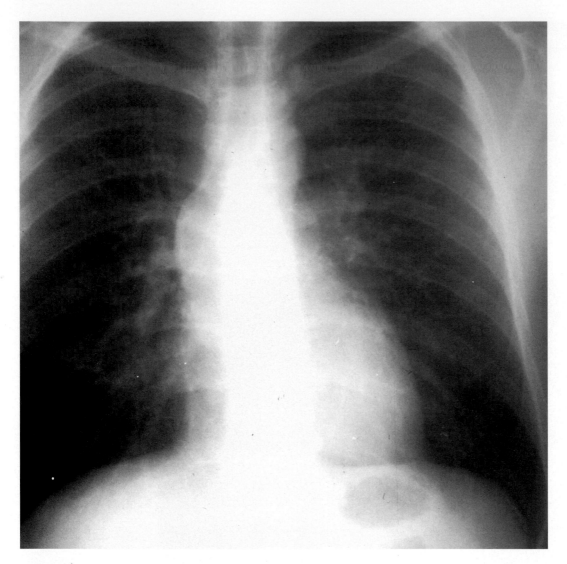

FIGURE 3-36   A 17-year-old with congenital aortic valve stenosis.
Note dilatation of the ascending aorta, increased convexity of the left
ventricle, and normal pulmonary vascularity. The systolic aortic gradient
was 100 mmHg.

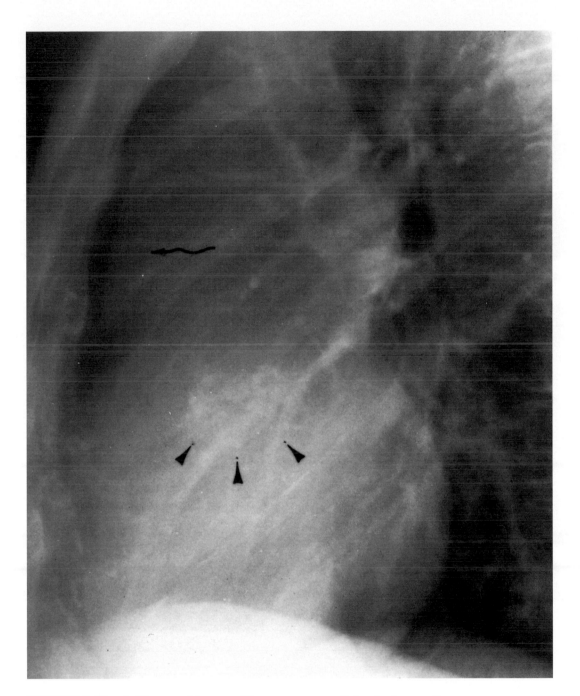

FIGURE 3-37   A 45-year-old man with severe congenital valvular aortic stenosis. The lateral view shows heavy amorphous calcification of the entire aortic valve (*arrowheads*), dilated ascending aorta (*arrow*), and left ventricular enlargement. (From Chen JTT: Radiology of valvular heart disease. *Appl Radiol* 1994; 23:11-19. Reproduced with permission from the publisher and author.)

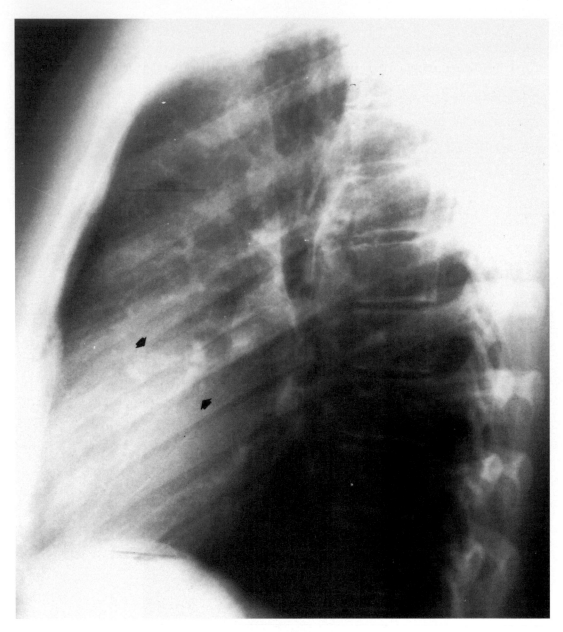

FIGURE 3-38   A middle-aged man with a calcified bicuspid aortic valve (*arrowheads*).

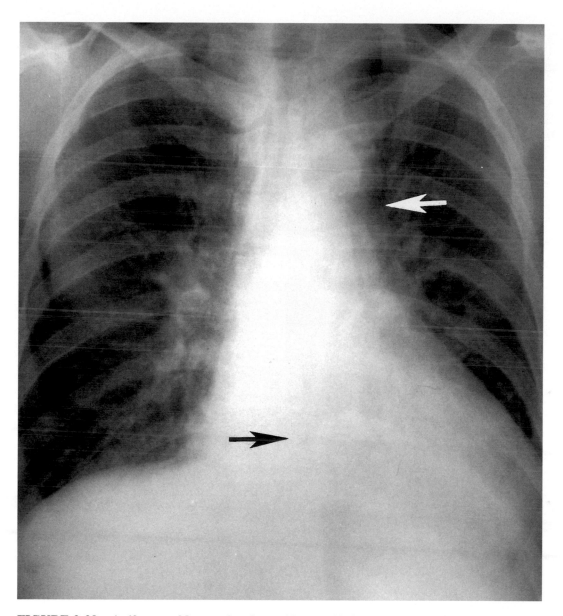

FIGURE 3-39   A 60-year-old man showing evidence of left ventricular
failure. The white arrow denotes the "3" sign of coarctation of the aorta;
the black arrow denotes the site of a heavily calcified aortic valve. He
underwent a two-stage operation with good results: coarctectomy followed
by aortic valve replacement.

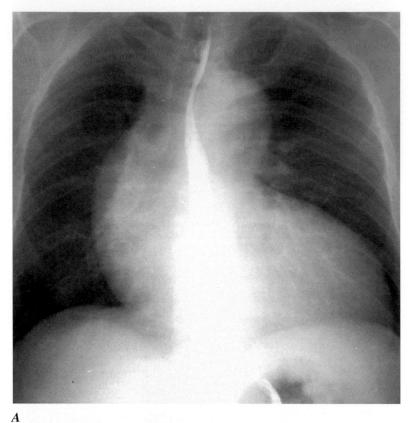

A

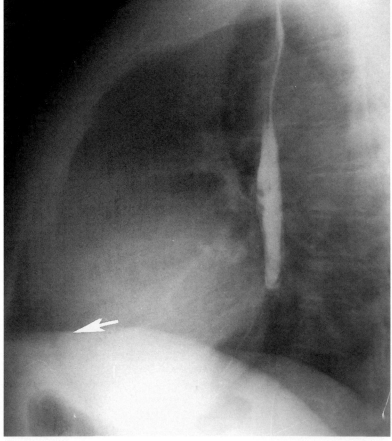

B

FIGURE 3-40 A 45-year-old man with Marfan syndrome, severe aortic regurgitation, and proximal aortic dissection into the pericardial cavity. Posteroanterior view (*A*) shows a huge left ventricle and aneurysmal dilatation of the ascending aorta. There is, however, no sign of left ventricular failure. (From Chen JTT: Radiology of valvular heart disease. *Appl Radiol* 1994; 23:11-19. Reproduced with permission from the publisher and author.) On the lateral view (*B*), one sees a small pericardial effusion (*arrow*).

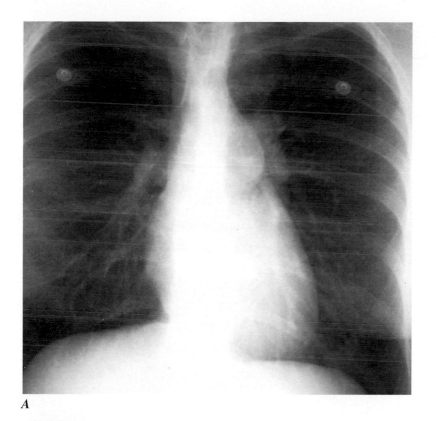

A

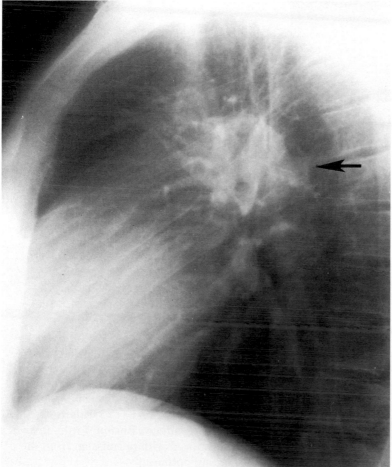

B

FIGURE 3-41   A 37-year-old woman with congenital valvular pulmonary stenosis. Posteroanterior view (*A*) shows dilatation of pulmonary trunk and left pulmonary artery as well as decreased size of the right pulmonary artery. Also note more flow to the left lung and less to the right. Lateral view (*B*) shows enlargement of right ventricle and pulmonary trunk as well as dilatation of the left pulmonary artery (*arrow*).

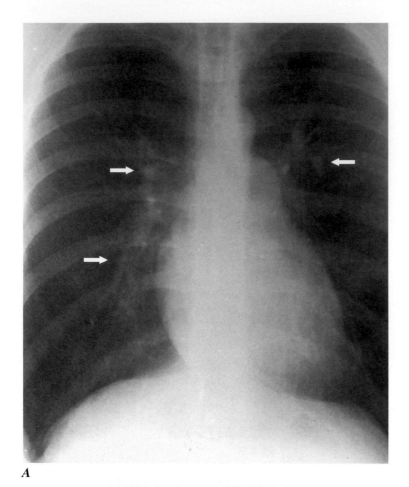

A

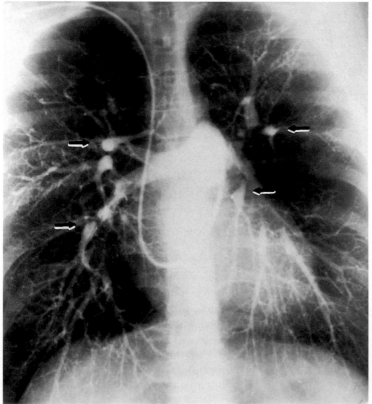

B

FIGURE 3-42   **A 23-year-old man with pulmonary artery branch stenoses. Postero-anterior (*A*) view shows enlargement of right ventricle and pulmonary trunk. The pulmonary vascularity is decreased, with multiple small rounded, oval-shaped, or triangular opacities (*arrows*) in both hilar and perihilar regions representing poststenotic dilatation of the distal pulmonary arteries. The pulmonary arteriogram (*B*) provides the explanation for the multiple perihilar opacities (*arrows*). (From Chen JTT: *Essentials of Cardiac Roentgenology.* Boston, Little, Brown, 1987. Reproduced with permission from the publisher and authors.)**

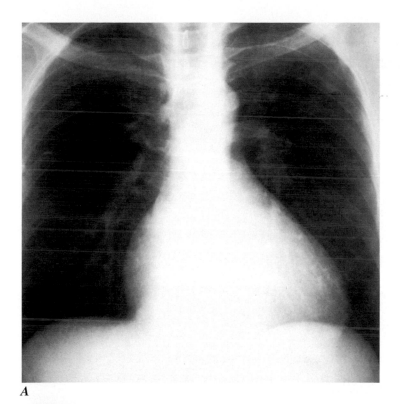

A

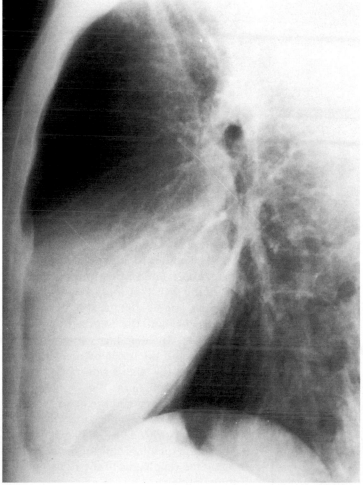

B

FIGURE 3-43 A 37-year-old man was admitted to the hospital because of a recent cerebral vascular accident. Deep-vein thrombosis was diagnosed by angiography. Echocardiography showed a classic picture of Ebstein's anomaly. Posteroanterior chest film (*A*) shows severe oligemia of both lungs and gross right-sided cardiomegaly. On the lateral view (*B*), one sees pure right-sided cardiomegaly and a very small hilar shadow.

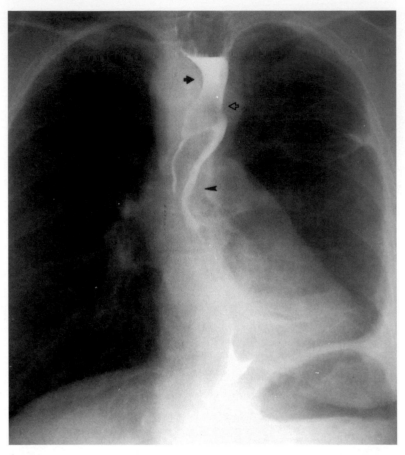

A

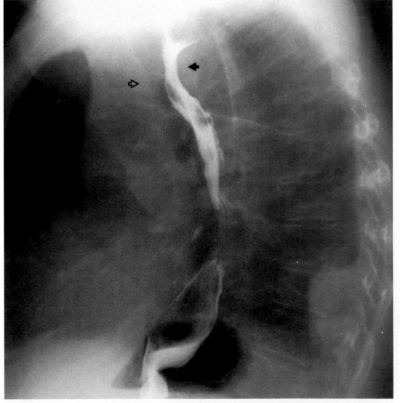

B

FIGURE 3-44 A 57-year-old woman
was seen primarily for carcinoma of
the tongue metastasizing to the lung.
Congenital double aortic arch was found
incidentally. With barium in the
esophagus, one sees bilateral indentation
on the trachea and the esophagus on the
PA view (*A*). The esophagus was indented
posteriorly and the trachea indented
anteriorly on the lateral view (*B*). The
solid arrow points to the higher, larger,
posterior right arch and the open arrow
points to the lower, smaller, anterior left
arch. The arrowhead on the PA view
points to the tortuous descending aorta
crossing the esophagus to the right side
of the midline.

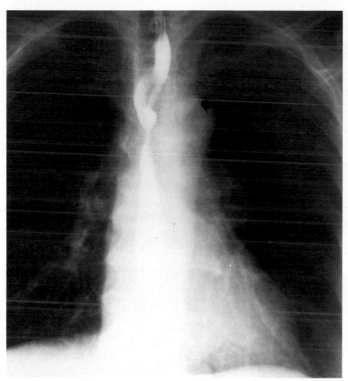

A

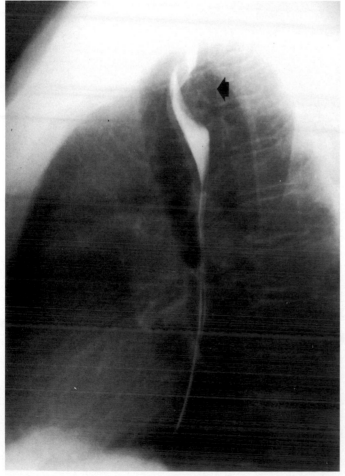

B

FIGURE 3-45 **A 64-year-old woman with ovarian carcinoma. A smooth oblique indentation on barium-filled esophagus (*arrowhead*) is seen in the PA view (*A*), from the left inferior to the right superior direction. In the lateral view (*B*), in addition to the indentation mentioned above, both the esophagus and the trachea are markedly displaced anteriorly (*arrow*). This is diagnostic of an aberrant right subclavian artery.**

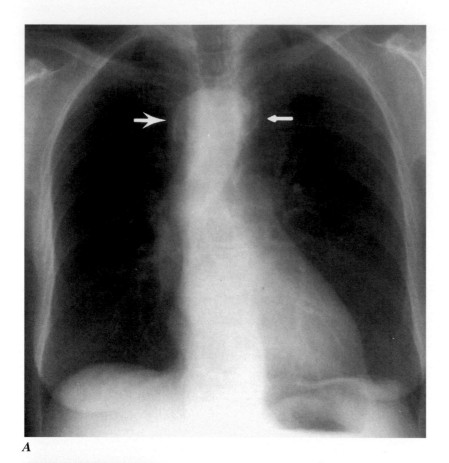

A

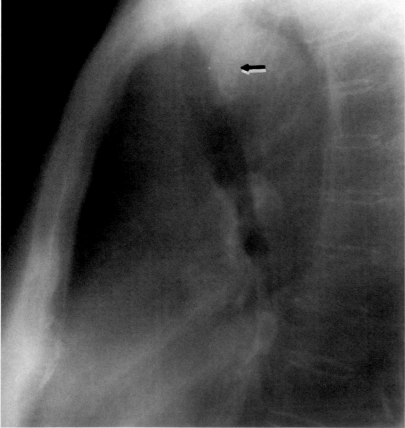

B

FIGURE 3-46   An asymptomatic woman was referred because of a "mediastinal mass." Typical findings of right-sided aortic arch with aberrant left subclavian artery are noted. On PA view (*A*), the trachea is deviated to the left side above the carina by the right arch (*large arrow*). The aortic diverticulum (*small arrow*) projects to the left of the midline but does not impinge on the left lateral border of the trachea because of its posterior location. On the lateral view (*B*), the trachea is displaced anteriorly by the large aortic diverticulum (*small arrow*) from which the aberrant left subclavian artery arises.

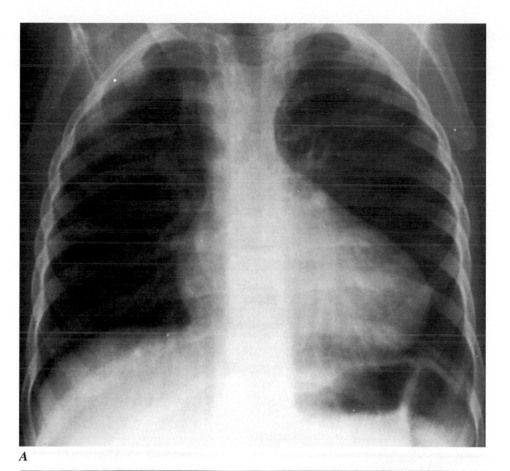

A

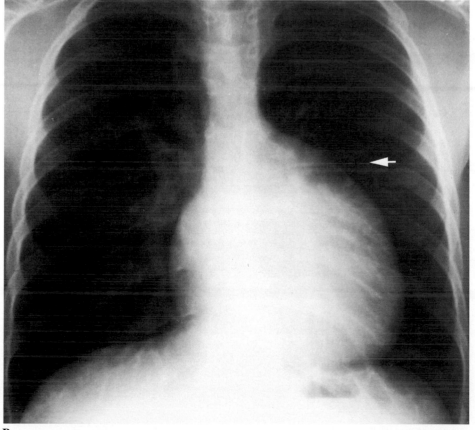

B

FIGURE 3-47 A teenage boy with tetralogy of Fallot demonstrating some common sequelae following complete repair. Before surgery (*A*), a typical boot-shaped heart and a right-sided aortic arch were noted. There was also decreased pulmonary vascularity. Postoperatively (*B*), a bulge over the right ventricular outflow tract (*arrow*) was noted. The heart was moderately enlarged, particularly the right ventricle. The vascularity was now slightly increased. These findings reflect (1) pulmonary insufficiency and (2) residual VSD, now shunting blood left to right.

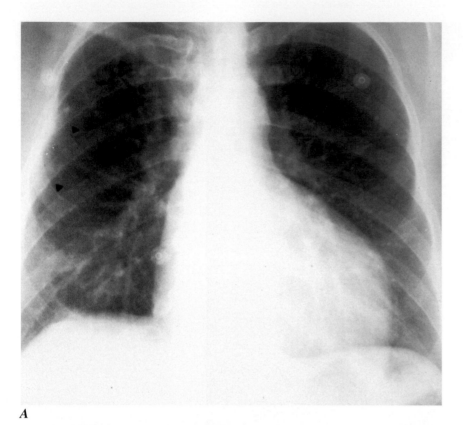

A

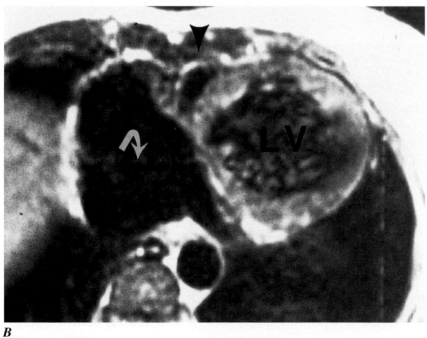

B

FIGURE 3-48   A 41-year-old woman with tricuspid atresia and right Blalock-Taussig shunt. PA view (*A*) shows markedly decreased flow on the left and less diminished flow on the right. Multiple areas of notching are noted in the right upper ribs (*arrowheads*). Other typical findings of tricuspid atresia include (1) flattening of the right atrial border, (2) concavity of the pulmonary trunk, (3) prominence of the left ventricle and the aorta. Transaxial magnetic resonance imaging (*B*) shows an enlarged left ventricle (LV), a hypoplastic right ventricle (*arrowhead*), and a large ASD shunting blood right to left (*curved arrow*).

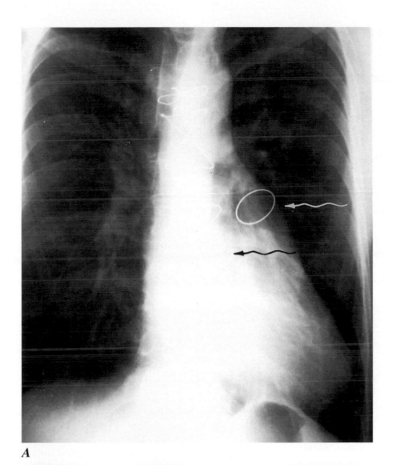

A

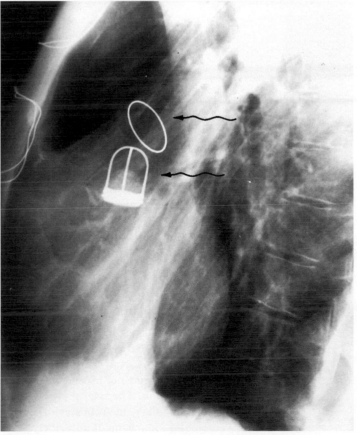

B

FIGURE 3-49   A 24-year-old man showing a satisfactory postoperative status of type I truncus arteriosus. Posteroanterior (*A*) and lateral (*B*) views show a normal cardiovascular appearance except for wires from a median sternotomy, a Hancock valve in the pulmonary position (*upper arrow*) and a Starr-Edwards valve in the aortic position (*lower arrow*).

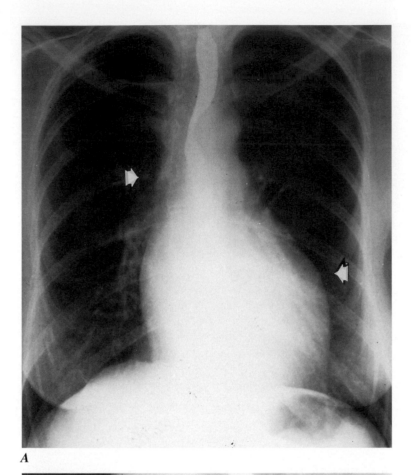

A

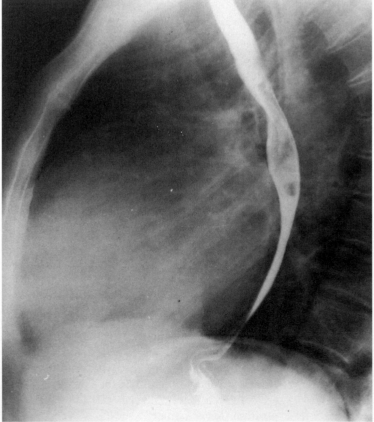

B

FIGURE 3-50   A 44-year-old woman with L-loop transposition of the great arteries presenting as "congestive heart failure from long-standing, severe mitral regurgitation." In reality, she had tricuspid regurgitation and right ventricular failure with pulmonary edema (not shown), which responded to treatment promptly. Two days later, on PA view (*A*), there was a cephalic flow pattern but edema had resolved. Note the peculiar left cardiac contour; a bulge inferiorly (*lower arrow*) and a straight border superiorly. This represents the left-sided right ventricle giving rise to the ascending aorta. The upper arrow denotes the absent image of ascending aorta in its normal position. The lateral view (*B*) shows left atrial enlargement posteriorly and right ventricular enlargement anteriorly.

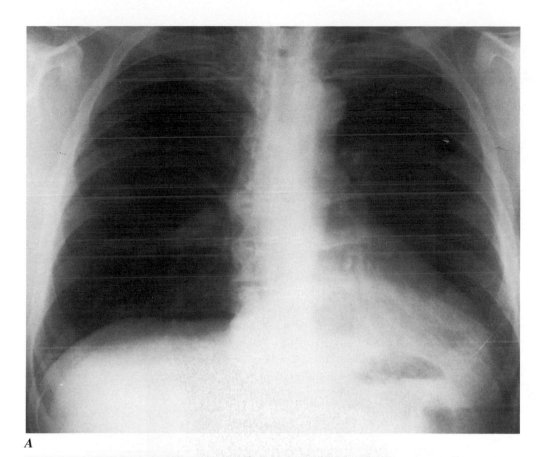

A

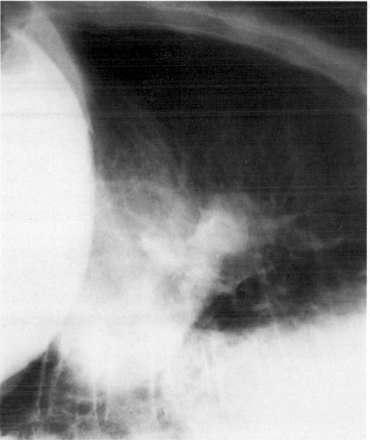

B

FIGURE 3-51   This 70-year-old man was seen because of chest pain. His PA chest radiograph (*A*) shows the heart to be situated mainly to the left of the midline. This is suggestive of congenital absence of the left side of the pericardium. A supine lateral view using horizontal x-ray beams (*B*) shows a striking backward drop of the whole heart. This is explained by the absence of normal anchorage to the sternum provided by the left side of the pericardium. (From Larsen RL, Behar VS, Brazer SR, et al: Chest pain presenting as ischemic heart disease: Absence of the pericardium. *N C Med J* 1994; 55:306–308. Reproduced with permission from the publisher and author.)

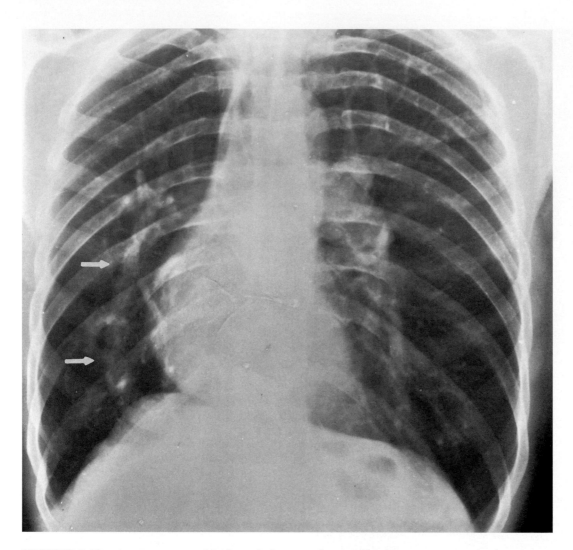

**FIGURE 3-52   A young man with the scimitar syndrome showing
(1) hypoplasia of the right pulmonary artery and hence small right
hemithorax, (2) a scimitar-like common collecting vein (*arrows*) draining
oxygenated blood from right lung to inferior vena cava (IVC), (3) increased
flow to the left lung due to a partial anomalous pulmonary venous
connection, and (4) bilateral bilobed lungs.**

REFERENCES

1. Chen JTT: The chest roentgenogram and cardiac fluoroscopy. In Schlant RC, Alexander RW, O'Rourke RA, et al (eds): *Hurst's The Heart*, 8th ed. New York, McGraw-Hill, 1994, 357–374.
2. Steiner RM, Gross GW, Flicker S, et al: Congenital heart disease in the adult patient: The value of plain film chest radiology. *J Thorac Imaging* 1995; 10:1–25.
3. Chen JTT: *Essentials of Cardiac Roentgenology*. Boston, Little, Brown, 1987.
4. Chen JTT: Radiology of valvular heart disease. *Appl Radiol* 1994; 23:11–19.
5. Chen JTT: The significance of cardiac calcifications. *Appl Radiol* 1992; 21:11–19.
6. Larsen RL, Behar VS, Brazer SR, et al: Chest pain presenting as ischemic heart disease: Absence of the pericardium. *N C Med J* 1994; 55:306–308.

CHAPTER 4

CARDIOVASCULAR ULTRASOUND

Joel M. Felner, M.D.

Vipul B. Shah, M.D.

Randolph P. Martin, M.D.

CARDIOVASCULAR ultrasound has shown continued growth over the last twenty-five years. This has involved not only technological advances but also widespread application of this imaging technique to the diagnosis and management of many cardiovascular conditions. Ultrasound has taken a premier role in the noninvasive workup of patients with presumed or known cardiovascular conditions.[1] In 1995, cardiovascular ultrasound included two-dimensional echocardiography, M-mode echocardiography, spectral and color Doppler ultrasound, transesophageal echocardiography, stress echocardiography, and the newly introduced fields of contrast echocardiography and intravascular ultrasound. Over the last two and a half decades, this technique has proven to be extremely useful not only for diagnosis but also for patient management. The fact that this test is noninvasive—or minimally invasive for transesophageal echocardiography—and can be performed portably or urgently has led to its widespread utilization not only in inpatient and outpatient cardiac or internal medicine settings, but also in the operating rooms, intensive care units (ICUs), and other critical care areas of numerous medical complexes.

Cardiovascular ultrasound has proven extremely useful in the evaluation of global and regional left ventricular function.[2] Not only has resting transthoracic echocardiography been shown to be a hallmark for the evaluation of global and regional left and right ventricular functions, but widespread applications now have validated the role of echocardiography with exercise or pharmacologic stress for the diagnosis and prognosis of coronary artery disease. When coupled with hemodynamic information given by Doppler, the structural information given by echocardiographic imaging has led to the application of cardiovascular ultrasound for valvular stenotic and regurgitant lesion [3] A natural extension of this has been the role of transesophageal echocardiography in evaluating native and prosthetic valve function, both in the operating room and in outpatient-inpatient settings. Transesophageal echocardiography has led to improved diagnostic and management capabilities for such conditions as cardiac source of embolus, aortic dissection, endocarditis, and unexplained hypotension, especially in critical care areas such as ICUs.[4]

The continued maturation of cardiovascular ultrasound has centered on improved quantification and image enhancement. In an era of increasing cost consciousness and emphasis on outcomes, cardiovascular ultrasound is strongly positioned to play a pivotal role as an important noninvasive imaging modality that directly influences patient management.

It is the purpose of the illustrations in this chapter to highlight some important clinical conditions commonly encountered in a busy cardiovascular ultrasound environment. Intravascular ultrasound is discussed and illustrated in Chap. 9.

MITRAL VALVE ABNORMALITIES

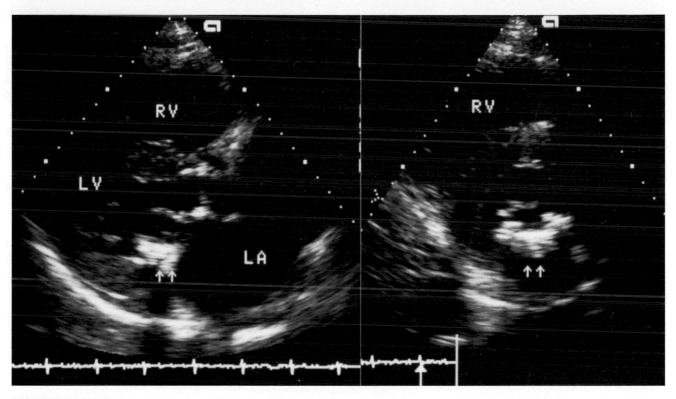

FIGURE 4-1 **A 64-year-old woman with diabetes and renal disease presented with a loud systolic murmur. Echocardiography was performed to evaluate the etiology of the murmur. The left-hand figure is a parasternal long-axis view showing the left ventricle (LV), right ventricle (RV), and left atrium (LA). The two arrows point to an echo-dense structure along the posterior mitral annulus, which represents dense posterior mitral annular calcific changes. The right-hand figure is a parasternal short-axis view, again showing, as outlined by the two white arrows, dense posterior mitral annular calcific changes. Such changes are common in the elderly and in patients with renal disease; they can cause mitral regurgitation.**

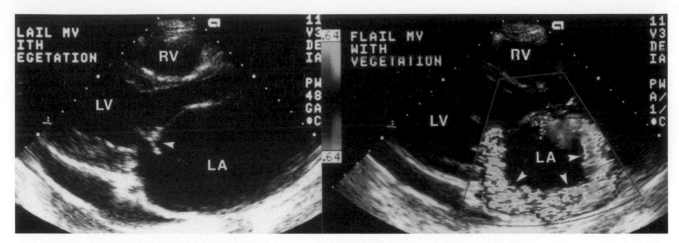

FIGURE 4-2   A 36-year-old woman with a history of 1/6 systolic murmur presented with fever, chills, congestive heart failure, and a 5/6 holosystolic murmur best heard at the apex. Echocardiography was performed to evaluate the etiology of the murmur and rule out valvular vegetations. The left-hand figure is a parasternal long-axis view showing the left ventricle (LV), the right ventricle (RV), and the left atrium (LA). The arrowhead points to a prolapsing echo-dense structure attached to the anterior leaflet of the mitral valve, which is compatible with a vegetative lesion. Note that the left atrium is dilated, which argues for some chronicity of the mitral regurgitation. The right-hand figure is a systolic frame obtained with color Doppler, which shows a posteriorly directed jet of severe mitral regurgitation with a rotation of nearly 360° within the left atrium. The anterior leaflet of the mitral valve in this patient has a significant flail portion calling for operative intervention.

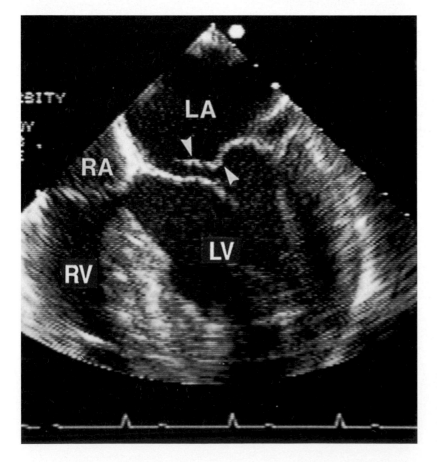

FIGURE 4-3   A 54-year-old man with a long-standing history of mitral valve prolapse presented with worsening symptoms of congestive heart failure and a 5/6 holosystolic murmur. Transesophageal echocardiography was performed to evaluate the etiology of the mitral regurgitation murmur. This transesophageal echocardiography was taken in a horizontal (0°) plane and shows the left atrium (LA), left ventricle (LV), right atrium (RA), and right ventricle (RV). The open-ended arrows point to a flail portion of the posterior leaflet, which is elongated and hooded. This is compatible with ruptured chordae to the posterior leaflet and would be responsible for significant mitral regurgitation.

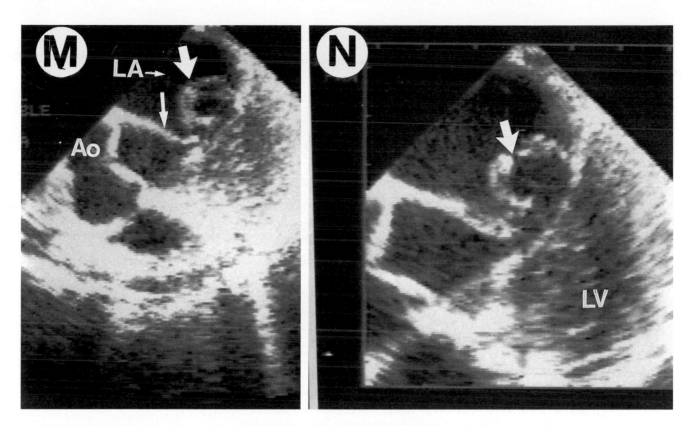

FIGURE 4-4 A 48-year-old woman presented to the emergency room in acute pulmonary edema. She had a loud systolic murmur heard throughout the precordium and an electrocardiogram consistent with an acute myocardial infarction. Transesophageal echocardiography was performed to determine the cause of the systolic murmur. A modified horizontal view of the mitral valve in systole (*M*) shows that the posterior leaflet (*large arrow*) is curled and has prolapsed into the left atrium (LA). The anterior leaflet (*small arrow*) is in its normal position. An enlargement of the mitral valve (*N*) shows the distorted and prolapsed posterior leaflet (*arrow*). The position and configuration of the leaflet is consistent with a rupture of the posterior papillary muscle. An eccentric, severe, mitral regurgitant jet was demonstrated by color-flow Doppler. Ao = aorta; LV = left ventricle.

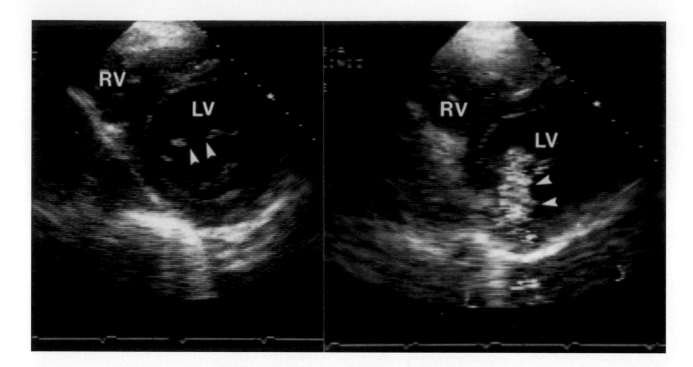

FIGURE 4-5 A 28-year-old woman presented with a loud 4/6 holosystolic murmur. As a young child, she had an atrial septal defect (ASD) repaired. Echocardiography was performed to evaluate the adequacy of repair and the etiology of the mitral regurgitation. The left-hand figure is a parasternal short-axis view showing the left ventricle (LV) and right ventricle (RV). The open-ended arrows point to a gap in the anterior leaflet of the mitral valve. The right-hand figure is a color Doppler interrogation showing a large, wide jet of mitral regurgitation. These findings are compatible with a cleft mitral valve. Cleft valve can occur as an isolated finding but is usually associated with primum ASDs.

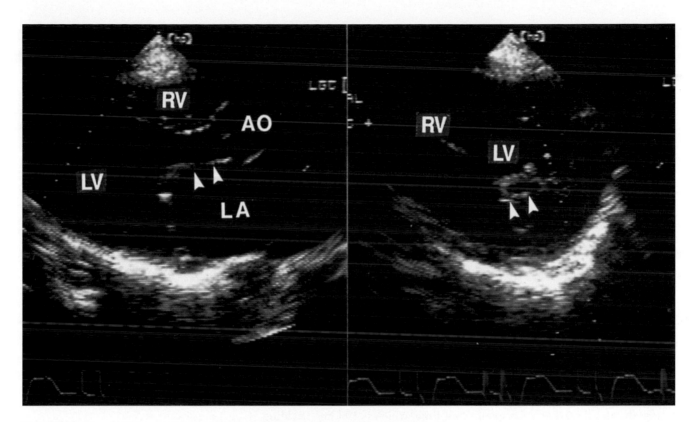

FIGURE 4-6   A 28-year-old Haitian woman presented with symptoms of shortness of breath on exertion. Physical examination revealed a loud opening snap and a 4/6 diastolic decresendo rumble. Echocardiography was performed to evaluate the presence and severity of rheumatic mitral valve disease. The left-hand figure is a parasternal long-axis view showing the left ventricle (LV), right ventricle (RV), aorta (AO), and left atrium (LA). The open-ended arrows point to the anterior leaflet of the mitral valve, which has a "hockey stick" deformity. This image was obtained during diastole. The posterior leaflet is thickened and relatively immobile. The right-hand image shows a parasternal short-axis view. The two white arrows point to the narrowed orifice of the mitral valve. This patient, who was found to have a valve area of 1.0 cm², is being considered for surgical intervention or balloon valvuloplasty.

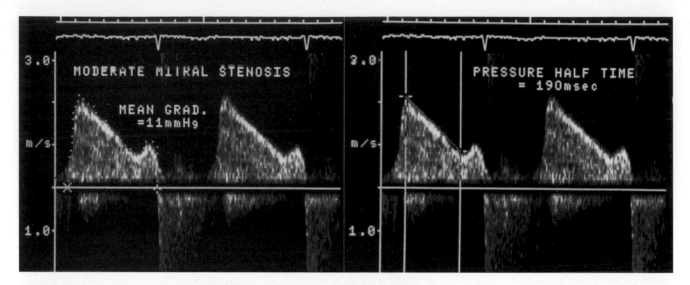

FIGURE 4-7   A 32-year-old woman with a past history of rheumatic fever presented with worsening dyspnea on exertion. She was sent for two-dimensional echocardiography and cardiac Doppler to evaluate the presence and severity of mitral valve stenosis. These figures illustrate continuous-wave Doppler interrogation of mitral inflow taken from the apex. The left-hand figure shows a diastolic mitral flow, with preserved atrial kick. There is a resting mean gradient of 11 mmHg. The right-hand figure shows calculation of pressure half-time, which is 190 ms. Dividing the constant 220 by 190 yields a valve area of 1.15 cm^2. This is compatible with moderate to approaching significant mitral stenosis. This patient was exercised in the echocardiography lab, where the mean gradient rose to 20 mmHg. The patient underwent mitral valve intervention.

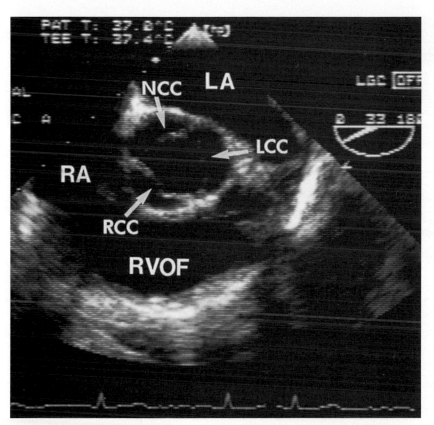

AORTIC VALVE ABNORMALITIES

FIGURE 4-8   This multiplane transesophageal evaluation of the aortic valve was obtained to rule out a cardiac source of embolus. The image was obtained at a rotation angle of 33° and shows a normal trileaflet aortic valve. The noncoronary cusp (NCC) is noted in relation to the interatrial septum. The left coronary cusp (LCC) and right coronary cusp (RCC) also appear delicate and are normal. The left atrium (LA), right atrium (RA), and right ventricular outflow tract (RVOF) are clearly identified. This patient had a normal aortic valve.

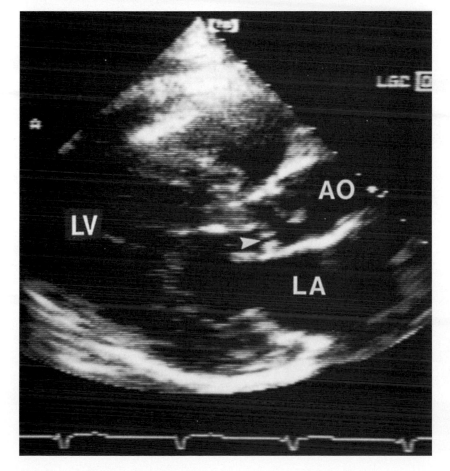

FIGURE 4-9   A 28-year-old man presented with harsh systolic murmur at the upper left sternal border, and echo was performed to rule out valvular aortic stenosis. This parasternal long-axis view shows bright extra echoes in the left ventricular outflow tract, below the aortic valve. The bright extra echoes represent a subvalvular ring. Left ventricle (LV), left atrium (LA), and aorta (AO) are labeled.

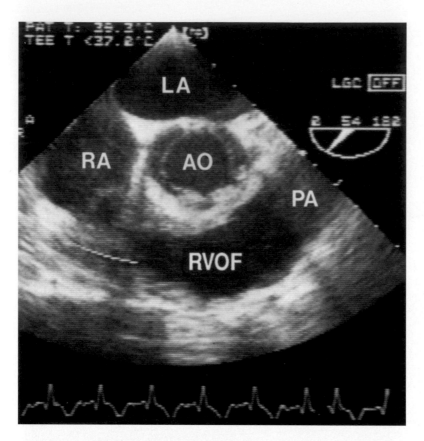

FIGURE 4-10   Upon examination, this 22-year-old man was found to have a loud systolic murmur possibly associated with endocarditis. Transesophageal echocardiography was performed to evaluate the aortic valve. The images, obtained with a multiplane probe at a rotation angle of 54°, show a bicuspid aortic valve with irregular thickening anteriorly. The aortic orifice (AO) is shown, with the left atrium (LA), right atrium (RA), right ventricular outflow tract (RVOF), and pulmonary artery (PA) labeled. The irregular areas of thickening anteriorly along the aortic valve are felt to represent sclerotic changes and not a vegetative lesion. The patient's blood cultures were negative.

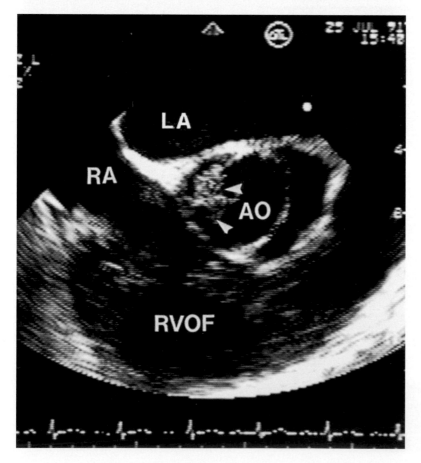

FIGURE 4-11   A 37-year-old woman presented with fever, chills, embolic events, and a long-standing history of systolic ejection click and murmur. Transesophageal echocardiography was performed to determine whether or not a vegetative lesion was present. The irregular bright extra echoes outlined by the open-ended arrows represent a vegetative lesion attached to one of the aortic cusps, which was functionally bicuspid. The left atrium (LA), right atrium (RA), and right ventricular outflow tract (RVOF) are identified and labeled. In any patient with a congenitally malformed valve who is felt to have endocarditis, it is important to perform transesophageal echocardiography in order to rule out the remote possibility of secondary extension of an aortic infection into the subvalvular apparatus or intervalvular fibrosis.

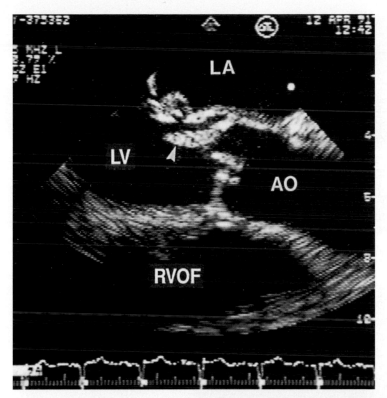

FIGURE 4-12 A 48-year-old man presented with fever, chills, and positive blood cultures. Transesophageal echocardiography was performed to evaluate the presence and location of his vegetative lesion. These images show a vertical (90°) view of the left-ventricular outflow tract (LVOF), left atrium (LA), ascending aorta (AO), and right ventricular outflow tract (RVOF). The white arrowhead points to a prolapsing structure, felt to be a vegetative lesion, attached to the posterior aortic leaflet. Just posterior to that is a buckled portion of the anterior leaflet of the mitral valve, which represents a subvalvular abscess. This patient, therefore, had two vegetative lesions and required extensive surgical debridement and repair.

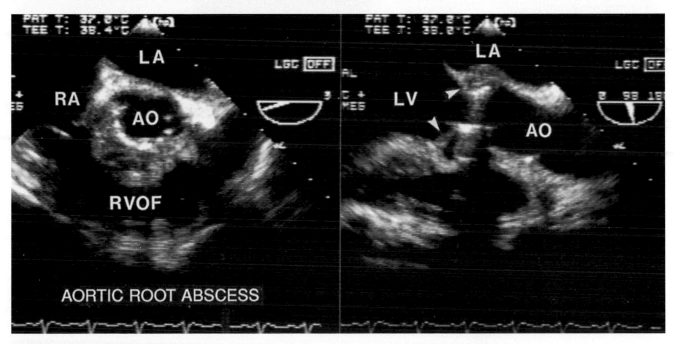

FIGURE 4-13 A 48-year-old man presented with signs and symptoms of endocarditis. The patient had had an aortic valve replacement 3 years earlier with a porcine tissue prosthesis. The left-hand image shows a 10° rotation with a multiplane probe. The aortic orifice (AO) is seen in the region of the sewing ring. Anterior to that and between the anterior sewing ring and the right-ventricular outflow tract (RVOF) is a homogeneous group of echoes measuring 1.5 cm in thickness; this is highly suggestive of a ring abscess. The left atrium (LA) and right atrium (RA) are labeled. The right-hand images show a vertical plane interrogation of 98°. The open-ended arrows point to a ring abscess. This patient underwent emergency surgery.

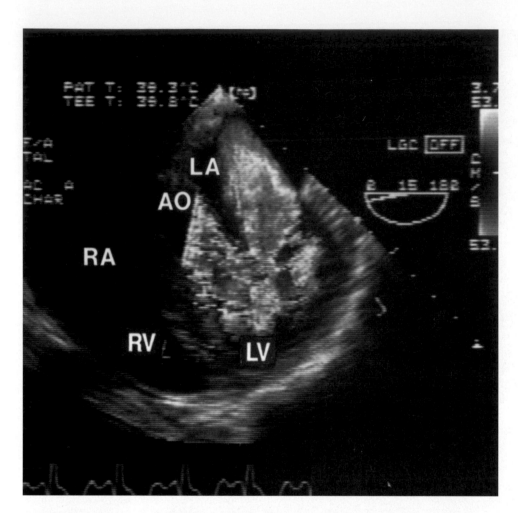

FIGURE 4-14   Transesophageal echocardiography was performed in a patient with presumed severe aortic regurgitation to evaluate the structure and integrity of the aortic valve. This transesophageal echocardiogram, performed in the horizontal plane at 0° during diastole, reveals severe aortic regurgitation with significant diastolic mitral regurgitation in the left atrium (LA). The right atrium (RA), right ventricle (RV), and left ventricle (LV) are identified. Significant diastolic mitral regurgitation can occur in the setting of severe acute aortic regurgitation when left ventricular diastolic pressures exceed left atrial pressures. (*See color Plate 14.*)

TRICUSPID VALVE ABNORMALITIES

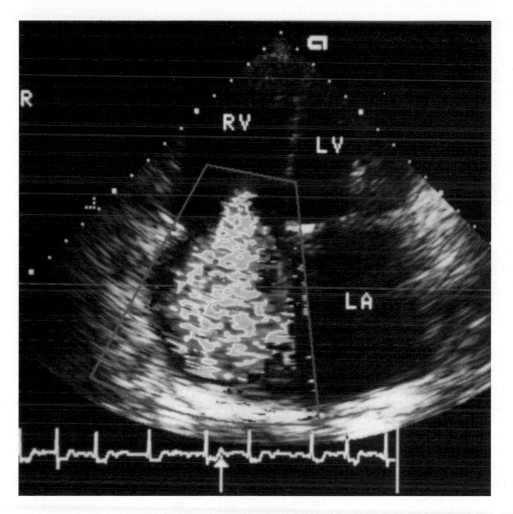

FIGURE 4-15   A 46-year-old woman who had had multiple pulmonary emboli presented in the echocardiography lab for evaluation of the size, shape, and function of her right ventricle and/or the severity of tricuspid regurgitation. She had bounding neck veins and a pulsatile liver. This apical transthoracic echocardiogram was obtained, showing the right ventricle (RV), left ventricle (LV), and left atrium (LA). Severe tricuspid regurgitation is noted by the mosaic color. Continuous-wave Doppler interrogation of this jet showed a peak flow velocity of 4.5 m/s. This gave an estimated minimum right ventricular systolic pressure of 95 mmHg, which was nearly systemic. Continuous-wave Doppler has been shown to be useful in estimating right ventricular systolic pressure. (*See color Plate 15.*)

PROSTHETIC VALVE ABNORMALITIES

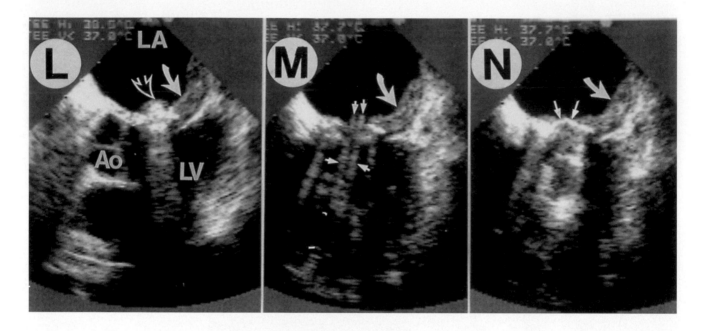

FIGURE 4-16   A 38-year-old man with a prosthetic valve (St. Jude Medical) in the mitral position had recently stopped his anticoagulants and presented with left-sided weakness and slurred speech. Transesophageal echocardiography was performed to evaluate the etiology of the stroke. An image in the horizontal (0°) plane (*L*) shows the mitral valve prosthesis (*open arrowhead*) with its reverberations extending into the left ventricle (LV) and a large elongated thrombus in the left atrium (LA) adjacent to it (*arrow*). An image in the horizontal (90°) plane in diastole (*M*) shows the two disks (leaflets) in open position (*vertical arrowheads*) and the disk's two parallel reverberations extending into the left ventricle (*horizontal arrowheads*). The thrombus, on the atrial surface, is in contact with the posterior stent of the prosthesis (*large arrow*). In systole (*N*), both disks (*arrows*) of the prosthesis are in the closed position, producing a shadow (reverberations) on the left ventricular side of the prosthesis. The large arrow identifies the (LA) thrombus. Ao = aorta.

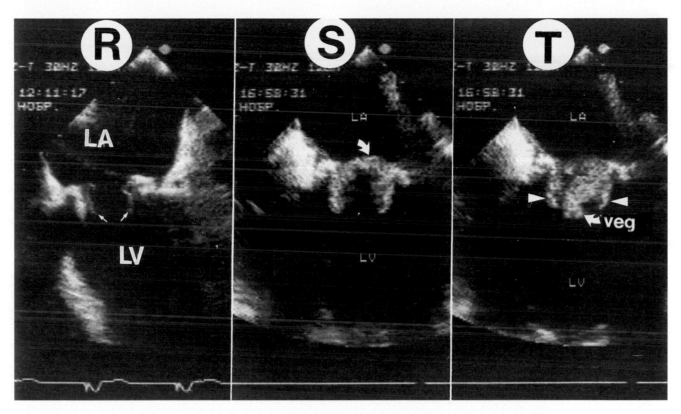

FIGURE 4-17 A 38-year-old man with a porcine mitral valve bioprosthesis presented with signs and symptoms suggestive of infective endocarditis. Transesophageal echocardiography was performed to evaluate the valve for possible vegetations. The first view (*R*), taken in the horizontal (0°) plane, was obtained at the time of discharge 3 years earlier, after the mitral valve prosthesis was first implanted. It shows two of the three leaftlets (*arrows*) in the open position (*diastole*) inside the stents of the bioprosthesis. Note that the leaflets are thin, without evidence of thrombus or vegetation. Transesophageal echocardiograms (*S* and *T*), also in the horizontal (0°) plane, were taken on admission to evaluate the prosthesis. The first of these (*S*) shows a vegetation (*arrow*) on the left atrial (LA) side of the prosthesis, at the onset of diastole; the second (*T*) shows the vegetation (veg) as it prolapses through the prosthesis in middiastole. The large infective mass occludes a large portion of the orifice as it descends into the mitral inflow tract at the level of the stent, demonstrating its significant mobility. The arrowheads identify two of the stents.

AORTIC PATHOLOGY

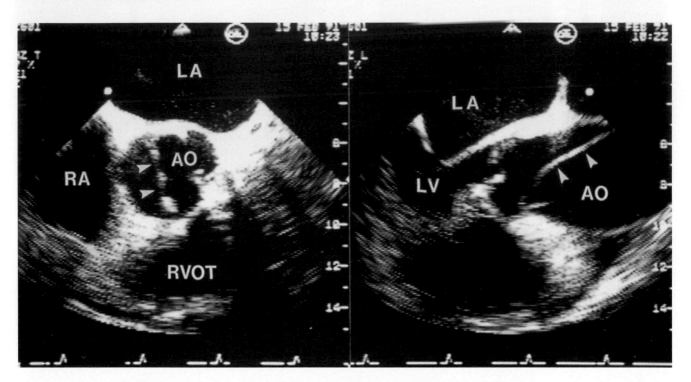

FIGURE 4-18   A 48-year-old man presented with significant chest pain that was sudden in onset and described as ripping or tearing. Although an earlier attack had quickly abated, the pain returned 2 days later. It was at this point that the patient sought medical attention. Transesophageal echocardiography was performed to rule out aortic dissection. The left-hand image is a horizontal or zero-plane image showing an intimal flap (*white arrowhead*) in the immediate supravalvular aorta (AO). The left atrium (LA), right atrium (RA), and right ventricular outflow tract (RVOT) are labeled. The right-hand image is a vertical or 90° image, with the large intimal flap originating from just superior to the aortic valve near the right coronary ostium; it is highlighted by the two white arrowheads. The false aortic lumen (AO) is identified and labeled. The left ventricle (LV) is also labeled. (See also Chap. 10.)

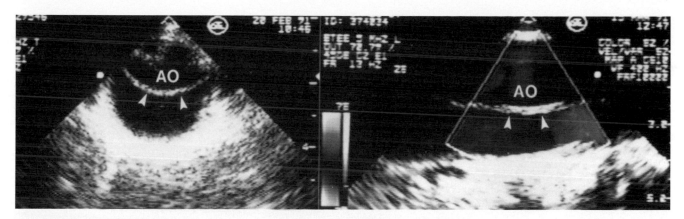

FIGURE 4-19   A 74-year-old patient was admitted with significant chest discomfort, described as at the mid-chest and radiating through to the back, waxing and waning. Because a faint aortic regurgitation murmur was heard, transesophageal echocardiography was performed after acute myocardial infarction had been ruled out. This transesophageal echocardiogram shows views of the descending thoracic aorta. The left-hand panel is a horizontal or zero-plane image, showing an intimal flap in the descending thoracic aorta (AO). The right-hand panel is a vertical or 90° view at the same level, again showing the intimal flap. This patient's ascending aorta was normal. This is a classic type III thoracic aortic dissection. (See also Chap. 10.)

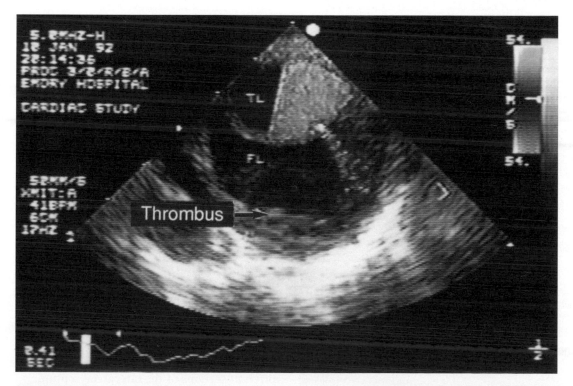

FIGURE 4-20   This transesophageal echocardiogram was obtained in a patient who was suspected of having a descending thoracic aneurysm and a possible dissection. These images show a type III dissection in the setting of a large dilated descending thoracic aorta. The true lumen is labeled (TL) and is easily distinguished from the false lumen (FL). Within the false lumen there is stagnant flow and thrombus. Communication between the true and false lumens is identified by the blue color Doppler. (*See color Plate 16.* See also Chap. 10.)

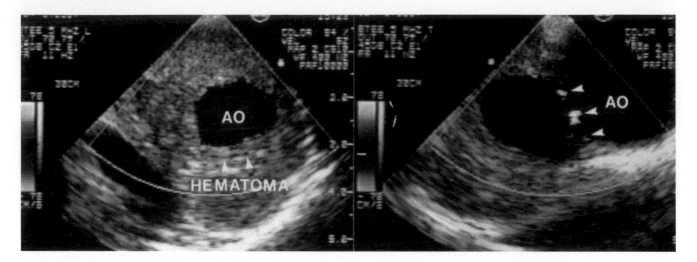

FIGURE 4-21   Single-plane transesophageal echocardiography was performed in the middle of the night on an 18-year-old man who had been involved in an automobile accident and had presumably sustained a deceleration injury. This single-plane transesophageal echocardiogram was obtained at the level of the proximal descending thoracic aorta (*left-hand figure*) and 3.0 cm caudal to that (*right-hand figure*). The left-hand figure shows a large hematoma with a small aortic lumen (AO). The right-hand figure shows the point of disruption of the aortic wall (*multiple white arrowheads*). These images were compatible with a contained rupture and transection of the descending thoracic aorta. Operative repair was performed, and the patient survived. (See also Chap. 10.)

CONGENITAL HEART DISEASE

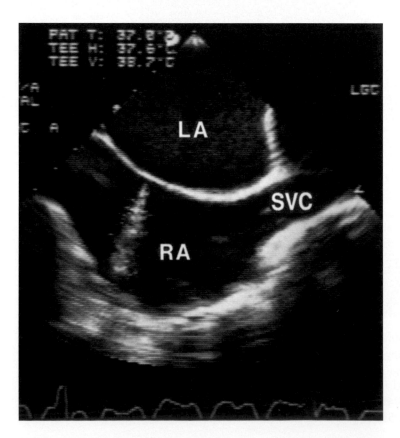

FIGURE 4-22   An 18-year-old woman was believed to have secundum atrial septal defect (ASD). Transthoracic echocardiography did not reveal substantial shunting; therefore transesophageal echocardiography was performed. These images reveal a vertical or 90° axis, showing what appears to be an intact interatrial septum between the left atrium (LA) and right atrium (RA). However, there is clearly a left-to-right shunt, noted by the blue jet of color Doppler. It is important to remember that while no defect in the interatrial septum is seen on this plane, advancing or retracting the transesophageal echocardiographic probe will interrogate different sections of the interatrial septum. When this was done, a small but definite ASD was noted. The patient had no signs of marked pulmonary hypertension, and she and her family elected to be followed despite advice that operative closure should be undertaken. (*See color Plate 17.*)

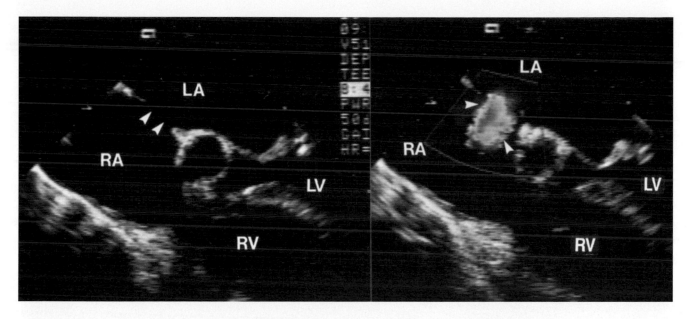

FIGURE 4-23   This patient, a 32-year-old woman, presented with atrial arrhythmias and increasing shortness of breath. Cardiovascular evaluation revealed a loud 2/6 systolic murmur with a wide and fixed split second heart sound. Transesophageal echocardiography was performed to look for an atrial septal defect. The left-hand image was obtained with a horizontal zero plane and shows a large ASD in the secundum septum *(white arrowheads)*. The left atrium (LA), right atrium (RA), right ventricle (RV), and left ventricle (LV) are identified. The right-hand panel shows obvious left-to-right shunting, as witnessed by the broad color Doppler jet. This jet measured 1.5 cm, compatible with a significant shunt. Transesophageal echocardiography is extremely useful in detecting the presence of an ASD, classifying its type, and locating the pulmonary veins. This patient had a simple secundum ASD and underwent successful surgical repair. (*See color Plate 18.*)

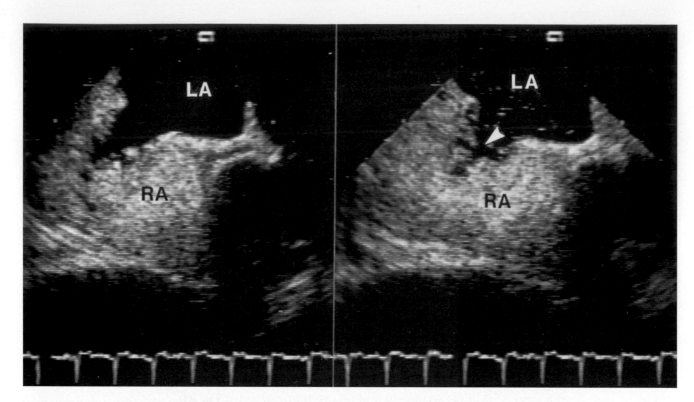

FIGURE 4-24 Contrast saline injection performed during transesophageal echocardiography on a patient with presumed secundum atrial septal defect (ASD). The contrast saline injection shows obvious negative contrast effect in the left-hand panel, as blood from the left atrium (LA) moves toward the right atrium (RA). The RA is opacified by contrast saline, and the unopacified blood from the left atrium creates a negative jet (*arrowhead*). The right-hand panel does show positive contrast crossing from the right atrium to the left atrium. This is a very sensitive sign of an ASD.

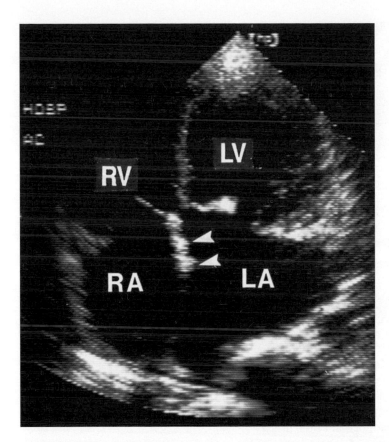

FIGURE 4-25   A 28-year-old man had undergone surgery for congenital heart disease and was being evaluated for adequacy of repair. An apical four-chamber view shows a bright group of extra echoes in the region of the interatrial septum *(white arrowheads)*. This represents a previous patch repair of a primum ASD. It appears that the tricuspid valve (just below the label RV) is abnormally positioned. This patient did have a common AV valve canal that was also repaired. The left atrium (LA) is large and is identified. The left ventricle (LV), right ventricle (RV), and right atrium (RA) are labeled.

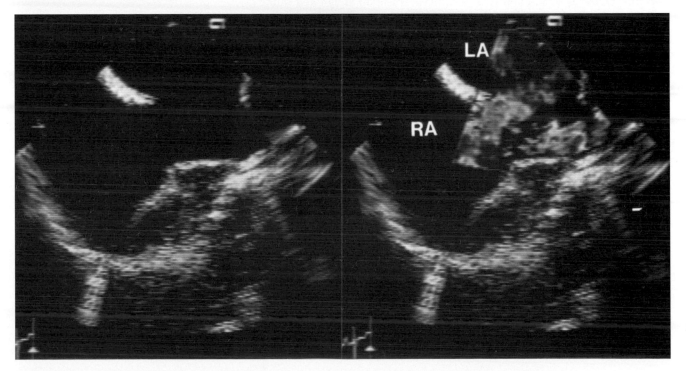

FIGURE 4-26   A 22-year-old man was studied to evaluate the presence and type of a presumed atrial septal defect. The patient was found to have left-axis deviation on his electrocardiogram. The left-hand panel is a vertical image of the interatrial septum, showing an area of echo dropout. The right-hand panel shows left-to-right shunting at the high atrial septal level with communication between the left atrium and the superior vena cava through a large sinus venosus ASD.

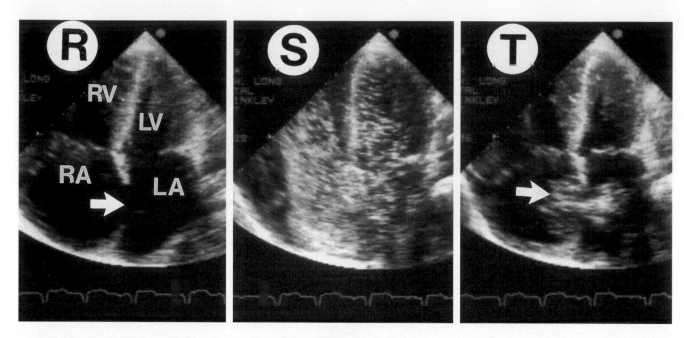

FIGURE 4-27 A 40-year-old woman presented with sudden onset of
shortness of breath and pleuritic chest pain. Two-dimensional transthoracic
echocardiography in the apical four-chamber position, together with an
intravenous contrast saline injection, was performed to evaluate her symptoms.
Prior to saline injection *(R)*, the right ventricle (RV) and right atrium (RA)
are slightly dilated and dropout of echoes in the midportion of the atrial
septum *(arrow)* is seen. Following peripheral injection of agitated saline *(S)*,
the RA and RV are opacified by contrast-containing blood. "Bubbles" flowing
into the left atrium (LA) and left ventricle (LV) confirm a right-to-left shunt.
The contrast *(arrow)*, is seen *(T)* as it straddles the large atrial septal defect.
Color-flow Doppler demonstrated severe tricuspid regurgitation with an
estimated pulmonary artery systolic pressure of 75 mmHg.

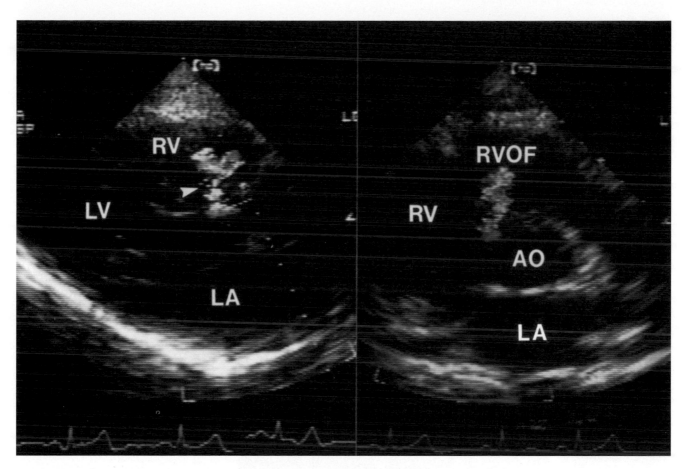

FIGURE 4-28   A harsh 4/6 systolic ejection murmur was heard in a
28-year-old asymptomatic man along the left upper sternal border.
The patient was actively engaged in athletics and had no complaints.
Echocardiography was performed to evaluate the murmur. The left-hand
panel shows a long-axis parasternal view of an obvious perimembranous
ventricular septal defect (VSD) *(arrowhead)*. Color Doppler (imaged in
black and white) shows left-to-right shunting at that level. The left ventricle
(LV), right ventricle (RV), and left atrium (LA) are labeled. The right-hand
panel is a parasternal short-axis view at the same level, again showing a
perimembranous VSD. The fact that the right ventricle is not dilated argues
against any significant shunting. The patient was reassured and instructed
in bacterial endocarditis prophylaxis.

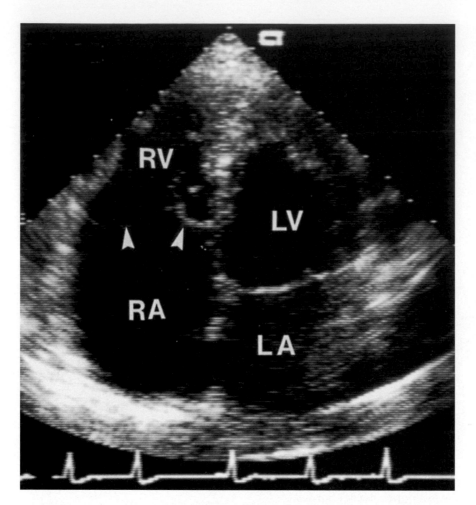

FIGURE 4-29   This is an apical four-chamber view taken from a patient who was imaged to rule out Ebstein's anomaly. It shows marked apical displacement of the tricuspid apparatus *(white arrowheads)* into the right ventricle (RV), leading to a large right atrium (RA) with atrialization of the ventricle. The left ventricle (LV) and left atrium (LA) are labeled.

CORONARY ARTERY DISEASE

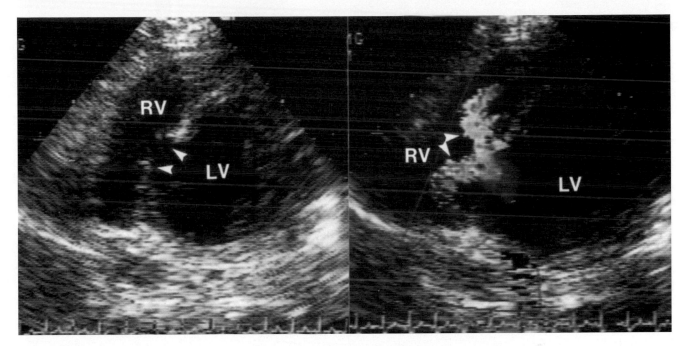

FIGURE 4-30 Four days after sustaining a large inferior myocardial infarction, this patient developed a loud holosystolic murmur with signs of acute cardiac decompensation. An emergency transthoracic echocardiogram was obtained to look for a possible flail mitral valve. The left-hand panel shows a parasternal short-axis view at the midventricular level. The white arrowheads point to the inferior septum, with an obvious area of discontinuity compatible with a large inferior VSD. The right-hand panels show obvious left-to-right shunting through this VSD. The right ventricle (RV) and left ventricle (LV) are labeled. The patient survived emergent surgery.

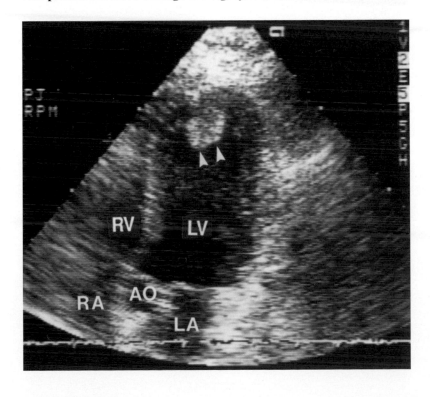

FIGURE 4-31 Three months after an anterior myocardial infarction, this 65-year-old male presented with a questionable embolic event. Transthoracic echocardiography was performed to evaluate the possibility of a left ventricular mass. This apical four-chamber view shows a large 2.0-cm circular echo-dense mass in the apex, as outlined by the white arrowheads. This is compatible with a sizable mural thrombus, which is projecting into the left ventricle (LV). Left ventricular thrombi that are mobile or project into the cavity are prone to embolize. The right ventricle (RV), right atrium (RA), aorta (AO), and left atrium (LA) are labeled.

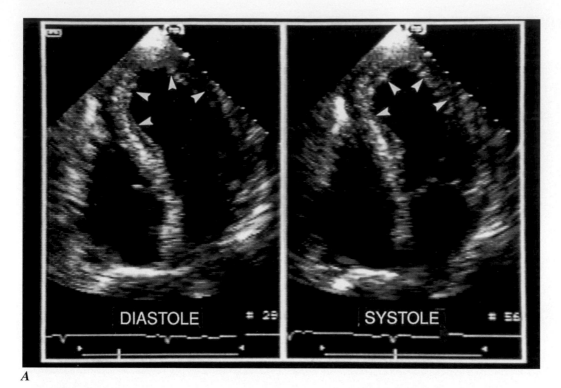

A

FIGURE 4-32   This 48-year-old man had had a myocardial infarction and underwent two-dimensional echocardiography to evaluate global and regional left ventricular function. *A.* Four-chamber view of the left ventricle taken during diastole (*left-hand panel*) and systole (*right-hand panel*). White arrowheads outline an area of large akinesis. There is very little inward systolic motion of the apical-septal, true apex, and apical-lateral walls during systole. *B.* An apical two-chamber view. *C.* An apical five-chamber view, again showing a large area of akinesis.

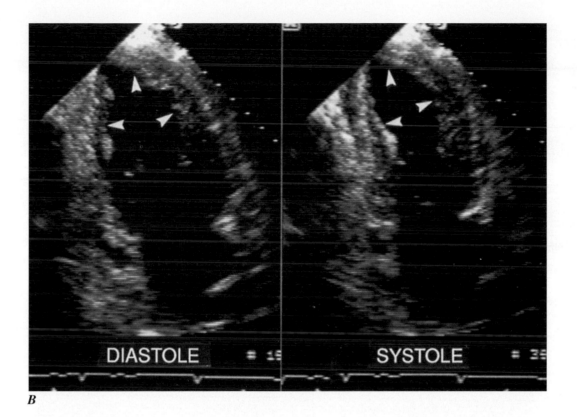

B

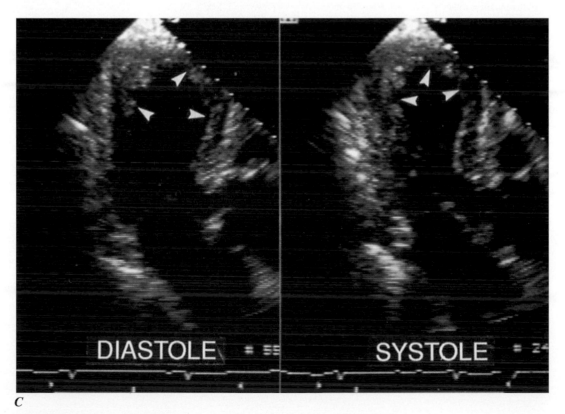

C

FIGURE 4-32 *(Continued)*

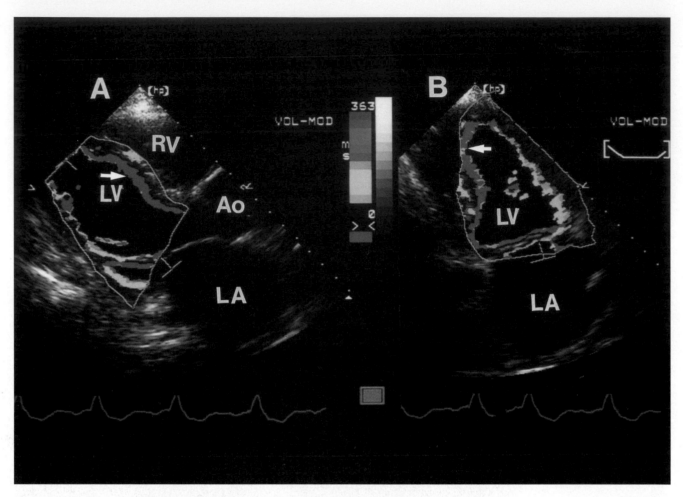

FIGURE 4-33 A 51-year-old man with a previous myocardial infarction presented with atrial fibrillation. Two-dimensional transthoracic echocardiography, with the parasternal long axis (*A*) and apical two-chamber (*B*) views shown, was performed to determine left atrial size and left ventricular contractility. A color display communicating time and motion was used to facilitate the assessment of left ventricular (LV) regional wall motion. This technique provides better visualization of the extent and synchrony of endocardial contraction and expansion throughout the cardiac cycle. The arrows point to the endocardial wall segments that move in a direction opposite to their expected motion; i.e., they are dyskinetic, consistent with the past history of a myocardial infarction. A large left atrium (LA) is present. RV = right ventricle; Ao = aorta. (*See color Plate 19.*)

INTRACARDIAC MASSES

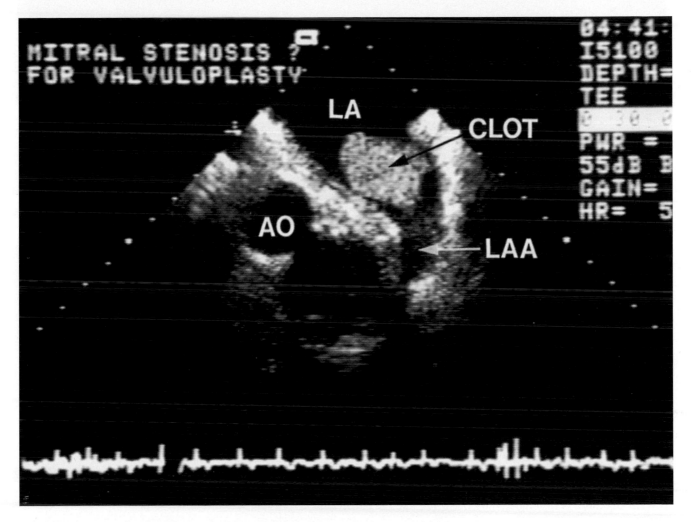

FIGURE 4-34   This patient, a 38-year-old nurse underwent transesophageal echocardiography prior to being considered for balloon mitral valvuloplasty. The echocardiography was performed to evaluate the mitral valve apparatus and rule out left atrial appendage thrombus. This horizontal plane image shows a large thrombus at the mouth of the left atrial appendage, which is labeled "CLOT." There is also stagnant "smoke" in the left atrial appendage (LAA). This patient is not a candidate for mitral balloon valvuloplasty. The patient underwent mitral valve replacement and thrombus removal. The left atrium (LA) and aorta (AO) are labeled.

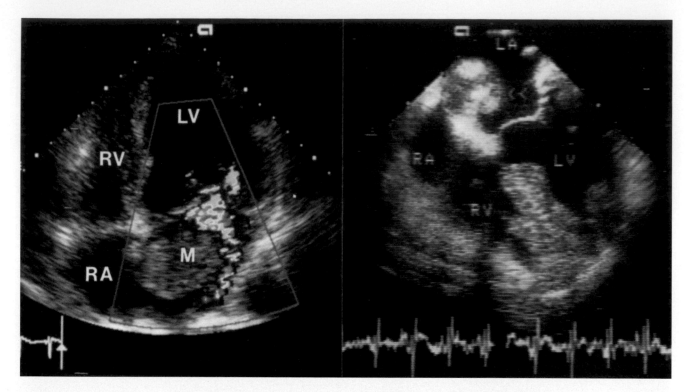

FIGURE 4-35   A 48-year-old woman presented with a recent embolic event to her left foot. At the time of embolectomy, a tissue diagnosis of left atrial myxoma was made. Transthoracic and transesophageal echocardiography was performed. The left-hand panel shows an apical four-chamber view obtained by transthoracic echocardiography. A large left atrial myxoma (M) is shown, within the left atrium occupying most of the volume of the left atrium. Color Doppler (shown in black and white) outlines the edge of the myxoma during diastole. The left ventricle (LV), right ventricle (RV), and right atrium (RA) are labeled. Transesophageal echocardiography was performed to further evaluate the site and size of attachment. This study shows that the left atrial myxoma is attached at the region of the foramen ovalis. The LA myxoma is highlighted by the white open arrowheads.

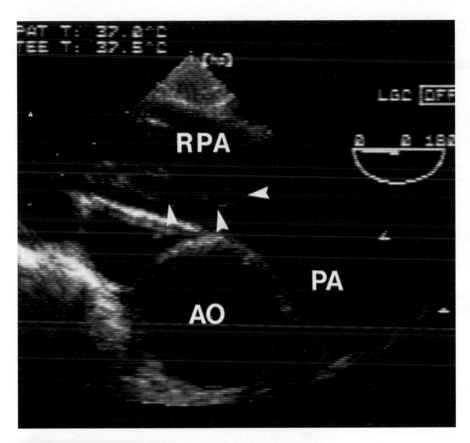

FIGURE 4-36 Emergency transesophageal echocardiography was performed on this patient, who had had a hip replacement and then suffered cardiac arrest. With resuscitation, the patient did regain normal cardiac rhythm and echocardiography was performed as an emergent procedure to rule in or out the presence of a saddle embolus. This 0° view shows an elongated (3-cm) mass within the right pulmonary artery, as outlined by the white arrowheads. The right pulmonary artery (RPA) appears dilated, as does the main pulmonary artery (PA). This mass was a portion of a previously embolized saddle embolus that showered both the right and left branch pulmonary arteries. Unfortunately this patient did not survive. The aorta (AO) is outlined.

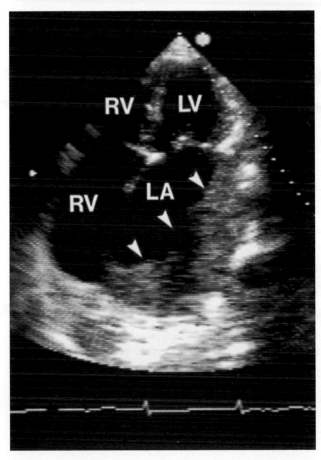

FIGURE 4-37 This 68-year-old man was admitted after a massive cerebrovascular accident (CVA). Echocardiography was performed to rule out intracardiac source of embolus. This apical four-chamber view shows a large, layered mural thrombus within the left atrium, as outlined by white arrowheads. The left atrium (LA) is massively dilated. The mitral valve shows obvious echo features of significant mitral stenosis. The right atrium (RA) and right ventricle (RV) are labeled. This patient, unfortunately did not survive his CVA. Transthoracic echo can detect left atrial thrombi if they are in the body of the left atrium. Small left atrial thrombi, especially if they are within the left atrial appendage only, are best detected by transesophageal echocardiography, which has a greater than 95 percent accuracy in detecting left atrial appendage thrombi. Transthoracic echocardiography detects less than 5 percent of left atrial thrombi if they occupy only the appendage and less than 50 percent of thrombi in the body of the left atrium.

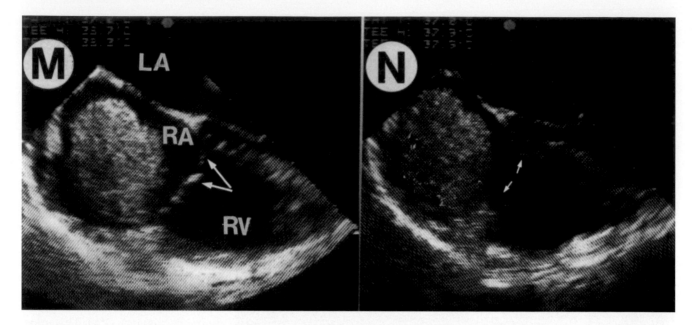

FIGURE 4-38 A 38-year-old woman presented with fatigue, peripheral edema, and large A waves in the jugular venous pulse. After transthoracic echocardiography uncovered a tumor, transesophageal echocardiography was performed to further evaluate the mass. Horizontal right atrial (RA) and right ventricular (RV) views (*M* and *N*) in systole and diastole, respectively, show a large tumor filling the entire right atrium. Hypoechoic vacuolations along the margins of the mass are consistent with myxoma. The site of attachment to the interatrial septum cannot be seen in this imaging plane. The tumor remains in the RA and does not prolapse across the tricuspid valve (*arrows*) into the RV, in contrast to most myxomas. There was minimal motion of this tumor within the RA. LA = left atrium.

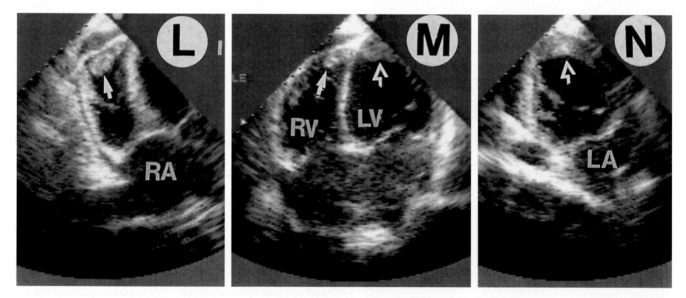

FIGURE 4-39 A 44-year-old man with chronic alcoholism presented with shortness of breath and pleuritic chest pain. Echocardiography was performed to determine whether or not a cause for the suspected pulmonary embolus could be found. A two-dimensional transthoracic echocardiogram in the apical four-chamber view demonstrated biventricular thrombi. The first view (*L*), angled to best delineate the right ventricle (RV), shows an apical thrombus (*arrow*). The thrombus is large and protrudes into the RV cavity. Clots that protrude into the cavity are likely to produce emboli. The second view (*M*) shows thrombi at the apices of both the RV (*arrow*) and left ventricle (LV) (*open arrow*). The third view (*N*), angled to best delineate the LV, shows the left ventricular thrombus. This thrombus is relatively flat and adherent to the wall. Flat, immobile clots have less tendency to embolize and may be mistaken for a thickened endocardial wall. RA = right atrium; LA = left atrium.

PERICARDIAL PATHOLOGY

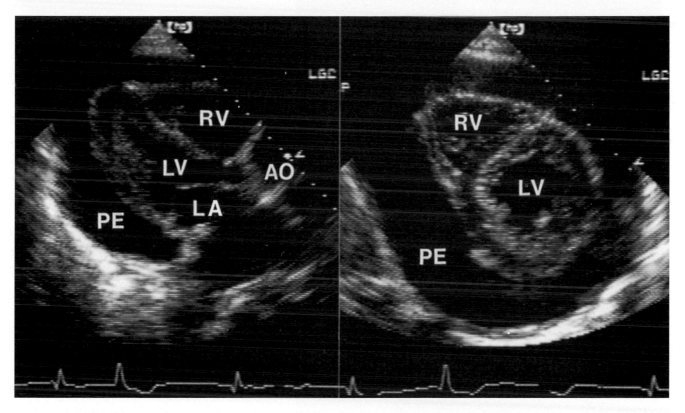

FIGURE 4-40   **This 38-year-old patient with kidney disease presented with increasing shortness of breath, neck vein distention, and marked cardiomegaly on chest x-ray. Echocardiography was performed to look for a pericardial effusion and evaluate its size. The left-hand panel shows a parasternal long axis outlining a large pericardial effusion (PE). The right ventricle (RV), left ventricle (LV), left atrium (LA), and aorta (AO) are outlined. The right-hand panel shows a short-axis view of the pericardial effusion, which is evenly distributed around the right ventricle (RV) and left ventricle (LV). There were no obvious echocardiographic features of tamponade.**

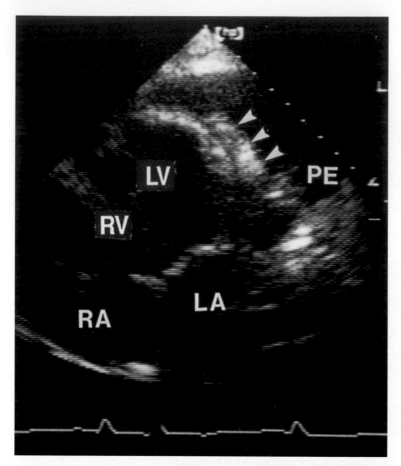

FIGURE 4-41 This 42-year-old woman with known metastatic melanoma presented with marked shortness of breath, marked neck vein distention, and signs of tamponade. A transthoracic echocardiogram was obtained to evaluate the presence or absence of tamponade and showed a large bright mass attached to the visceral pericardium (*outlined by white arrowheads*) within a very large pericardial effusion. This was felt to be a melanoma mass and proved to be so at autopsy. The patient did, however, undergo successful pericardiocentesis, only later to succumb to her disease. The pericardial effusion (PE), left ventricle (LV), right ventricle (RV), right atrium (RA), and left atrium (LA) are outlined and labeled.

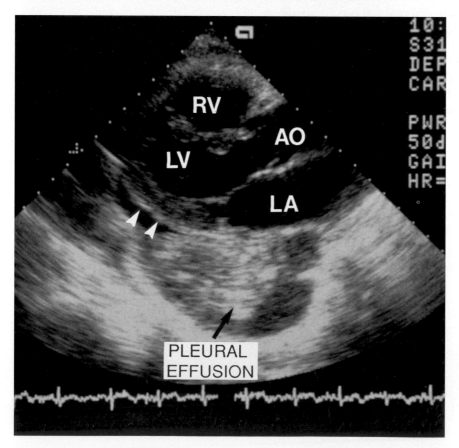

FIGURE 4-42 This 64-year-old man underwent coronary artery bypass grafting 6 weeks before he presented with increasing shortness of breath and signs of a possible pericardial effusion on chest x-ray. A parasternal long-axis view was obtained, showing a very small pericardial effusion (*white arrowheads*) and a large, organized pleural effusion (*black arrow*). The right ventricle (RV), left ventricle (LV), left atrium (LA), and aorta (AO) are labeled.

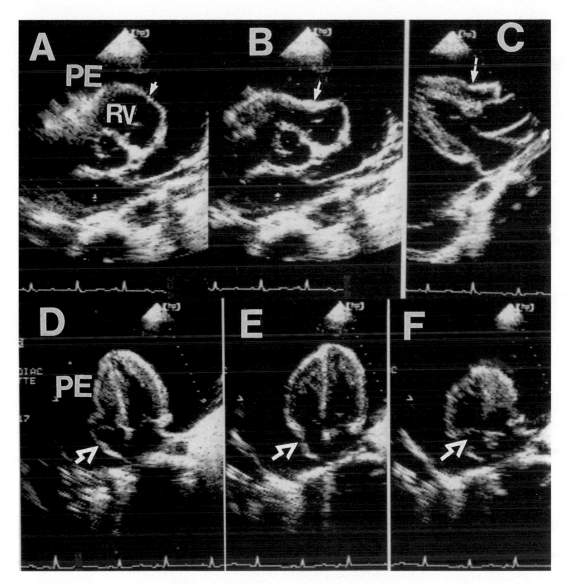

FIGURE 4-43   A 43-year-old man with known Hodgkin's lymphoma was admitted to the hospital with marked shortness of breath and distended neck veins 4 weeks after radiation therapy. An echocardiogram was obtained to evaluate an enlarged cardiopericardial silhouette on the chest x-ray. A two-dimensional transthoracic echocardiagram shows a large pericardial effusion (PE) almost completely surrounding the heart. Of the parasternal short-axis views (A and B), the first (A), at onset of diastole, shows a normal right ventricular (RV) free wall (arrow). The second (B), in early diastole, shows slight indentation of the RV free wall (arrow). A parasternal long axis view in middiastole (C) shows marked indentation of the RV free wall (arrow). Apical four chamber views (D, E, and F) show progressive collapse (open arrows) of the right atrial free wall during diastole. Finally, the right atrial wall appears normal at the beginning of diastole (D) and then progressively invaginates (E and F). This echocardiogram is virtually diagnostic of cardiac tamponade.

CARDIOMYOPATHY

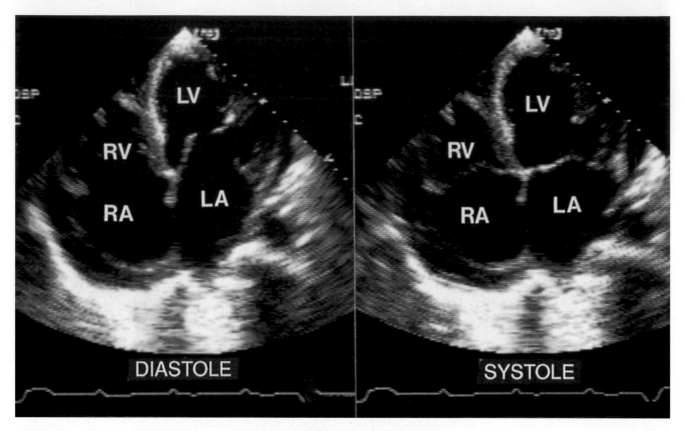

FIGURE 4-44 A 34-year-old woman was seen 2 weeks after the delivery of her second child; she was experiencing increasing shortness of breath. Cardiomegaly was noted on chest x-ray. Two-dimensional echocardiography performed to evaluate left ventricular size, shape, and function. The left-hand panel shows an apical four-chamber view during diastole, with obvious four-chamber enlargement and probably significant left and right ventricular dysfunction. The left ventricle (LV), right ventricle (RV), right atrium (RA), and left atrium (LA) are labeled. The right-hand panel shows systole. There is obviously a marked decrease in global systolic ejection fraction. It was felt that this patient had developed a peripartum cardiomyopathy.

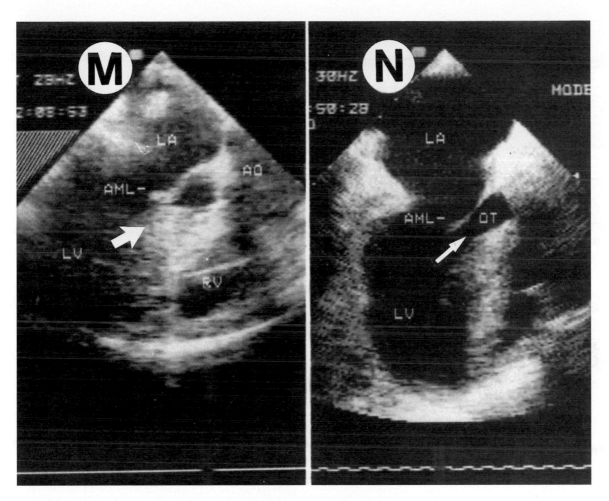

FIGURE 4-45 A 48-year-old man with hypertrophic obstructive cardiomyopathy was to undergo septal myectomy. An intraoperative transesophageal echocardiogram was ordered to provide the surgeon with visualization of the hypertrophied septum so as to determine the extent of the myectomy and to uncover any potential complications (e.g., ventricular septal defect). The preoperative study (*M*) shows the marked septal hypertrophy (*arrow*), which virtually obliterates the left ventricular outflow tract. The postoperative study (*N*) shows the significant reduction in the thickness of the septum and the increase (*arrow*) in the left ventricular outflow tract (OT). LA = left atrium; LV = left ventricle; RV = right ventricle; AO = aorta; AML = anterior mitral leaflet.

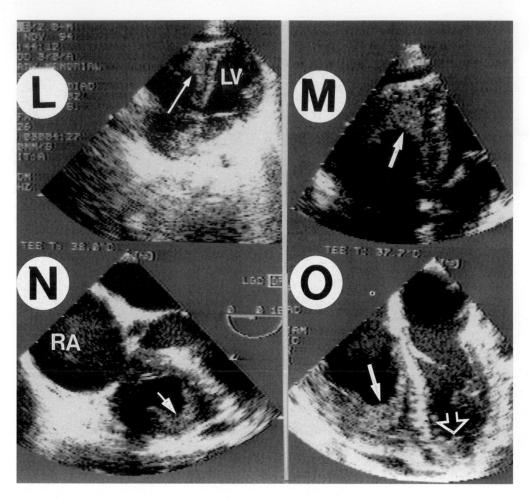

FIGURE 4-46 A 23-year-old man presented with a 3-month history of dyspnea or exertion. Workup revealed 25 percent eosinophils in the peripheral smear. Echocardiography was performed to help determine the etiology of the shortness of breath and marked eosinophilia. A transthoracic echocardiogram (*L*) from the apical four-chamber view demonstrates a mass filling the right ventricular apex (*arrow*); this is characteristic of endocardial fibrosis seen in the hypereosinophilic syndrome. An enlargement of this view (*M*) shows the configuration of the echogenic area (*arrow*) along the apical endocardium. Transesophageal echocardiography was performed to further evaluate the endocardium and determine whether there was involvement of other chambers. Transesophageal echocardiograms in the horizontal (0°) plane are also seen. The first of these (*N*), angled toward the right heart, shows the fibrotic mass filling the apex of the right ventricle (*arrow*). A true four-chamber view (*O*) shows that, in addition to the mass in the right ventricle (*arrow*), there is a small mass at the apex of the left ventricle (*open arrow*). The right ventricle is the chamber primarily involved in this patient and the apex is virtually obliterated, a characteristic finding in this type of restrictive cardiomyopathy. The patient underwent surgical removal of the endocardial fibrous tissue from the right ventricular cavity only and had no evidence of recurrence on the 6-month follow-up echocardiogram. RA = right atrium.

MISCELLANEOUS

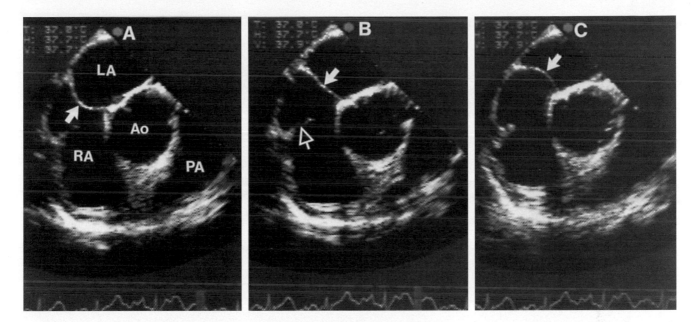

FIGURE 4-47   A 36-year-old woman presented with a stroke.
Transesophageal echocardiography was performed to look for an embolic
source. This transesophageal echocardiogram illustrates an atrial septal
aneurysm, or "floppy septum." It demonstrates how the redundant septal
tissue bulges back and forth between the left atrium (LA) and right atrium
(RA). In diastole (A), the redundant aneurysmal septum (*arrow*) moves
toward the RA. At end-diastole (B), the interatrial septum (*arrow*) is in a
neutral position. In systole (C), the floppy septum (*arrow*) reverses its
direction and moves toward the LA. Ao = aorta; PA = pulmonary artery.

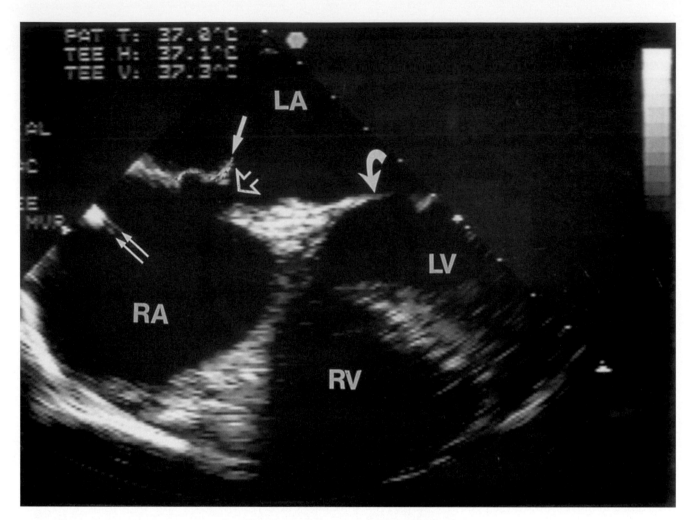

FIGURE 4-48   A 33-year-old woman with known rheumatic heart disease was admitted to undergo balloon mitral valvuloplasty. A transthoracic echocardiogram had previously revealed that the stenotic mitral valve was amenable to this procedure; i.e., the leaflets were not very calcified and no mitral regurgitation was present. Transesophageal echocardiography was performed to aid the interventional cardiologist in the sizing and placement of the balloon during valvuloplasty and for prompt assessment of the mitral valve as well as detection and quantification of mitral regurgitation and the degree of intactness of the atrial septum. In this modified four-chamber horizontal view, the transseptal balloon catheter (*double arrow*) is shown at the lateral edge of the right atrium (RA) just after its recoil through the interatrial septum. The membrane of the foramen ovale (*arrow*) has been torn by the balloon catheter, creating a large atrial septal defect (*open arrow*). The proximal portion of the anterior mitral leaflet (*curved arrow*) is identified. A moderate left-to-right shunt at the atrial septum was a result of the procedure. LA = left atrium; RV = right ventricle.

REFERENCES

1. ACC/AHA guidelines: American College of Cardiology/American Heart Association Task Force for the Clinical Application of Echocardiography. *Circulation* 1990; 82:2323–2345.
2. Felner JM, Martin RP: The echocardiogram. In: Schlant RC, Alexander RW, O'Rourke RA, et al. (eds): *Hurst's The Heart*. 8th ed. New York, McGraw-Hill, 1994, pp 375–422.
3. Pearlman AS: Technique of Doppler and color flow Doppler in the evaluation of cardiac disorders and function. In: Schlant RC, Alexander RW, O'Rourke RA, et al. (eds): *Hurst's The Heart*. 8th ed. New York, McGraw-Hill, 1994, pp 2229–2251.
4. Seward JB, Khandheria BK, Freeman WK, et al: Multiplane Transesophageal echocardiography: Image orientation, examination technique, anatomic correlations and clinical applications. *Mayo Clin Proc* 1993; 68:523–551.

CHAPTER 5

NUCLEAR CARDIOLOGY

Lynne L. Johnson, M.D.

NUCLEAR cardiology provides the only well-documented and clinically available noninvasive modality to assess regional myocardial perfusion; therefore it has found widespread clinical usage.[1] Because only tracer doses of ionizing radiation are administered, the radiation burden to patients is extremely low. In addition to myocardial perfusion, global and regional left- and right-ventricular function can be assessed using radionuclide techniques. Measurement of global left-ventricular function (ejection fraction) from radionuclide data is calculated from change in counts and therefore does not suffer limitations associated with geometry-dependent models.

The two primary cardiac imaging modalities using radionuclides, single-photon myocardial perfusion imaging and ventricular function analysis (gated blood-pool scintigraphy and first-pass radionuclide angiography) were developed more than 20 years ago. Diagnostic imaging modalities with radionuclides have been used clinically in patient care for more than 15 years. Over this period of time, technology has evolved dramatically, including scintillation camera design and performance as well as the development of radiopharmaceuticals. In the United States in 1995, tomographic imaging of myocardial perfusion tracers is employed almost exclusively. Planar imaging is performed only when bedside portable imaging is necessary or when, for some physical reason, a patient cannot undergo tomographic imaging. Although thallium-201 is still widely used as a perfusion agent in myocardial imaging, the technetium-labeled myocardial perfusion agents are finding increasing use because of the better nuclear properties of technetium-99m compared to thallium-201 plus the additional ability to acquire information on regional and global left-ventricular function. This additional information on ventricular function can be provided either by gated tomography and/or by acquiring, in dynamic imaging mode, the serial passage of the bolus of radiotracer through the central circulation, i.e., first-pass radionuclide angiography. Experimentally, myocardial uptake of both thallium-201 and technetium-99m sestamibi is dependent on both regional myocardial blood flow and active metabolic processes of the myocytes; theoretically, therefore, both agents access both flow and myocardial viability. There are data supporting the use of both agents for assessing myocardial viability.

The diagnostic accuracy of tomographic perfusion imaging using either thallium-201 or agents labeled with technetium-99m has been well documented in the literature.[2,3] Although there are several artifactual causes for false-positive scans, most of these are readily identifiable and can either be corrected with software (motion correction) or prevented by applying appropriate stress modalities (vasodilator stress in patients with left bundle branch block).

Myocardial perfusion imaging combined with infusion of a pharmacologic agent, e.g., dipyridamole, adenosine, or dobutamine, has found increasing clinical use, especially in patients who are elderly or cannot perform adequate treadmill exercise.[4] Dobutamine increases the rate pressure product and in this regard simulates exercise, whereas the vasodilators evoke flow heterogeneity in beds with reduced flow reserve and in some cases can provoke ischemia through a "steal" mechanism.

In addition to diagnostic applications, myocardial perfusion imaging has been shown to have important prognostic value.[5,6] Scan findings associated with increased incidence of cardiovascular events include defect extent, defect reversibility, and signs of stress-induced left ventricular dysfunction. The use of perfusion imaging to identify patients at increased risk for cardiovascular events has been applied particularly to patients who have had myocardial infarctions (MI) and those undergoing high-risk noncardiac surgery.

The major clinical indications for myocardial perfusion imaging include the following: chest pain evaluation; follow-up evaluation of patients with known coronary artery disease to assess efficacy of medical management or progression of disease; preoperative risk assessment in patients undergoing high-risk noncardiac surgery who have many clinical risk factors; post-MI evaluation to assess myocardium at further ischemic risk and the severity of left ventricular dysfunction; and assessment of myocardial viability in patients with coronary artery disease and moderate to severe left ventricular dysfunction to determine whether or not such a patient is a suitable candidate for myocardial revascularization.

The cases presented in this chapter are illustrative of some of the newer single-photon tomographic and gated tomographic techniques as well as thallium perfusion imaging.

CASE 1

HISTORY:

A 46-year-old man with treated systemic hypertension (HTN) as his only risk factor for coronary artery disease was referred for 2-day ^{99m}Tc-MIBI (sestamibi) treadmill stress testing to evaluate atypical chest pain.

STRESS-TEST PARAMETERS:

The baseline electrocardiogram (ECG) was normal. The patient exercised for 16 min 41 s of the Bruce protocol (17.3 METS)—achieving a peak HR of 178 bpm, BP of 200/80 mmHg—and stopping due to fatigue. There were no exercise-induced chest pain or ischemic ECG changes. Because of his excellent exercise performance and exercise scan, the patient did not return on day 2 for the resting scan.

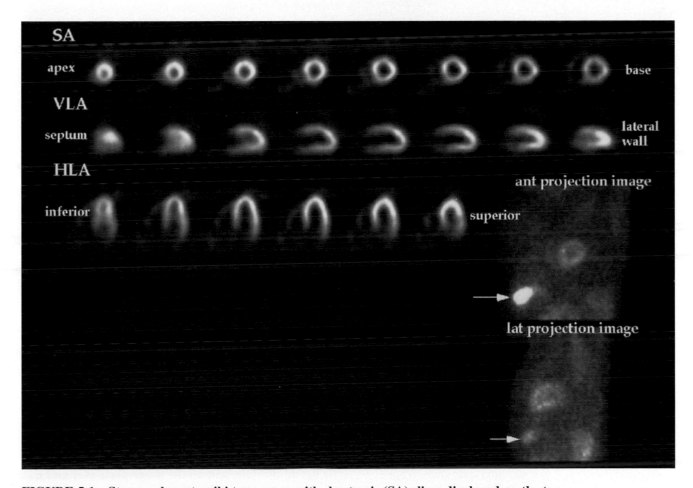

FIGURE 5-1   **Stress-only sestamibi tomogram with short-axis (SA) slices displayed on the top row, vertical long-axis (VLA) slices displayed in the middle row, and horizontal long-axis (HLA) slices displayed on the bottom row. There is normal (homogeneous) tracer uptake throughout the myocardium. The two projection images are displayed to show the biodistribution of sestamibi, which is excreted enterohepatically. The gallbladder (*arrow*) has more activity than the heart but is anatomically well enough separated from the heart that gallbladder activity is excluded from the cardiac reconstruction limits.**

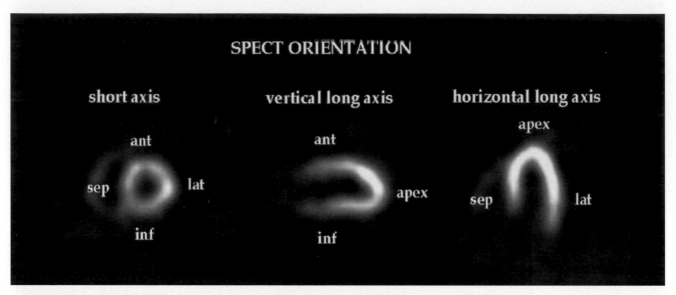

FIGURE 5-2 Representative mid-short axis, mid-vertical long axis, and mid-horizontal long-axis slices from the normal scan of Fig. 5-1. On the short-axis slices, the anterior wall is between about 10:30 and 1:30 o'clock, the lateral wall between 1:30 and 4:30, the inferior wall between 4:30 and 7:30, and the septum between 7:30 and 10:30. The septal and lateral segments can be further divided into anteroseptal and inferoseptal segments and the lateral into anterolateral and inferolateral segments. When the short-axis slices are divided into six sectors, each sector is of equal size.

FIGURE 5-3 Because of the high count rate achieved with sestamibi imaging, it is possible to gate the tomographic acquisition. The cardiac cycle is commonly divided into eight segments, and eight separate tomograms are displayed from each gated single photon emission computed tomography (SPECT) acquisition. These eight tomograms can then be viewed in cine format to evaluate regional wall motion. Shown across the tops of *A* and *B* are all short-axis slices from end-systole to end-diastole, and on the lower parts of *A* and *B*, the representative images at end-diastole (*A*) and end-systole (*B*) from the cine display. The eight tomograms are also summed to make the high-statistics tomographic slices, as shown in Fig. 5-1, which are then read for assessment of regional tracer uptake and bull's-eye display generation. ▶

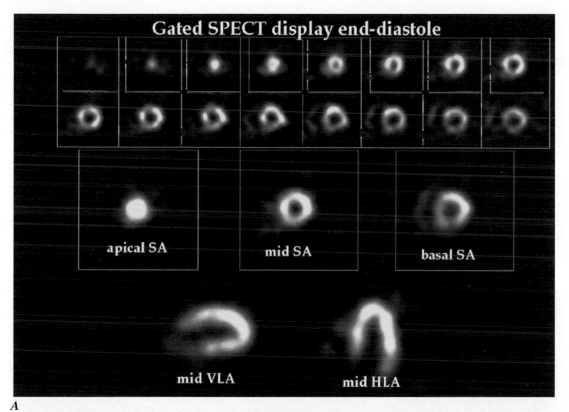

A

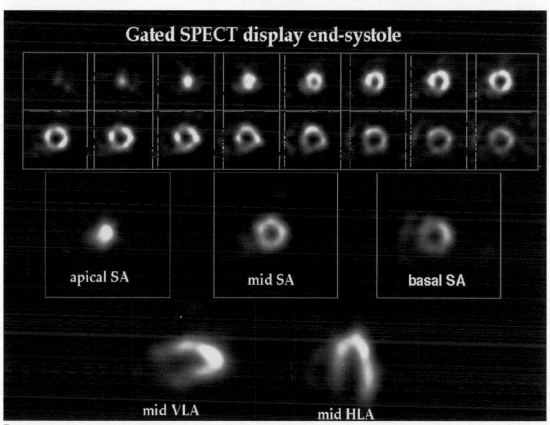

B

CASE 2

HISTORY:

This 79-year-old man had an MI in 1988 followed by four-vessel coronary artery bypass grafting (CABG). The patient's physician found new changes on his resting ECG and referred him for a treadmill stress thallium study.

STRESS-TEST PARAMETERS:

The patient exercised 3 min of the Bruce protocol (4.7 METS), achieving a peak HR of 154 bpm, BP of 164/90 mmHg, and stopping due to fatigue. The baseline ECG showed inferior Q waves, and there were no further changes with exercise.

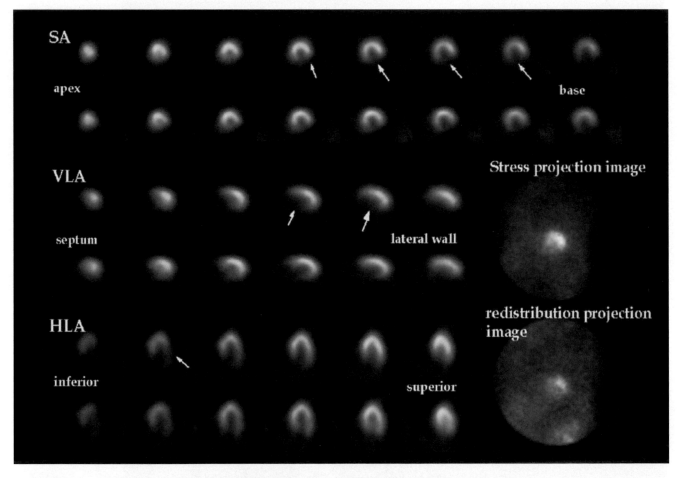

FIGURE 5-4   **The top row of each set of slices displays stress images, the bottom row redistribution images. SA = short axis, VLA = vertical long axis, HLA = horizontal long axis. The arrows point to an inferior perfusion defect seen on the early scan that did not change on the 4-h redistribution scan, consistent with the diagnosis of scar in the inferior wall. Because of the history of an inferior wall myocardial infarction, it was elected not to perform thallium reinjection on this patient.**

CASE 3

HISTORY:

This 33-year-old man had an anterior MI 8 years previously. Coronary angiography at the time of the MI showed a thrombus in the left anterior descending coronary artery (LAD), which lysed following thrombolytic therapy. No intimal disease of any of the coronary arteries was observed following thrombolytic therapy. Lipid and coagulation studies were normal. Long-term anticoagulation was instituted. He remained asymptomatic and continued to do construction work as before. His physician ordered a stress thallium study to evaluate functional capacity, left ventricular (LV) scar, chamber size, and to look for any evidence for further disease.

STRESS-TEST PARAMETERS:

The baseline ECG showed an intraventricular conduction delay (IVCD). The patient exercised for 13 min 24 s of the Bruce protocol (13.5 METS), achieving a peak HR of 183 bpm, peak BP of 180/70 mmHg, and stopping due to fatigue.

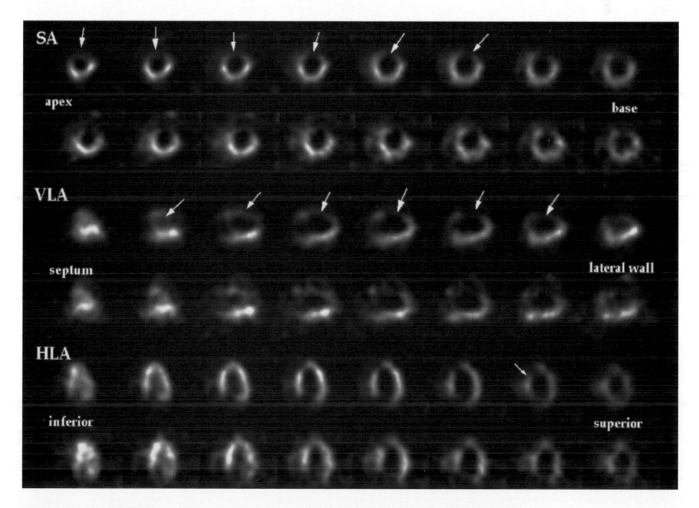

FIGURE 5-5   The top row of each set of slices displays stress images, the bottom row redistribution images. SA = short axis, VLA = vertical long axis, HLA = horizontal long axis. The LV is dilated. The arrows point to a large fixed anterior defect.

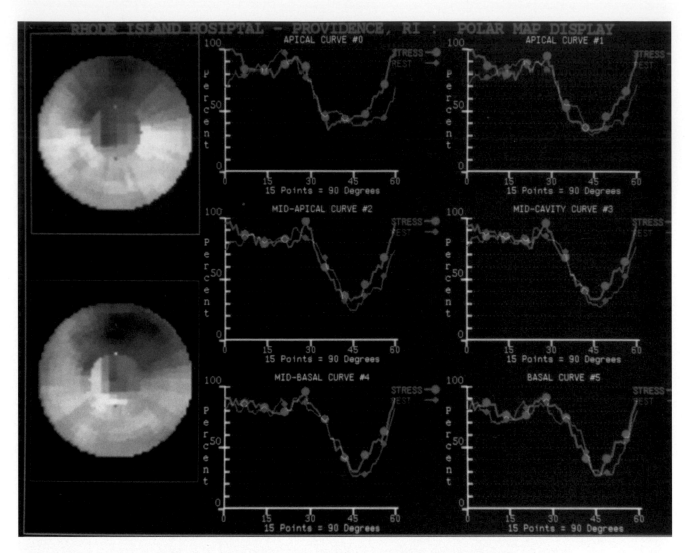

FIGURE 5-6 Polar map display of data from Fig. 5-5. The polar maps are created by telescoping the short-axis slices into a circular display in which the base is at the periphery of the circle and the apex in the center. Each map is scaled to the hottest pixel for that scan (either stress or rest). On the color display, the highest counts are represented as white and light yellow through shades of orange to brown and black (0 counts). The center of the polar map display is derived from count data from the apex of the left ventricle, proceeding outward to the base represented by the peripheral part of the circle. The polar map on the top is the stress map, and the one below is the rest map. Displayed to the right are six circumferential count profiles from representative short-axis slices from apex (*upper left corner*) to base (*bottom right corner*). Zero degrees is at 3 o'clock, and the maps go clockwise. The blue curve is stress, the red curve redistribution. As can be seen in these displays, the inferior wall counts are high, while the anterior wall counts are profoundly reduced to between 30 and 35 percent of peak counts and do not change between stress and redistribution, consistent with scar in the anterior wall. (*See color Plate 20.*)

CASE 4

HISTORY:

This 45-year-old man had an inferior MI and percutaneous transluminal coronary angioplasty (PTCA) of the left circumflex coronary artery (LCx) 3 months after his MI. One month following PTCA, he underwent 2-day stress and rest sestamibi imaging for evaluation of recurrent symptoms of chest pain.

STRESS-TEST PARAMETERS:

Resting ECG showed QS in aVL and tall R wave in V1. He exercised for 8 min 47 s of the Bruce protocol (7.5 METS), achieving a peak HR of 158 bpm, peak BP of 180/80 mmHg, and some stopping due to fatigue. The ECG showed ischemic changes.

CORONARY ANGIOGRAPHY:

Based on the results of this study, the patient underwent coronary angiography, which showed the following: 50 percent stenosis of distal LAD, 90 percent stenosis of the proximal LCx, 50 percent stenosis of a proximal ramus branch, 100 percent occlusion of the distal ramus branch, 45 percent stenosis of the mid-right coronary artery (RCA).

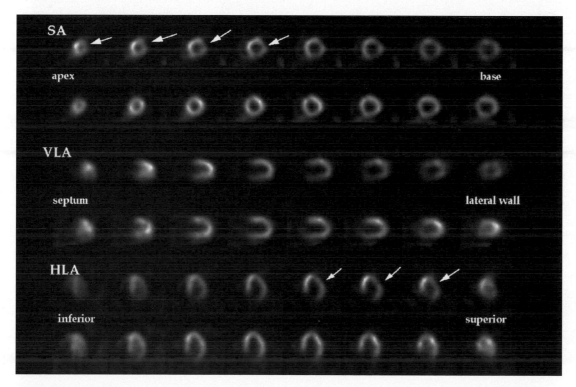

FIGURE 5-7 **The top row of each set of slices displays stress images, the bottom row rest images. SA = short axis, VLA = vertical long axis, HLA = horizontal long axis. The arrows point to a lateral wall defect that extends from about 1 o'clock to 5 o'clock, with fill-in following rest injection demonstrating reversible ischemia in the lateral wall, the usual distribution of the left circumflex artery.**

CASE 5

HISTORY:

This 57-year-old man had an MI followed by CABG 5 years previously. He was referred for stress thallium study because of recent-onset atypical chest pain thought clinically to be "indigestion."

STRESS-TEST PARAMETERS:

Baseline ECG showed nonspecific ST-T-segment abnormalities. The patient exercised for 7 min 18 s of the Bruce protocol (10.2 METS), achieving a peak HR of 148 bpm, peak BP of 200/80 mmHg, and stopping due to fatigue. The stress ECG was interpreted as nondiagnostic for ischemia because of the baseline abnormalities.

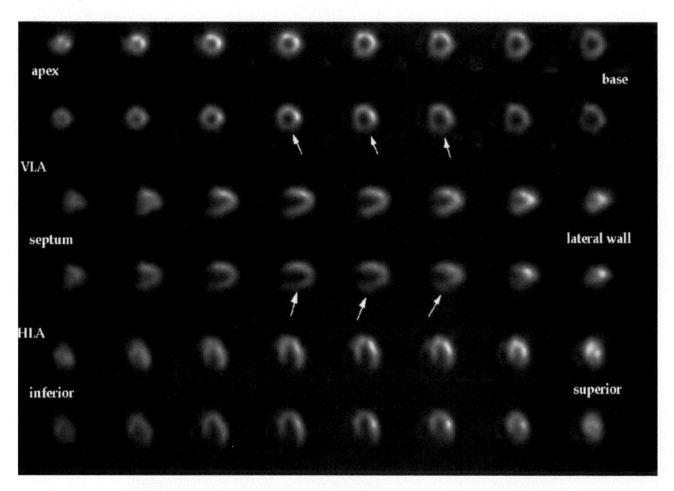

FIGURE 5-8   The top row of each set of slices displays stress images; the bottom row, redistribution images. SA = short axis, VLA = vertical long axis, HLA = horizontal long axis. The arrows point to an inferior defect, which is more apparent on the redistribution images than on the stress images and therefore represents an example of reverse thallium redistribution. The most likely etiology for this finding in this patient is a prior non-Q-wave inferior infarction.

CASE 6

HISTORY:

This 21-year-old woman who had undergone repair of tetralogy of Fallot (TOF) with renal failure underwent stress thallium imaging as part of prerenal transplant evaluation.

STRESS-TEST PARAMETERS:

Baseline ECG showed intraventricular conduction delay (IVCD). Patient exercised for 9 min 28 s of the Bruce protocol (10.2 METS), achieving a peak HR of 165 bpm, peak BP of 180/88 mmHg, and stopping due to fatigue. The stress ECG could not be interpreted for ischemia because of the IVCD.

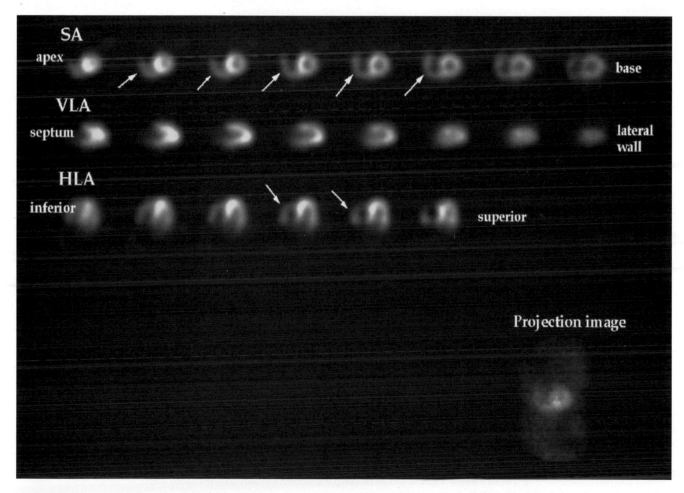

FIGURE 5-9 Only the exercise scan is displayed. SA = short axis, VLA = vertical long axis, HLA = horizontal long axis. The arrows point to the prominent right ventricle (RV). Although a normal-sized RV is frequently seen on sestamibi scans, because of the lower counts and lower energy of thallium, the normal thin-walled RV is not consistently seen on thallium tomographic slices. When it is seen as well as demonstrated in this case, it means that the RV is enlarged and/or hypertrophied.

CASE 7

HISTORY:

This 60-year-old woman (height, 5 ft, 5 in.; weight, 205 lb) was referred for stress thallium study for the evaluation of chest pain.

STRESS-TEST PARAMETERS:

The resting ECG was normal. The patient exercised for 5 min 5 s of the Bruce protocol (7.5 METS), achieving a peak HR of 167 bpm, peak BP of 190/100 mmHg, and stopping due to fatigue. There were no exercise-induced chest pain or ischemic ECG changes.

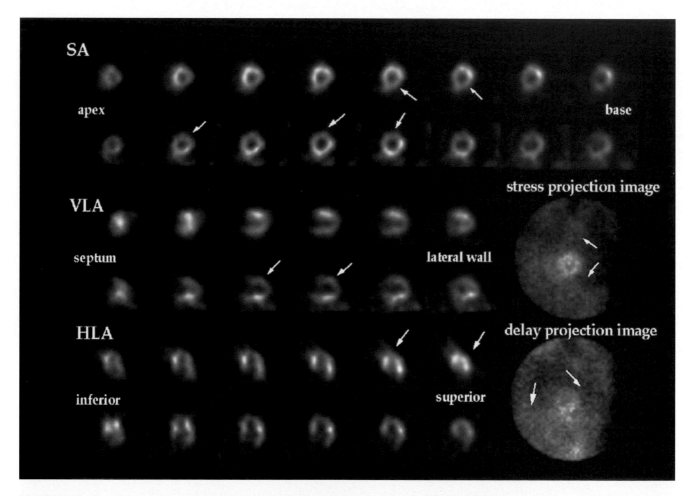

FIGURE 5-10   **The top row of each set of slices displays stress images; the bottom row, redistribution images. SA = short axis, VLA = vertical long axis, HLA = horizontal long axis. The arrows point to a lateral wall defect on the stress images and an anterior wall defect on the redistribution images. The projection images are helpful in identifying the breast-tissue planes on the two sets of images. From the projection images, it can be seen that the left breast position shifts dramatically between the early and delayed images. It is important to look at the raw projection image data in all patients but especially in women to avoid interpreting shifting breast tissue as ischemic defects.**

CASE 8

HISTORY:

This 34-year-old white woman had mitral valve prolapse and a strongly positive family history for coronary artery disease (CAD). She was referred to a cardiologist for the evaluation of chest pain. Despite her sex and youth, because of her family history and the nature of her chest pain, her physician referred her for stress perfusion imaging. Because of her known history of bilateral breast implants, a stress sestamibi study was performed.

STRESS-TEST PARAMETERS:

The resting ECG was normal. The patient exercised for 11 min 16 s of a Bruce protocol (13.5 METS), achieving a HR of 147 bpm, BP of 140/80 mmHg, and stopping due to fatigue. There was no exercise-induced chest pain or ischemia ECG changes.

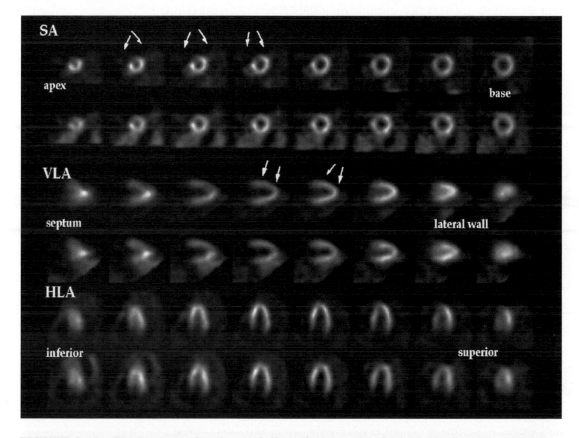

FIGURE 5-11   The top row of each set of slices displays stress images; the bottom row, rest images. SA = short axis, VLA = vertical long axis, HLA = horizontal long axis. The arrows point to a rounded, photopenic structure anterior and superior to the left ventricle, seen best on the short-axis slices. The fixed anterior defect caused by the implants is noted. The fixed defects in this case were attributed to soft tissue artifacts and the scan was read as normal. Confirming the reading of "normal" in this patient were the results of simultaneously acquired first-pass left ventricular ejection fraction (LVEF) values at rest (60 percent) and peak exercise (67 percent). Because of the higher energy of sestamibi compared to thallium, there is less soft tissue attenuation of photons; but even on sestamibi scans, breast tissue in women can present problems in scan interpretation.

CASE 9

HISTORY:

This 64-year-old man was referred for treadmill stress thallium study for the evaluation of chest pain. He had had an MI 8 years previously.

STRESS-TEST PARAMETERS:

Baseline ECG showed nonspecific ST-T-segment abnormalities. The patient was taking a beta blocker, calcium channel blocker, and ACE inhibitor. He exercised for 7 min of the Bruce protocol (9.5 METS), achieving a peak HR of 80 bpm, peak BP of 148/92 mmHg, and stopping due to dyspnea. The ECG showed no further changes from baseline.

CORONARY ANGIOGRAPHY:

The patient subsequently underwent coronary angiography, which showed the following: 85 percent proximal and 100 percent midstenoses of the LAD, 60 percent of a ramus branch, 100 percent of the proximal LCx, 75 percent proximal and 80 percent distal stenoses of the RCA.

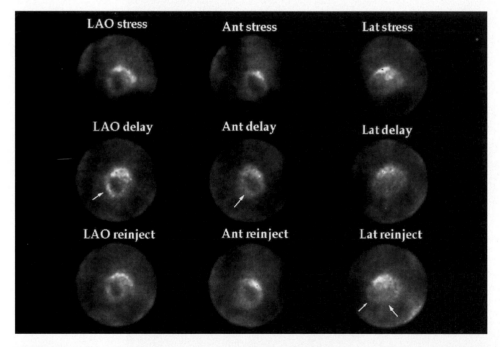

FIGURE 5-12.   The patient underwent planar thallium stress, delay, and reinjection imaging. The stress images show extensive perfusion defects involving the septal and inferoapical segments in the left anterior oblique (LAO) view, inferior wall and apex in the anterior view, and distal anterior wall and diaphragmatic walls in the lateral view. Arrows show redistribution into the septum and inferior walls at 4-h delayed imaging. Following reinjection of thallium and repeat imaging, the distal anterior wall and diaphragmatic walls show defect fill-in. Reinjection of 1 mCi of thallium following completion of redistribution imaging boosts blood thallium levels, allowing for more thallium activity to be taken up in viable myocardium with low resting blood flow (hibernating myocardium). The scan shows ischemia in multiple vascular territories.

CASE 10

HISTORY:

This 41-year-old woman (height, 5 ft 10 in.; weight, 290 lb) with insulin-dependent diabetes mellitus had a stent placement in the LAD. She was referred for stress thallium study for the evaluation of recurrent chest pain and underwent a dipyridamole study because she was unable to exercise.

STRESS-TEST PARAMETERS:

The exercise stress test was negative for clinical or ECG evidence of ischemia.

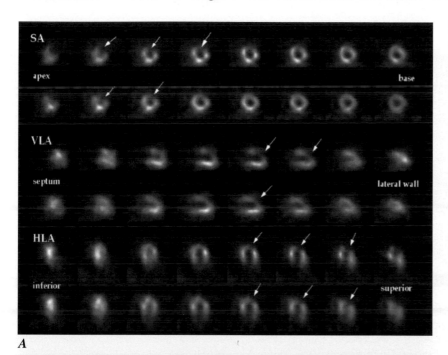

A

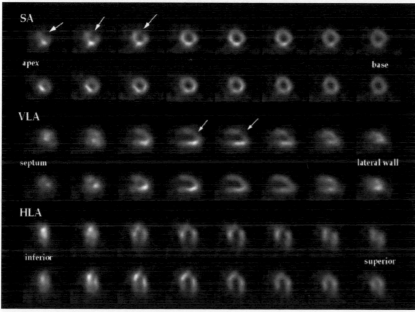

B

FIGURE 5-13   The top row of each set of slices (*A*) displays stress images; the bottom row, redistribution images. The top row in each set of slices (*B*) displays redistribution and the bottom row reinjection images. SA = short axis, VLA = vertical long axis, HLA = horizontal long axis. The arrows point to an anterior wall defect that does not change appreciably at 4-h delayed imaging. Following thallium reinjection (*B*), the anterior defect fills in completely. Although the defect was not extensive or severe, the information that it filled in completely following reinjection was important in this case to differentiate between an infarction and ischemia.

CASE 11

HISTORY:

This 78-year-old woman had a recent MI complicated by congestive heart failure. She underwent coronary angiography, which showed the following: 50 percent left main stenosis, 100 percent mid-LAD stenosis with reconstitution of the distal vessel via collaterals, 60 percent of OM1 (first obtuse marginal branch), 80 percent proximal RCA stenosis (dominant vessel), 60 percent of the posterior descending artery (PDA). To be evaluated for myocardial viability, the patient underwent thallium rest and redistribution scans. As part of a study comparing thallium and sestamibi as viability agents, she also underwent a resting sestamibi scan and a gated blood pool scan. All scans are displayed in the following figures.

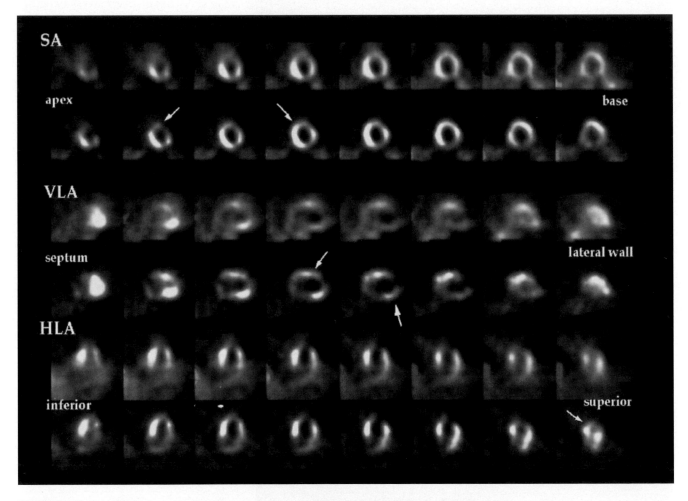

FIGURE 5-14   **The top row of each set of slices displays rest images; the bottom row, redistribution images. SA = short axis, VLA = vertical long axis, HLA = horizontal long axis. The early rest images show anterior, apical, and inferior defects. The arrows point to walls (anterior, anteroseptal distal, and inferior) that show redistribution at 4 h.**

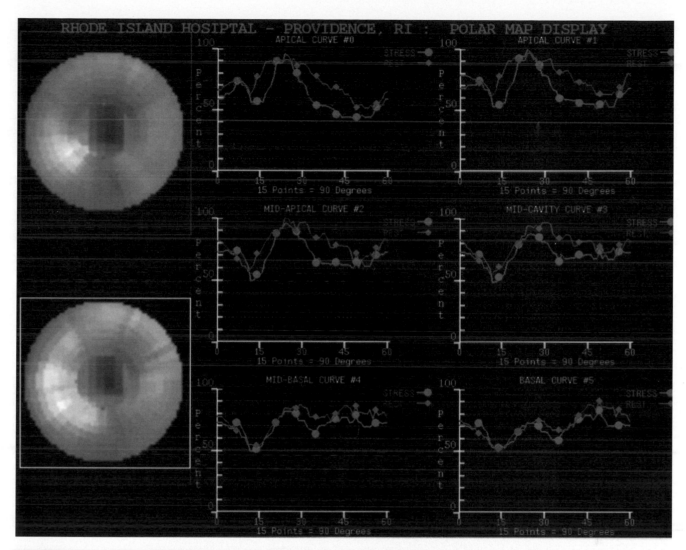

FIGURE 5-15 The polar display shows redistribution in the inferior wall (distal), as well as anterior and anteroseptal walls (distal). The apex, which is not displayed, was reduced to 25 percent of peak counts and did not change. The quantitative data reveal extensive myocardial viability based on the presence of redistribution following a rest injection of thallium as well as count levels above 50 percent of peak counts in most of the heart except the apex. (*See color Plate 21.*)

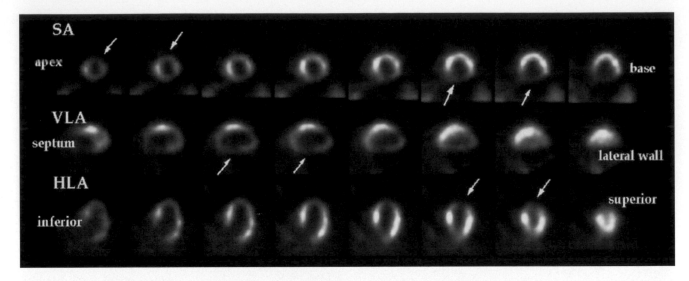

FIGURE 5-16   Tomographic scan performed following the injection of sestamibi at rest. The defects are identified in the same territories as on the thallium scans. Viability can be determined from the resting sestamibi scan using criteria similar to those applied to thallium scans— that is, counts above a certain percentage of peak represent viability.

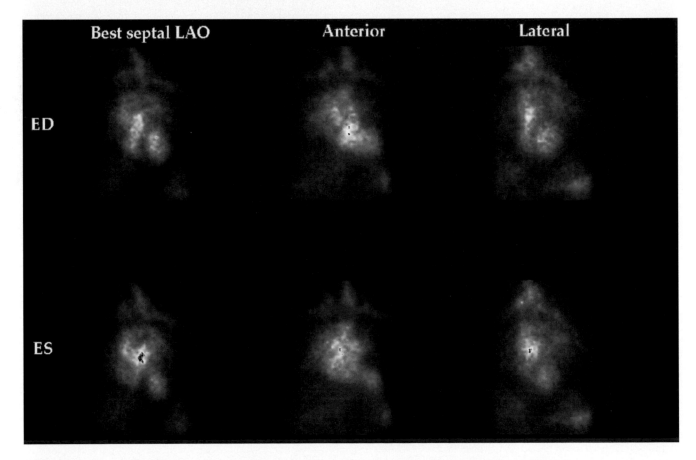

FIGURE 5-17   Gated blood pool scan performed at rest on the same patient showing a dilated left ventricle with global hypokinesis. The LVEF was calculated to be 25 percent. The dissociation between thallium or sestamibi count levels and wall motion in this case are due to either hibernation and/or stunning.

CASE 12

HISTORY:

This 68-year-old man with long-standing angina pectoris recently experienced a worsening of this condition and was referred for stress thallium study.

STRESS-TEST-PARAMETERS:

The patient was unable to exercise due to a knee problem so he underwent a dipyridamole stress test. Since the baseline ECG showed left ventricular hypertrophy (LVH) with secondary ST-T wave changes, the stress ECG could not be interpreted for ischemia. There were no symptoms of ischemia during dipyridamole administration.

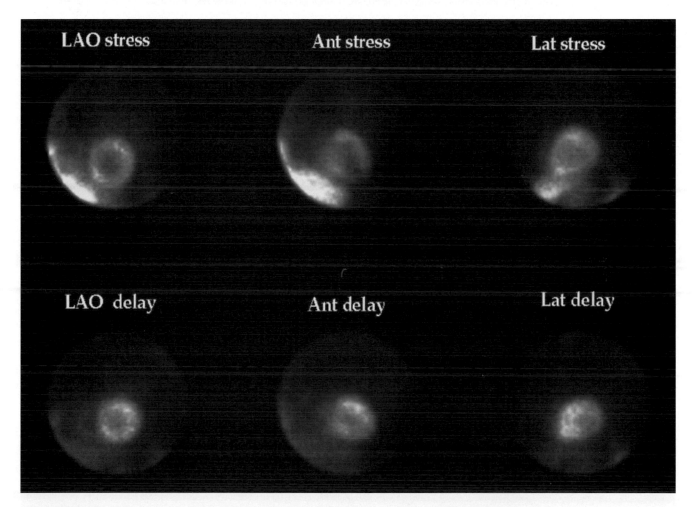

FIGURE 5-18   **The patient underwent stress and redistribution planar thallium imaging. The stress images show transient LV dilatation appreciated by comparing the size of the LV in the LAO and anterior views between the immediate poststress images and the 4-h delay images. There are extensive defects in multiple vascular territories on the early scans and, in addition to a dramatic decrease in LV chamber size at delayed imaging, the tracer distribution almost normalizes with the exception of the inferoapical segment in the anterior view. The increased thallium activity in the liver on the stress images is due to increased splanchnic blood flow caused by dipyridamole. This scan pattern is associated with severe multivessel and/or left main coronary artery disease and predictive of further ischemic events and increased risk of mortality. The patient refused coronary angiography.**

CASE 13

HISTORY:

This 85-year-old man with a history of hypertension had an MI 6 years previously with subsequent symptoms of congestive heart failure. Coronary angiography at that time revealed three-vessel coronary disease (70 percent proximal LAD, 50 percent D2, 50 percent proximal LCx, 80 percent OM2). He was readmitted with another MI and worsening heart failure and referred for stress perfusion imaging for post-MI evaluation.

STRESS-TEST PARAMETERS:

The patient underwent a dipyridamole stress perfusion test because he was unable to exercise. This was combined with sestamibi imaging as a 2-day protocol. Baseline ECG showed left ventricular hypertrophy (LVH) with frequent ventricular premature depolarizations (VPDs). The test induced no chest pain, and the ECG was uninterpretable for ischemia.

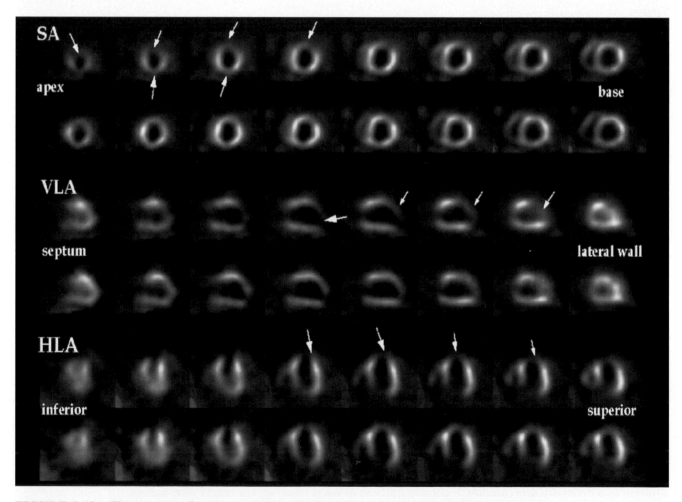

FIGURE 5-19   The top row of each set of slices displays stress images; the bottom row, rest images. SA = short axis, VLA = vertical long axis, HLA = horizontal long axis. The LV is enlarged and the RV easily seen on the sestamibi images, although it is probably normal in size and thickness. The arrows point to both anterior and inferior defects on the poststress images, with some defect fill-in following the rest injection.

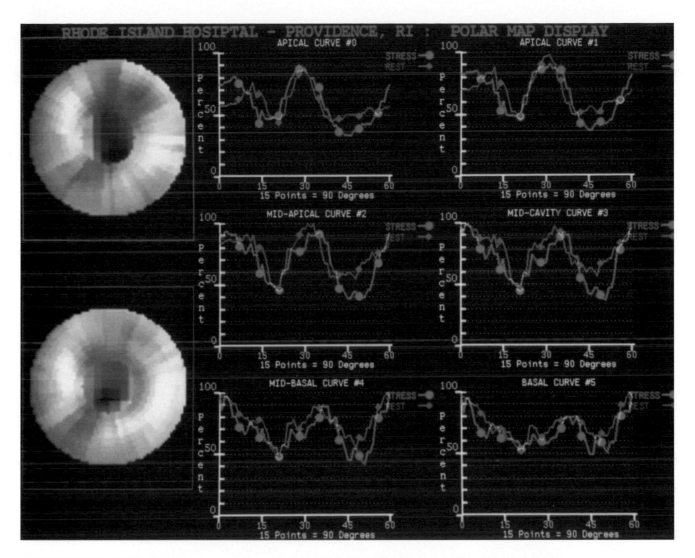

FIGURE 5-20   **Polar display from the same patient. The two defects are seen as the two dips in the curves, and the difference between the blue and red curves distally corresponds to the defect fill-in seen on the scans. Profiles from the apex are not included in this display. The apex shows the most severe count reduction, and the defect is fixed. (*See color Plate 22.*)**

CASE 14

HISTORY:

This 61-year-old woman was referred for stress thallium study for the evaluation of new-onset chest pain. Her risk factors for coronary artery disease include hypertension and a positive family history.

STRESS-TEST PARAMETERS:

The patient underwent dipyridamole stress testing because she was unable to exercise. Baseline ECG showed nonspecific ST-T abnormalities. During dipyridamole administration, the patient developed chest pain thought clinically to be angina and developed ischemic ECG changes.

CORONARY ANGIOGRAPHY:

As a result of this test, the patient underwent coronary angiography, which showed the following: 50 percent proximal and 90 percent mid stenoses of the LAD, 100 percent stenosis of the proximal LCx with reconstitution of the distal vessel via jeopardized collaterals, and 90 percent proximal stenosis of a dominant RCA.

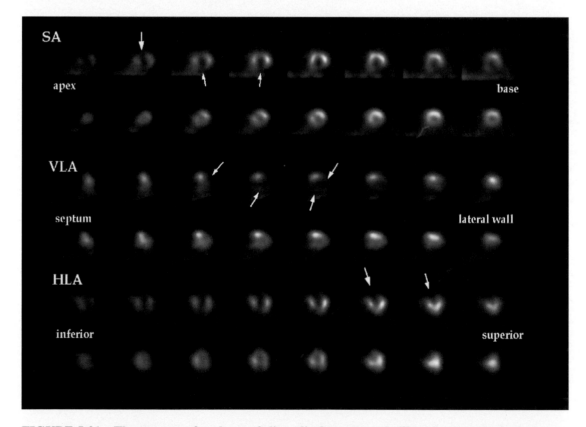

FIGURE 5-21 **The top row of each set of slices displays stress thallium images; the bottom row, redistribution images. SA = short axis, VLA = vertical long axis, HLA = horizontal long axis. There is transient ischemic dilatation of the left ventricle on the stress images in addition to extensive reversible defects in both the LAD (anterior, anteroseptal, apex) and RCA territories. The outward splaying of the apical aspect of the septal and lateral walls in the HLA slices is consistent with ischemic aneurysmal dilatation of the apex.**

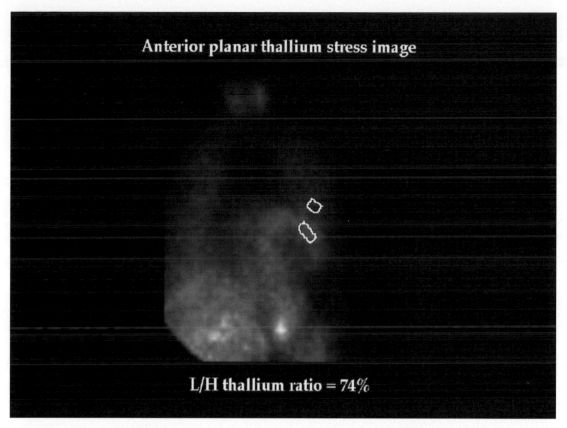

FIGURE 5-22   The thallium lung/heart ratio on the stress planar image acquired before the tomogram showed a value of 0.74, which is very high (normal is less than 0.5) and occurs along with transient ischemic dilatation of the LV, as an indicator of stress-induced LV dysfunction.

CASE 15

HISTORY:

This 70-year-old man had had two episodes of exertional chest fullness that cleared rapidly on both occasions. On a routine visit to his physician, Q waves were seen on leads V2 and V3 that had not been present on the previous visit, so patient was referred for stress thallium study to evaluate the extent of coronary artery disease.

STRESS-TEST PARAMETERS:

The baseline ECG showed an anterior MI of indeterminate age and T-wave inversions in the anterolateral leads. The patient exercised 4 min and 9 s of the Bruce protocol (6.5 METS), achieving a peak HR of 138 bpm, peak BP of 182/90 mmHg, and stopping because of fatigue and dyspnea. In the 2 min of recovery, he developed chest fullness, which resolved spontaneously by minute 6 of recovery. The ECG was uninterpretable for ischemia due to baseline abnormalities.

CORONARY ANGIOGRAPHY:

Angiography showed a 95% lesion of the LAD involving the take-off of D1. LV gram showed severe hypokinesis of the anterolateral and apical segments with LVEF of 35%. The patient underwent angioplasty of the LAD lesion. Based on the thallium scan showing predominantly ischemia and viability in the LAD territory, it was thought that the LV dysfunction was largely due to stunning and/or hibernation and it was expected that there will be significant improvement in LVEF following revascularization.

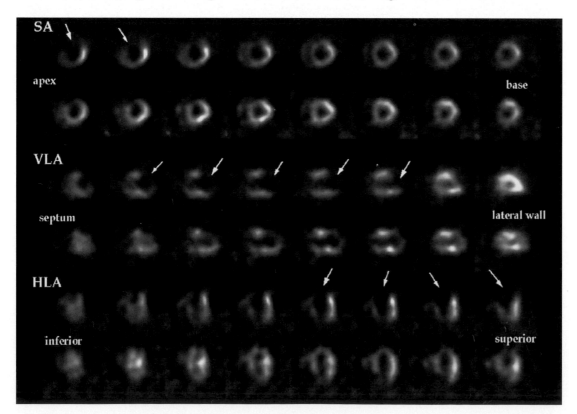

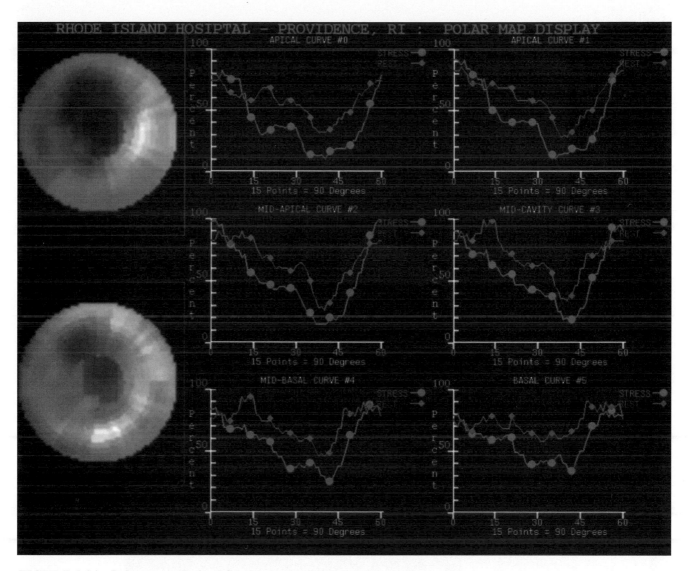

FIGURE 5-24   Polar maps derived from scan data of the patient in Fig. 5-23. *(See color Plate 23.)*

◀ **FIGURE 5-23**   The top row of each set of slices displays stress thallium images; the bottom row, redistribution images. SA = short axis, VLA = vertical long axis, HLA = horizontal long axis. There is impressive transient ischemic dilatation of the left ventricle on the stress images with outward splaying of the distal septal and lateral walls seen on the VLA slices. This is consistent with ischemic aneurysmal dilatation of the apex. Extensive, largely redistributing defects involving the inferior, septal, and anterior walls as well as the apex are also seen on the polar maps (Fig. 5-24. *See also color Plate 23).*

CASE 16

HISTORY:

This 69-year-old man was referred for stress perfusion study to evaluate new-onset exertional chest pain. The study was performed as a stress and rest two-day sestamibi protocol.

STRESS-TEST PARAMETERS:

The baseline ECG was normal. The patient exercised for 4 min and 21 s of the Bruce protocol (7.1 METS), achieving a peak HR of 88 bpm, peak BP of 142/74 mmHg, and stopping due to exhaustion and a drop in systolic BP from 142 to 122. The ECG showed ischemic changes.

CORONARY ANGIOGRAPHY:

On the basis of the results of this test, the patient underwent coronary angiography, which showed the following: 70 percent stenosis of the proximal and mid-LAD, 60 percent stenosis of the proximal RCA and 80 percent of the PDA, and 99 percent stenosis of the right posterolateral branch.

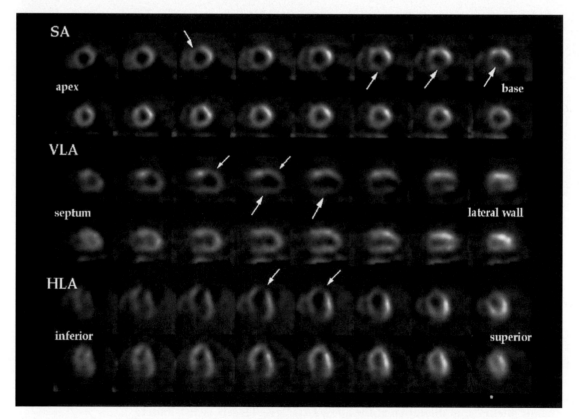

FIGURE 5-25   The top row of each set of slices displays stress images; the bottom row, rest images. SA = short axis, VLA = vertical long axis, HLA = horizontal long axis. There is transient ischemic dilatation of the left ventricle on the stress images and, in addition, reversible perfusion defects involving both the anterior and inferior walls and apex, as shown by the arrows, demonstrating reversible ischemia in the distribution of the LAD and RCA.

CASE 17

HISTORY:

This 50-year old man had an MI 4 years earlier and was now being evaluated for new-onset atypical chest pain. He was referred for a stress perfusion study, which was performed as a 2-day protocol stress and rest sestamibi study.

STRESS-TEST PARAMETERS:

Baseline ECG showed inferior Q waves. The patient exercised for 9 min and 59 s of the Bruce protocol (10.2 METS), achieving a peak HR of 176 bpm, peak BP of 180/70 mmHg, and stopping because of fatigue. There were no ischemic ECG changes.

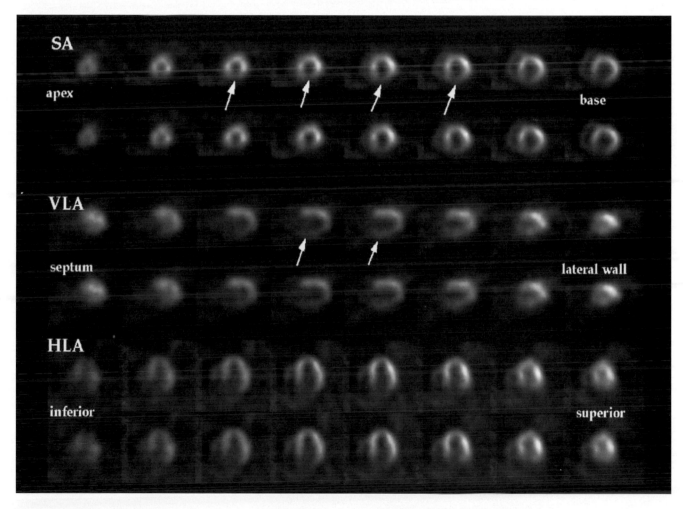

FIGURE 5-26   **The top row of each set of slices displays stress images; the bottom row, rest images. SA = short axis, VLA = vertical long axis, HLA = horizontal long axis. A fixed inferior defect (*arrows*) is seen on the slices and the polar map display in Fig. 5-27.**

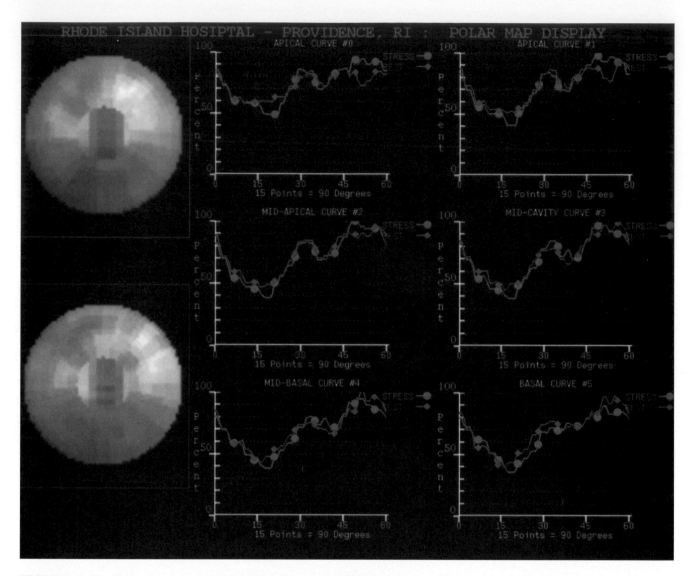

FIGURE 5-27   Polar map showing fixed inferior wall defect. *(See color Plate 24.)*

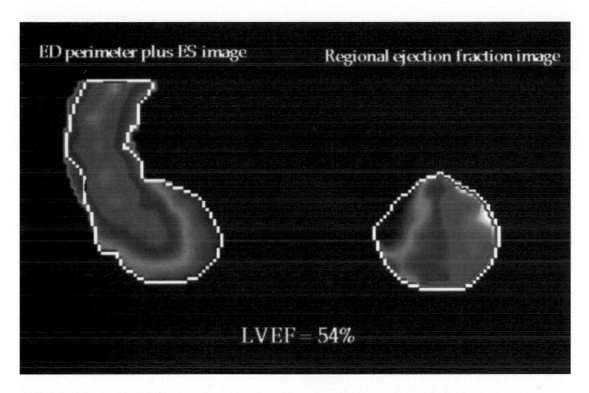

FIGURE 5-28   During the injection of the rest dose of sestamibi, a dynamic first-pass acquisition was performed for measurement of LVEF and evaluation of wall motion. This figure shows the first-pass study with low-normal LVEF and mild inferior hypokinesis seen on both the combined ED perimeter and ES image and on the regional ejection fraction image, in which regional ejection fractions in the LV region are color-coded with yellow, being the highest, through shades of red to purple, blue, green, and black. ED = end-diastolic; ES = end-systolic. (*See color Plate 25.*)

CASE 18

HISTORY:

The patient is a 47-year-old man who had an anterior MI 3 years previously. This was followed by a PTCA of the LAD, which was repeated 3 months prior to this referral. The patient developed recurrent chest pain after the most recent PTCA; 2-day stress and rest sestamibi imaging protocol was ordered to evaluate vessel patency.

STRESS-TEST PARAMETERS:

The baseline ECG showed nonspecific ST-T-segment abnormalities. The patient exercised 8 min and 32 s of the Bruce protocol (10.2 METS), achieving a peak HR of 123 bpm, peak BP of 150/86 mmHg, and stopping due to chest pain. The stress ECG was nondiagnostic for ischemia due to baseline abnormalities.

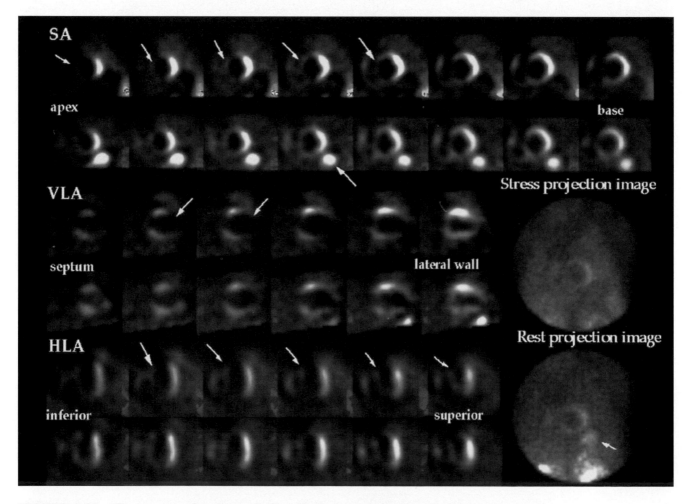

FIGURE 5-29   The top row of each set of slices displays stress images; the bottom row, rest images. SA = short axis, VLA = vertical long axis, HLA = horizontal long axis. There are extensive fixed defects involving the anterior wall, anterior septum, apex, and inferior walls. The rest projection image shows the biodistribution of sestamibi with intestinal uptake. Uptake in a loop of bowel in the upper abdomen is adjacent to heart and can be seen in the SA and VLA slices but does not interfere with scan interpretation.

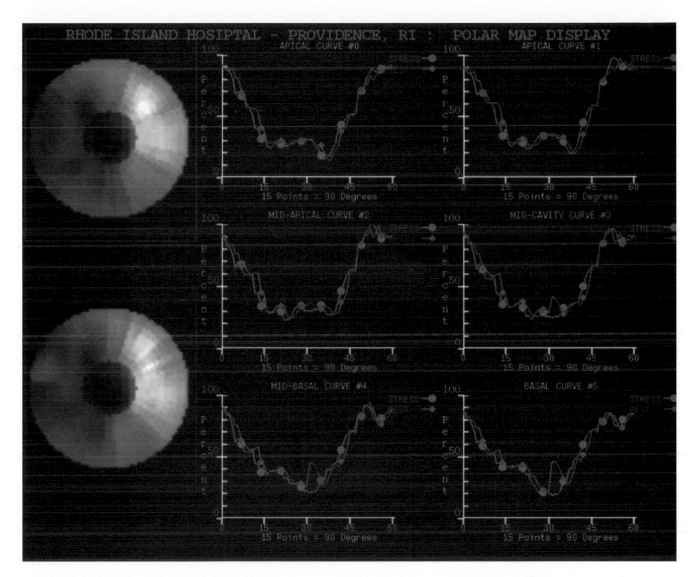

FIGURE 5-30 The polar map also demonstrates an extensive and severe fixed defect in the inferior wall and anteroseptum; the apical defect was also severe with 16 percent of peak activity. *(See color Plate 26.)*

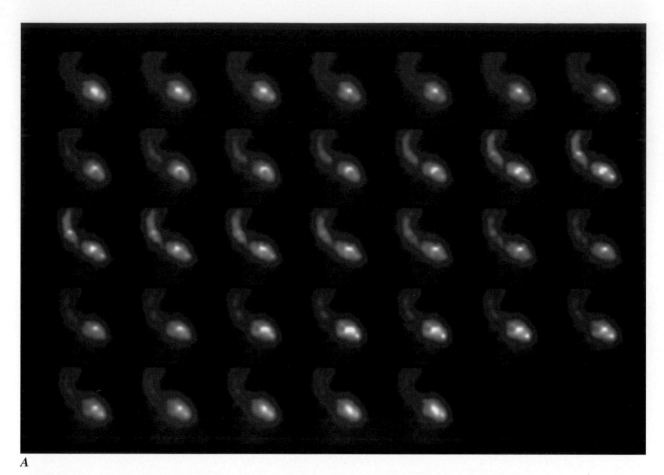

A

FIGURE 5-31 During the injection of the rest dose of sestamibi, a dynamic first pass acquisition was performed for measurement of LVEF and evaluation of wall motion. Individual frames from the LV (*A*) and RV (*B*) acquisition and a single static regional wall motion image of the first-pass study (*C*) are displayed. The most normally contracting wall is the basal anterolateral wall, and the global LVEF is moderately reduced at 38 percent.

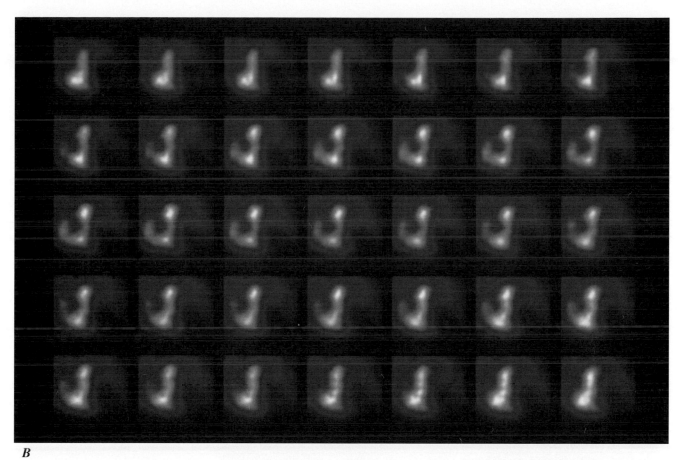

B

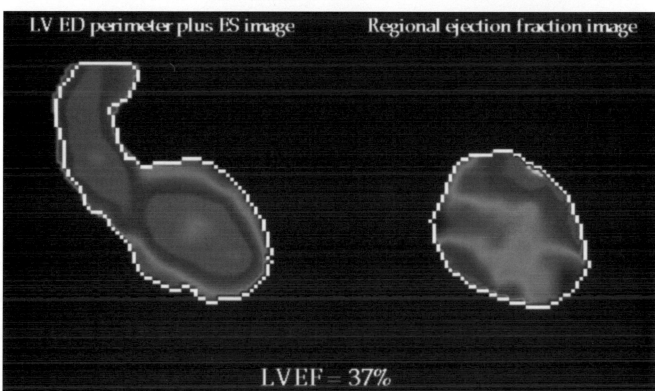

LV ED perimeter plus ES image   Regional ejection fraction image

LVEF = 37%

C

FIGURE 5-31 (*Continued*)

CASE 19

HISTORY:

This 23-year-old obese woman on birth-control pills underwent a lung scan to evaluate sharp chest pain of acute onset resulting from pulmonary embolism.

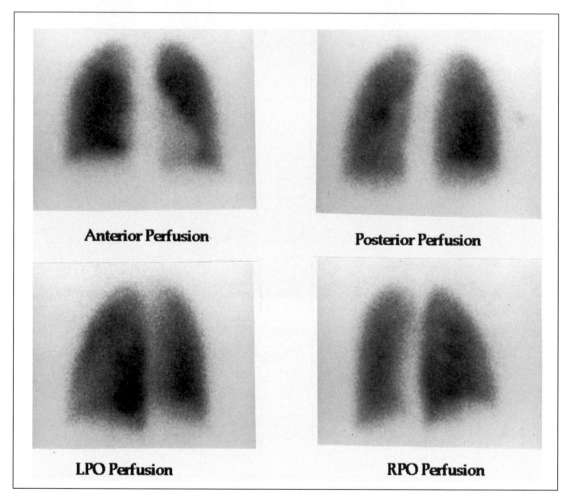

FIGURE 5-32   Perfusion lung scans in four views. LPO = left posterior oblique. RPO = right posterior oblique. The patient was injected with ^{99m}Tc-labeled macroaggregated albumin and imaged immediately after injection. The scans were interpreted as showing normal perfusion to all lung segments, thereby making pulmonary embolism very unlikely. (See also Chap. 11.)

CASE 20

HISTORY:

This 60-year-old woman was admitted to the hospital with acute onset of dyspnea and hypoxemia. She underwent a lung scan to evaluate for pulmonary embolism.

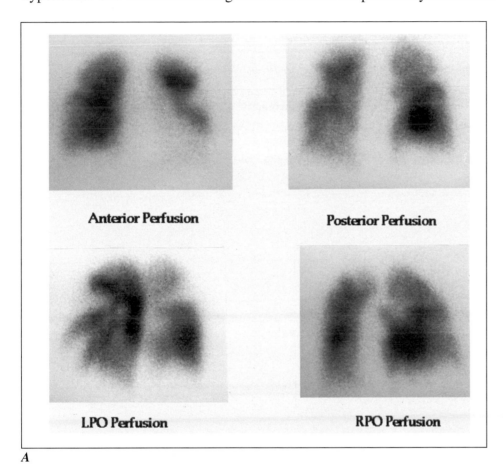

Anterior Perfusion

Posterior Perfusion

LPO Perfusion

RPO Perfusion

A

FIGURE 5-33 *A* and *B*. Perfusion lung scans in four views. LPO = left posterior oblique; RPO=right posterior oblique. The patient was injected with ^{99m}Tc-labeled macroaggregated albumin and imaged immediately after injection. The patient then inhaled a radioactive gas,^{133}Xe, followed by early (initial breath), equilibrium (about 2 min), and washout imaging. The perfusion scans show multiple segmental defects. The ventilation scans were interpreted as normal without evidence of gas trapping. This scan was interpreted as indicating a high probability of pulmonary emboli. The patient underwent pulmonary angiography, which confirmed the diagnosis. (Courtesy of Dr. Pat Spencer and Dr. Richard Noto.) (See Chap. 11.)

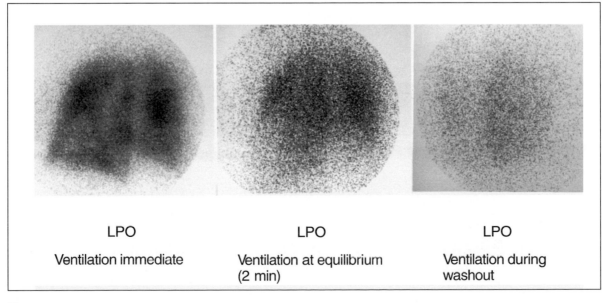

LPO

Ventilation immediate

LPO

Ventilation at equilibrium (2 min)

LPO

Ventilation during washout

B

REFERENCES

1. Johnson LL, Pohost GM: Nuclear cardiology. In: Schlant RC, Alexander RW, O'Rourke RA, et al (eds): *Hurst's the Heart*, 8th ed. New York, McGraw-Hill, 1994, pp 2218–2323.

2. Van Train KF, Berman DS, Garcia EV, et al: Quantitative analysis of stress thallium-201 myocardial scintigrams: A multicenter trial. *J Nucl Med* 1986; 27:17–25.

3. Van Train KF, Garcia EV, Maddahi J, et al: Multicenter trial validation for quantitative analysis of same-day rest-stress technetium-99m-sestamibi myocardial tomograms. *J Nucl Med* 1994; 35:609–618.

4. Verani MS: Pharmacologic stress myocardial perfusion imaging. *Curr Probl Cardiol* 1993; 18:481–528.

5. Brown KA: Prognostic value of thallium-201 myocardial perfusion imaging: A diagnostic tool comes of age. *Circulation* 1991; 83:363–381.

6. Stratmann HG, Williams GA, Wittry MD, et al: Exercise technetium-99m sestamibi tomography for cardiac risk stratification of patients with stable chest pain. *Circulation* 1994; 89:615–622.

CHAPTER 6

MAGNETIC RESONANCE IMAGING

Gerald G. Blackwell, M.D.

Gerald M. Pohost, M.D.

MAGNETIC resonance imaging (MRI) is increasingly being applied to the diagnostic evaluation of patients with diseases involving the heart and vascular tree.[1] This technology is unique because, during a single examination, clinically relevant information can be obtained to evaluate cardiac morphology, function, quantitative flow, and the integrity of the cerebral and peripheral vasculature. Research is being carried out in several major medical centers worldwide in an attempt to furnish diagnostically useful information in the areas of myocardial perfusion, noninvasive angiography of the proximal coronary arterial tree, and metabolic information using in vivo spectroscopic methods to evaluate high-energy phosphate and lipid metabolism. Successful integration of some or all of these studies would provide a true "one-stop shop" to comprehensively assess cardiovascular diagnostics noninvasively in a cost-effective manner.[2] This exciting technology is being successfully introduced into training programs for cardiovascular specialists and should lead to even more effective applications in the future.

Medical MRI exploits the physical principle of magnetism to provide high-resolution images of the distribution of hydrogen nuclei throughout the body.[3] The hydrogen atom has a microscopic magnetic charge associated with the "spin" of its positively charged proton. Hydrogen nuclei are abundantly distributed throughout the body (more than 70 percent of the body is made up of hydrogen nuclei), primarily in the form of water and fat. When exposed to an external magnetic field, the billions of hydrogen nuclei in the human organism can be aligned so as to produce a measurable net magnetic moment.[4] Utilizing magnetic field gradients, radiofrequency energy, and sophisticated computer power, one can obtain high-resolution three-dimensional images of both static hydrogen atoms (soft tissue) and moving structures (vascular conduits and flowing blood).

There are several major advantages to MRI that should be noted: (1) The technique is noninvasive, exposing the patient to no ionizing radiation and requiring no intravascular contrast injection. (2) These noninvasive images can be acquired in any desired tomographic plane, allowing three-dimensional examination of morphology and physiology.[5] (3) Tissue contrast in MRI, on the other hand, is related to multiple factors including hydrogen density, motion (blood flow), the intrinsic magnetic characteristics of the tissue, and acquisition parameters as defined by the operator. (4) There are very few contraindications to MRI, and image quality is independent of body habitus, making the technology practical for use in most patients[6] (Tables 6-1 and 6-2). These advantages are now routinely applied in the clinical care of patients with cardiovascular diseases.

Table 6-3 lists disease states in which MRI has already been shown to be indicated as a first-line diagnostic test. This includes patients with stable thoracic aortic disease of any type, complex congenital heart disease, constrictive pericardial disease, and those who require assessment of paracardiac masses.[7] Magnetic resonance angiography also has an established role in the assessment of runoff vessels in patients with severe

TABLE 6-1
Contraindications to Magnetic Resonance Imaging[a]

Pacemakers

Cardioverters/defibrillators

Cerebral aneurysm clips

Magnetically activated implants or foreign bodies

Pre-6000 series Starr-Edwards prostheses

[a]Sternal wires, coronary artery stents, and most prosthetic heart valves are safe for MRI.

TABLE 6-2
Sources of Artifact in Magnetic Resonance Images

Motion artifact

Patient motion (nongatable; reduced by ultrafast imaging strategies)

Cardiac motion (reduced by ECG gating)

Respiratory motion (reduced by respiratory gating)

Irregular cardiac rhythms (misregistration artifacts; reduced by arrhythmia-rejection software)

Metallic implants (distortion of homogeneous magnetic field)

Turbulent blood flow patterns (can be diagnostically useful in stenotic and regurgitant valvular disease as well as for detecting intracardiac shunts)

Table 6-3

Established Primary Indications for Cardiovascular Magnetic Resonance Imaging

Stable thoracic aortic disease

    Aneurysm

    Dissection

    Coarctation

Complex congenital heart disease

Constrictive pericardial disease

Paracardiac masses

Assessment of distal runoff vessels in patients with severe lower-extremity peripheral vascular disease

Table 6-4

Indications for which Cardiovascular Magnetic Resonance Imaging Provides Diagnostically Useful Information and Is Being Increasing Utilized

Assessment of global and regional left ventricular function

Assessment of global and regional right ventricular function

Valvular heart disease

Hypertrophic cardiomyopathy (especially atypical patterns)

Complicated effusive pericardial disease

Extracranial cerebral vascular disease

Abdominal aortic disease

Indications indicated from promising research studies

    Myocardial perfusion imaging

    Coronary angiography

    Assessment of cardiac viability

peripheral vascular disease in whom contrast angiography is frequently nondiagnostic.[8] Table 6-4 lists situations in which MRI has been shown to provide useful information and can therefore be used as an alternative diagnostic modality. These include the assessment of global and regional left ventricular function,[9,10] right ventricular function, valvular heart disease, complex effusive pericardial disease, and abdominal aortic disease. Magnetic resonance angiograms of the extracranial cerebral vasculature are now frequently being used in the diagnostic evaluation of patients with known or suspected cerebral vascular disease. Current research directions for cardiovascular MRI include the assessment of myocardial perfusion and acquisition of noninvasive MR angiograms of the proximal coronary arterial tree. It is to be expected that the role of cardiovascular MRI will continue to increase as the technology develops.

This chapter provides an introduction to information that can be obtained using MRI in patients having a spectrum of cardiovascular pathology. Conventional spin-echo (black blood pool) and gradient-echo (white blood pool, cine MRI) images are shown that were acquired using commercially available hardware and software. These figures were obtained in the daily operation of an MRI lab dedicated to the care of patients with cardiovascular diseases. The exquisite resolution of cardiovascular MRI can be captured in these figures, but it is important to recognize that—as in the case of cardiac catheterization, echocardiography, and nuclear imaging—functional information using MRI can best be depicted by cine loop displays of dynamic data sets. For a more detailed description of magnetic resonance methods and applications, the reader is referred to the reference list at the end of this chapter.[11]

BASIC PRINCIPLES OF MAGNETIC RESONANCE IMAGING

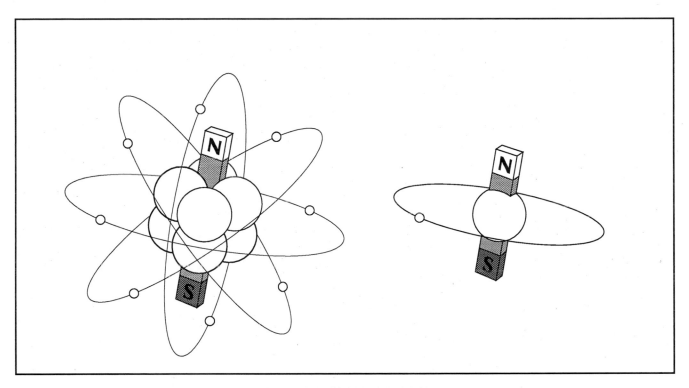

FIGURE 6-1   Medical magnetic resonance images display the distribution of hydrogen atoms throughout the body. A hydrogen nucleus is composed of a single proton, and the spin associated with this positively charged proton produces a microscopic electromagnetic field. In this diagram, the hydrogen nucleus is depicted as a bar magnet, having both north and south poles. For illustrative purposes, a more complex atom is shown alongside. (Reproduced from Blackwell G, Cranney G, Pohost G: *MRI: Cardiovascular System.* New York, Gower Medical Publishing, 1992. By permission.)

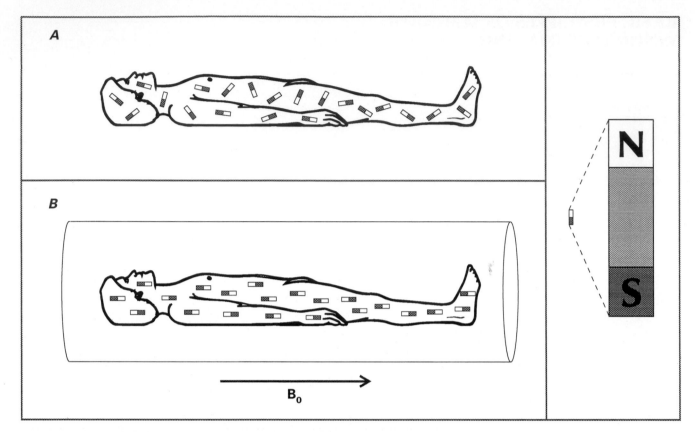

FIGURE 6-2   This figure represents the alignment of hydrogen nuclei within the human body in the absence of an external magnetic field (*A*) and in the presence of a homogeneous magnetic field (*B*). Nuclei are depicted as tiny bar magnets having north and south poles. In the absence of an external magnetic field, all nuclei are randomly aligned and there is no net magnetic moment. In the presence of a homogeneous magnetic field, the nuclei are required to align in a precise fashion and a magnetic moment is produced (B_0). It is this magnetic moment that is detectable with MRI. (Reproduced from Blackwell G, Cranney G, Pohost G: *MRI: Cardiovascular System*. New York, Gower Medical Publishing, 1992. By permission.)

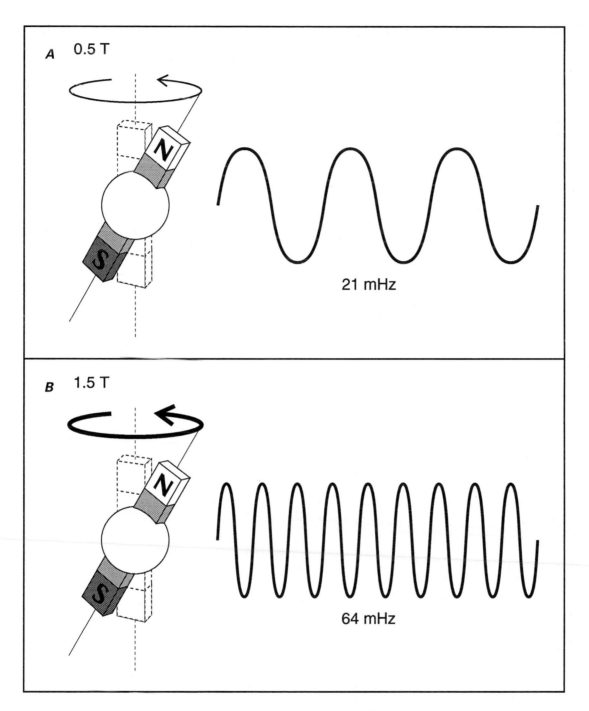

A   0.5 T

21 mHz

B   1.5 T

64 mHz

FIGURE 6-3   Hydrogen nuclei spin, or precess, at a specific frequency
which is dependent upon the force of the external magnetic field that
they are experiencing. The precession frequency of an individual nuclear
species is governed by laws of physics and is given by the Larmor equation.
In this figure, the top panel represents the precession frequency of hydrogen
nuclei when experiencing an external magnetic field strength of 0.5 tesla.
The precession frequency of all hydrogen nuclei will be just over 21 mHz.
The bottom panel shows the precession frequency of hydrogen nuclei
when experiencing an external magnetic field of 1.5 teslas. The precession
frequency is three times greater than in the previous example and is
approximately 64 mHz. (Reproduced from Blackwell G, Cranney G,
Pohost G: *MRI: Cardiovascular System*. New York, Gower Medical
Publishing, 1992. By permission.)

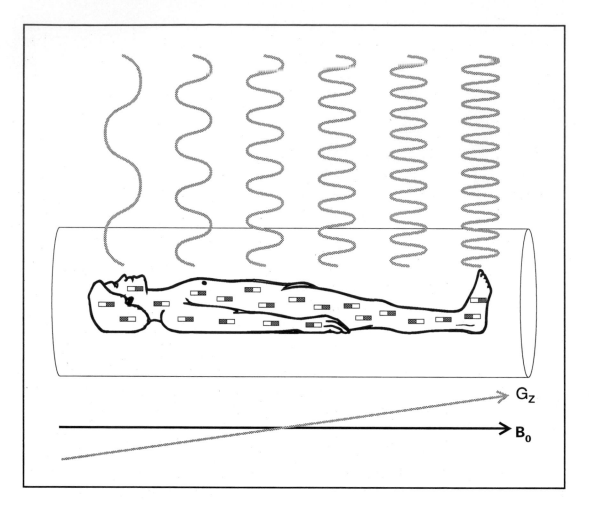

FIGURE 6-4 This illustration depicts the principle responsible for magnetic resonance imaging. Protons within the body are designated as tiny bar magnets with the white end being the north pole and the black end the south pole. These represent only a small fraction of the protons within the body. Please note that the preponderance of magnets is oriented with their north pole facing toward the head and their south pole toward the foot of the patient. This is due to the extrinsic magnetic field created by the large cylindrical magnet within which the patient is placed for an MRI study (B_0). The wavy lines above the patient depict radio waves at different frequencies. Note that the frequency increases as one goes from the patient's head to the patient's foot. These differences in radio frequency (RF) are related to the small differences in magnetic field going from head to foot created by the so-called magnetic field gradient (G_z). In this example, the imaging computer is programmed to recognize that lower frequency resonating protons come from the head, whereas higher frequency resonating protons come from the foot, with resonance frequencies in between representing the rest of the body. This spatially encoded approach uses these frequency differences to generate images in three dimensions. (Reproduced from Blackwell G, Cranney G, Pohost G: *MRI: Cardiovascular System*, New York, Gower Medical Publishing, 1992. By permission.)

AORTIC DISEASE

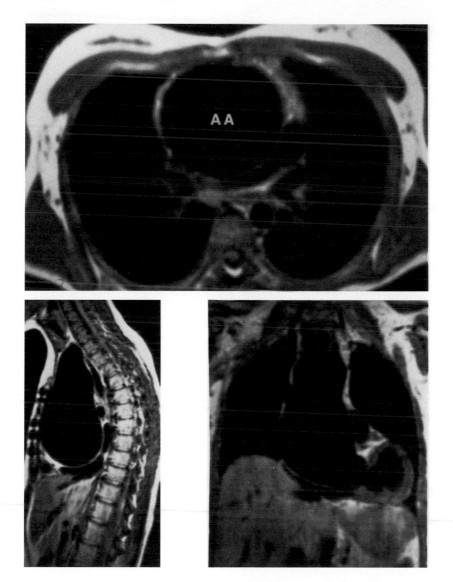

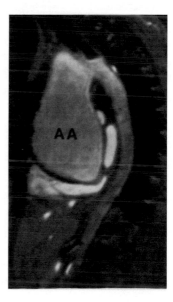

FIGURE 6-5   A 22-year-old female with aortic disease and an ascending aortic aneurysm. Transverse, sagittal, and coronal spin echo images and a left anterior oblique (LAO) cine-MRI demonstrate an ascending aortic aneurysm (AA). Note that the right pulmonary artery and left atrium are compressed by this massive aneurysm.

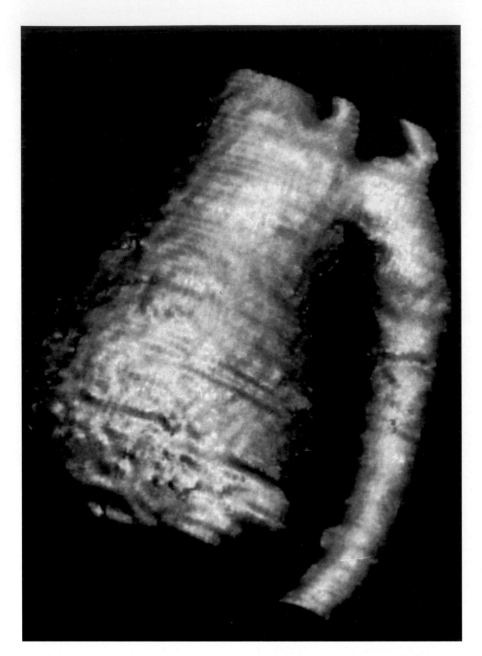

FIGURE 6-6 **Three-dimensional reconstruction of an ascending aortic aneurysm. Note massive aneurysmal enlargement of the ascending segment as well as involvement of the innominate artery. The distal arch and descending thoracic aorta are normal. Three-dimensional reconstruction of magnetic resonance tomograms provides unprecedented insight into aortic anatomy.**

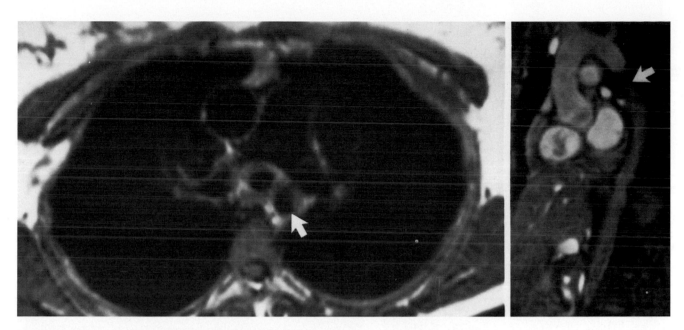

FIGURE 6-7   A 33-year-old female with hypertension. Axial spin echo *(left panel)* **and LAO gradient echo** *(right panel)* **demonstrate an aortic coarctation** *(arrows).* **Minimal luminal diameter in this region was 9 mm. The ascending aorta and aortic arch are of normal size. There is no significant poststenotic dilatation.**

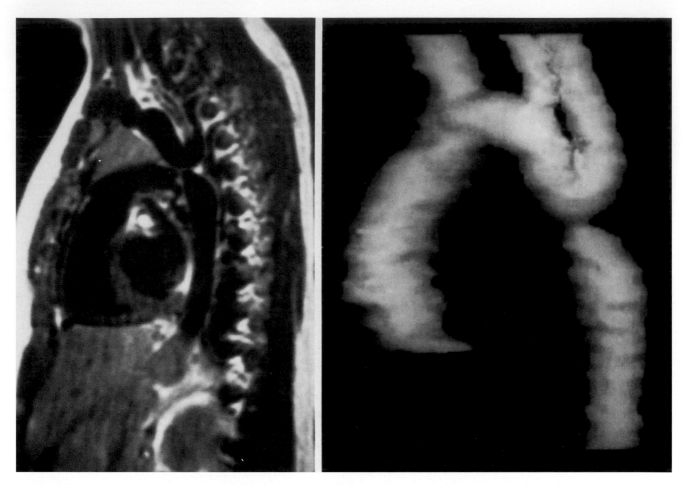

FIGURE 6-8 A 14-year-old boy with hypertension and decreased lower extremity pulses. Sagittal spin-echo *(left panel)* and three-dimensional reconstruction *(right panel)* clearly identify an aortic coarctation and its relationship to the arch vessels. Note the enlargement of the left subclavian artery. Magnetic resonance imaging can obviate the need for invasive angiography in young adults with coarctation.

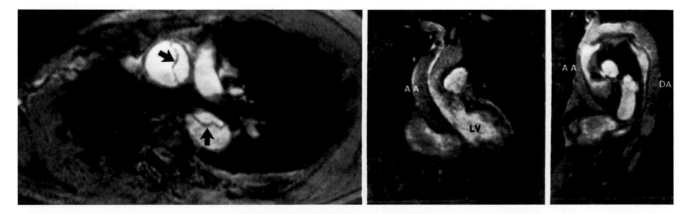

FIGURE 6-9 A 57-year-old man who presented with acute onset chest pain. A type I aortic dissection is clearly identified in the axial *(left panel)*, coronal ascending aortic *(middle panel)*, and LAO *(right panel)* cine-MRI frames. Arrows highlight the intimal flap on the transverse sections. The true and false lumens are well seen on the coronal ascending aortic and LAO images. AA = ascending aorta; DA = descending aorta; LV = left ventricle.

VENTRICULAR FUNCTION

Biplane Long Axis

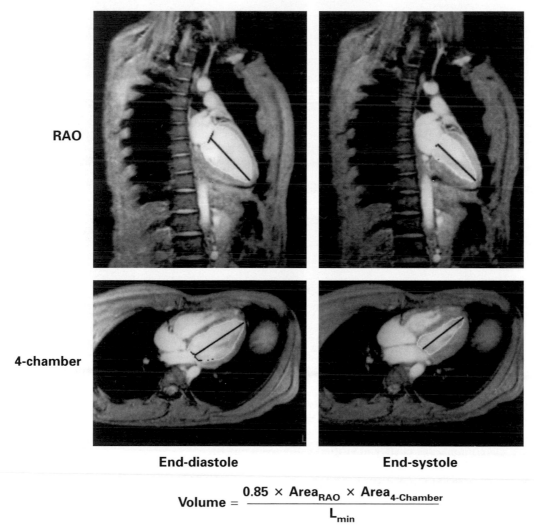

$$Volume = \frac{0.85 \times Area_{RAO} \times Area_{4\text{-Chamber}}}{L_{min}}$$

FIGURE 6-10   Biplane area length method for determining left ventricular volumes and ejection fraction using cine-MRI. End-diastolic and end-systolic frames from orthogonal imaging planes are obtained. Left ventricular areas are planimetered and the long axis length is measured to determine end-diastolic and end-systolic volume. Determination of ventricular volumes and ejection fraction using cine-MRI has been shown to provide rapid, accurate, and reproducible data. (From *Curr Probl Cardiol* 1994; 19:119–175. Reproduced with permission from the publisher and authors.)

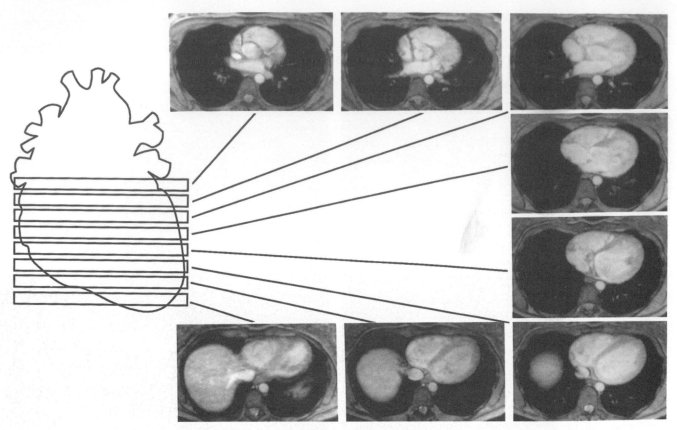

Volume = (area 1 + area 2 + ...area 8) × slice thickness × interslice factor

FIGURE 6-11 Determination of ventricular volumes and ejection fraction using a stacked set of axial tomograms and a Simpson's rule algorithm. This approach requires minimal geometric assumptions and is easy to acquire. Although the valve planes are clearly identified using axial images, partial volume effects are problematic and regional wall motion is more difficult to assess. (From *Curr Probl Cardiol* 1994; 19:119–175. Reproduced with permission from the publisher and authors.)

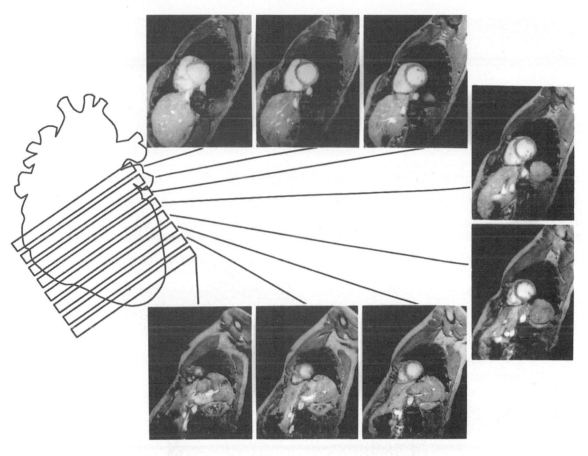

Volume = (area 1 + area 2 + ...area 8) × slice thickness × interslice factor

FIGURE 6-12 Determination of ventricular volumes and ejection fraction using a stacked set of short-axis tomograms and a Simpson's rule algorithm. This approach is excellent for assessing regional wall motion in all segments except the left ventricular apex. Through-plane motion at the cardiac base is a potential source of error. (From *Curr Probl Cardiol* 1994; 19:119–175. Reproduced with permission from the publisher and authors.)

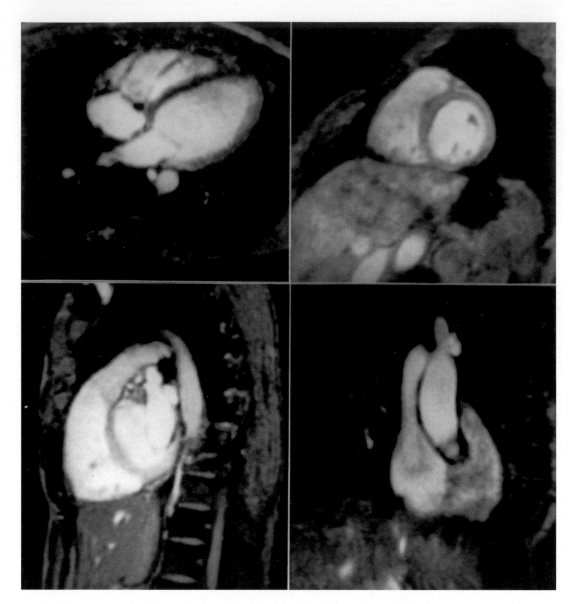

FIGURE 6-13 Magnetic resonance imaging is uniquely well suited for evaluation of the right ventricle. This figure shows four different views that are commonly employed in the assessment of right ventricular morphology and function. The top left-hand panel is a standard four-chamber view; the top right-hand panel is a short-axis view; the bottom left-hand panel is a right ventricular outflow-tract view, and the bottom right-hand panel is a right anterior oblique view of the right ventricle. Magnetic resonance imaging should be regarded as the gold standard for the assessment of right ventricular function. (From *Curr Probl Cardiol* 1994; 19:119–175. Reproduced with permission from the publisher and authors.)

ISCHEMIC HEART DISEASE

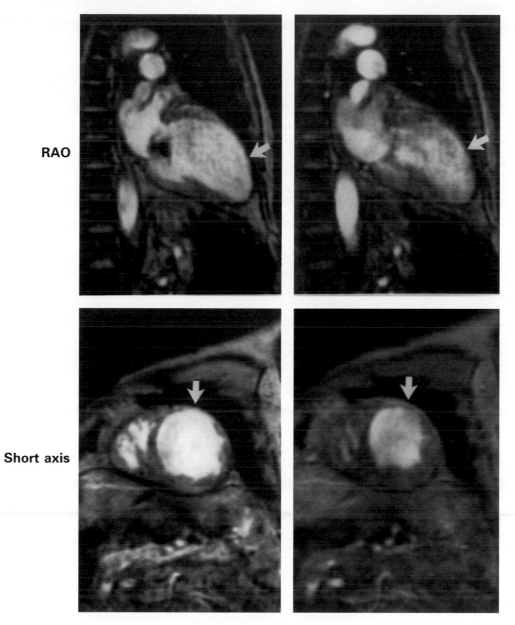

FIGURE 6-14 A 68-year-old man after occlusion of the proximal left anterior descending (LAD) coronary artery. Right anterior oblique (RAO) and short-axis gradient-echo images were obtained at end-diastole and end-systole. The current images were obtained several months postinfarction and demonstrate extreme wall thinning and chamber dilatation as remodeling of the left ventricle. The arrows demonstrate diastolic thinning and the absence of systolic wall thickening. Magnetic resonance imaging is very useful in following serial changes in left ventricular remodeling after acute myocardial infarction.

End-diastole   **End-systole**

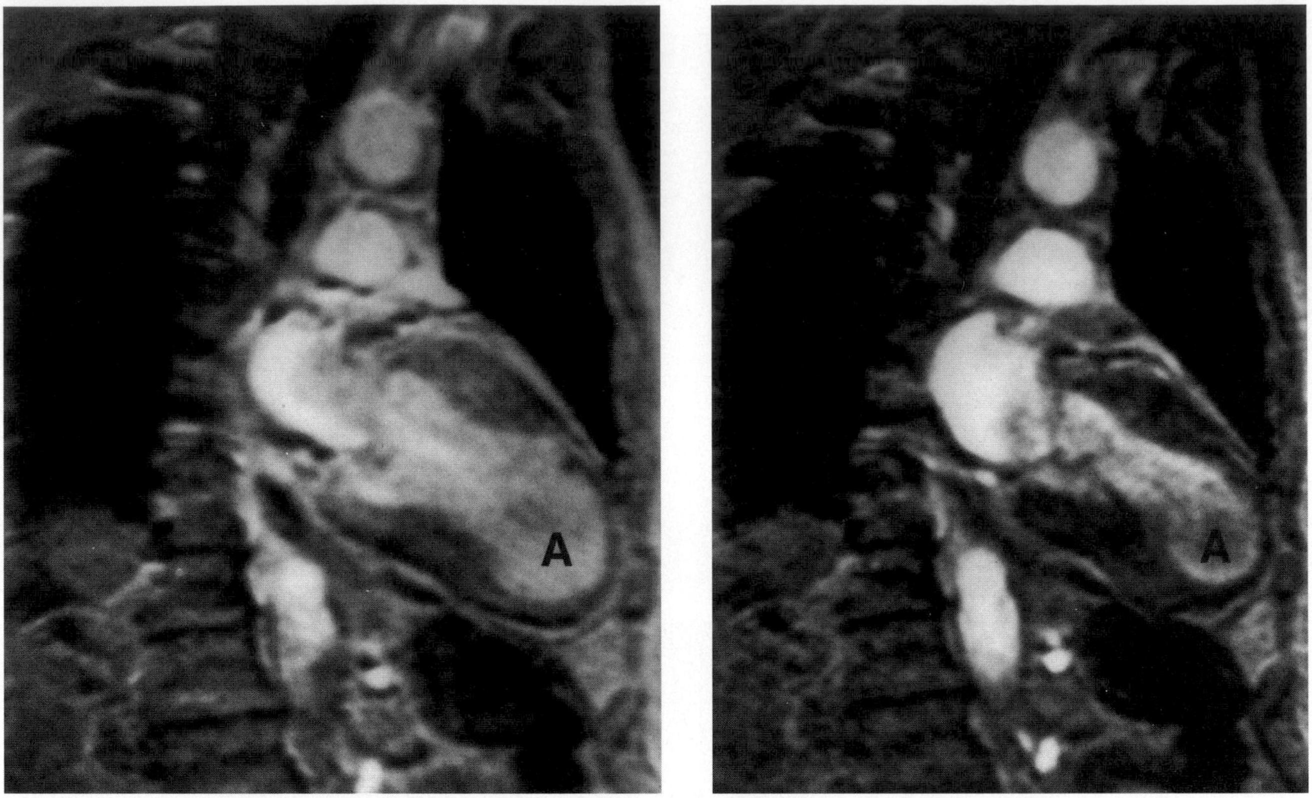

FIGURE 6-15   A 73-year-old man with known coronary artery disease and refractory ventricular arrhythmias. End-diastolic and end-systolic cine-MRI frames in an RAO projection demonstrate an extensive apical aneurysm. The ability to acquire images in multiple tomographic planes makes it possible to assess global ventricular function as well as regional ventricular function in the nonaneurysmal segment. This information is particularly useful when surgical aneurysmectomy is being considered. A = aneurysm.

4-chamber

Short axis

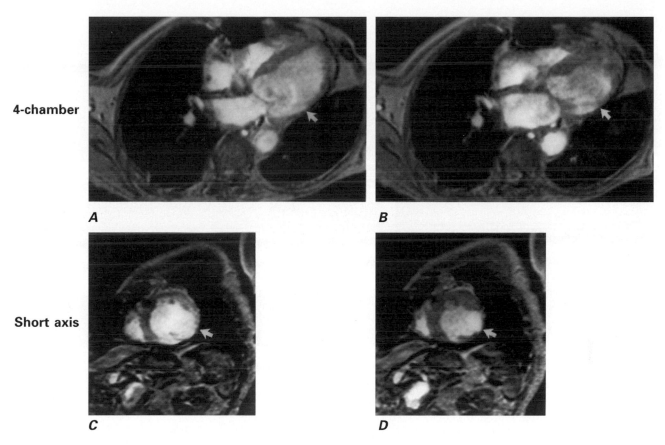

A   B

C   D

FIGURE 6-16   An 82-year-old white man with coronary artery disease after coronary artery bypass grafting who presented with progressive heart failure and complex ventricular arrhythmias. End-diastolic and end-systolic frames in the four-chamber and short-axis planes demonstrate extreme thinning of the inferior and posterolateral left ventricular segments as well as a dilated left ventricle. Diastolic thinning and the absence of systolic wall thickening is highly predictive of nonviable myocardium.

VALVULAR DISEASE

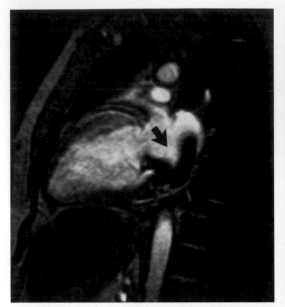 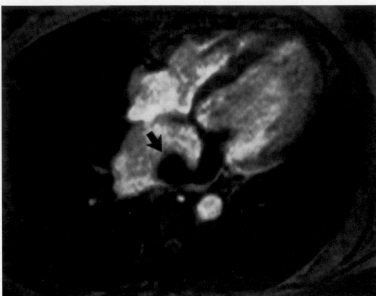

FIGURE 6-17   A 45-year-old man with subacute bacterial endocarditis
and acute congestive heart failure. A large, eccentric jet of mitral
regurgitation is identified which is directed against the posterolateral
left atrial wall. *Left-hand panel*: RAO cine-MRI frame. *Right-hand panel*:
four-chamber cine-MRI frame. Arrows delineate the extensive MRI
signal loss secondary to valvular regurgitation.

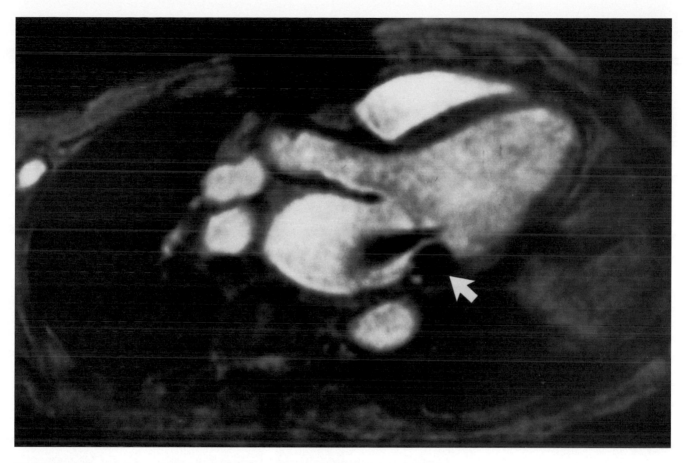

FIGURE 6-18   A 74-year-old woman with progressive shortness of breath.
Signal loss on MRI consistent with mitral annular calcification is identified
(arrow), with associated mitral regurgitation. This lesion is commonly
identified in elderly patients.

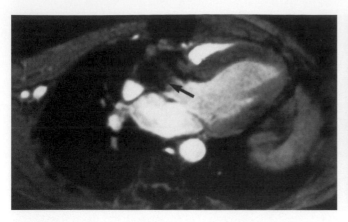
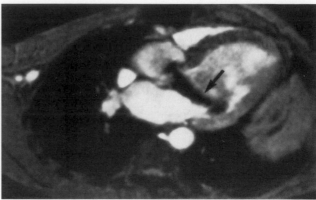

FIGURE 6-19   A 27-year-old man with combined aortic valve disease. Extensive MRI signal loss is located in the proximal ascending aorta on this systolic frame from a cine-MRI acquired in the left ventricular outflow-tract plane *(arrow, left panel).* The right-hand panel is a diastolic frame that demonstrates a large regurgitant lesion extending from the aortic valve to the posterior left ventricular free wall and impinging on the anterior mitral leaflet.

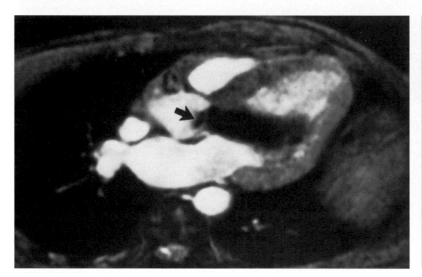
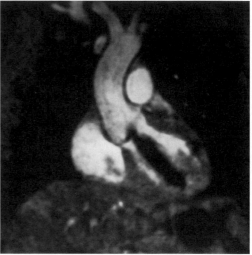

FIGURE 6-20   A 28-year-old man with severe aortic regurgitation secondary to a biscuspid aortic valve. Left ventricular outflow-tract view *(left panel)* demonstrates a large jet of aortic regurgitation that extends to the posterior wall of the left ventricle. A large proximal convergence zone *(arrow)* is identified and has been shown to correlate with severe aortic regurgitation. The coronal ascending aortic plane *(right panel)* provides an additional view of the regurgitant jet.

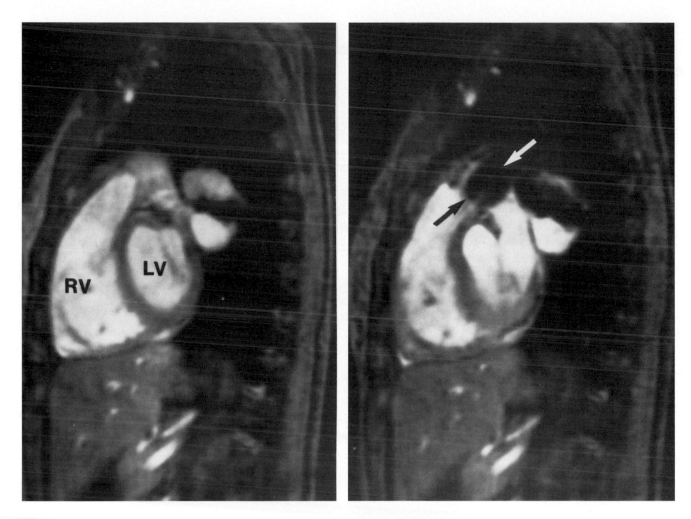

FIGURE 6-21   A 17-year-old woman with a loud systolic ejection murmur located in the second left interspace. End-diastolic *(left panel)* and systolic *(right panel)* cine-MRI frames from a right ventricular outflow-tract plane. The arrows in the systolic frame enclose MRI signal loss characteristic of valvular pulmonic stenosis. Magnetic resonance imaging can recognize valvular and subvalvular pulmonic stenosis and determine the effect of these lesions on right ventricular size and function. RV = right ventricle; LV = left ventricle.

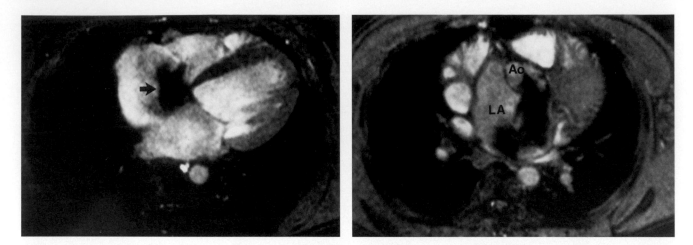

FIGURE 6-22   A 23-year-old man after pulmonary autograft repair of congenital aortic valve disease. Postoperatively, he developed signs of heart failure, and MRI demonstrates a fistula from the aorta to the left atrium. The right-hand panel demonstrates extensive MRI signal loss extending from the aorta (Ao) into the left atrium (LA). The left-hand panel demonstrates severe tricuspid regurgitation *(arrow).*

MYOCARDIAL AND PERICARDIAL DISEASE

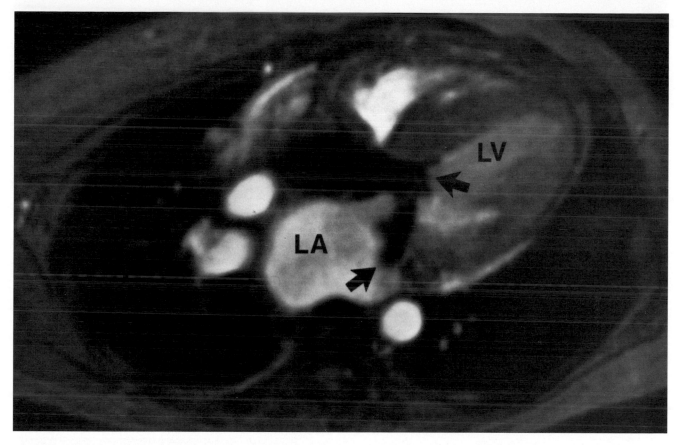

FIGURE 6-23   **A 42-year-old woman with progressive shortness of breath and paroxysmal atrial fibrillation. This left ventricular outflow-tract systolic cine-MRI frame demonstrates severe left ventricular hypertrophy with a septal predominance characteristic of hypertrophic cardiomyopathy. Extensive areas of signal loss are identified in both the left ventricular outflow tract (LVOT) and left atrium. The LVOT turbulence is caused by dynamic obstruction of the outflow tract, while the turbulence extending to the left atrium is secondary to mitral regurgitation. Left ventricular outflow tract obstruction and mitral regurgitation are frequent findings in patients with hypertrophic cardiomyopathy (*arrows*). Magnetic resonance imaging is useful in precisely identifying the location and extent of hypertrophy in atypical variants of hypertrophic cardiomyopathy. LA = left atrium; LV = left ventricle.**

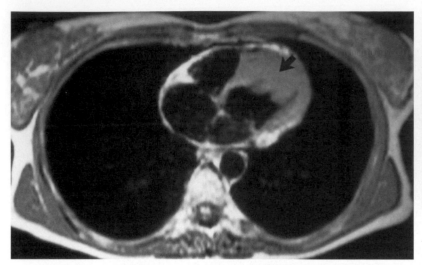
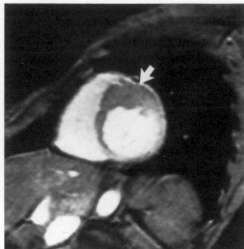

FIGURE 6-24 A 38-year-old woman with an atypical variant of hypertrophic cardiomyopathy. The axial spin-echo image *(left panel)* demonstrates extensive left ventricular hypertrophy *(black arrow)*. On the short axis gradient-echo image *(left panel),* extensive hypertrophy can be seen to be localized to the anterior left ventricular segment *(white arrow).*

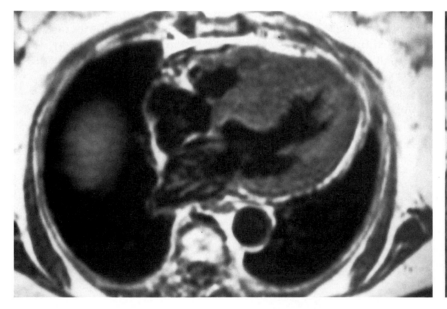
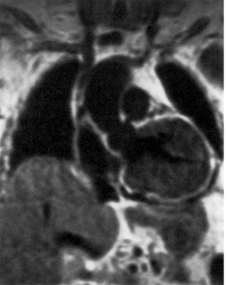

FIGURE 6-25 A 71-year-old woman with long-standing hypertension and symptoms of progressive heart failure. Severe concentric left ventricular hypertrophy and a small left ventricular cavity typically associated with diastolic dysfunction are identified on these axial and coronal spin-echo images. Cine-MRI demonstrated normal systolic function. Accurate distinction between systolic and diastolic forms of heart failure is often required to guide optimal therapy.

End-diastole   **End-systole**

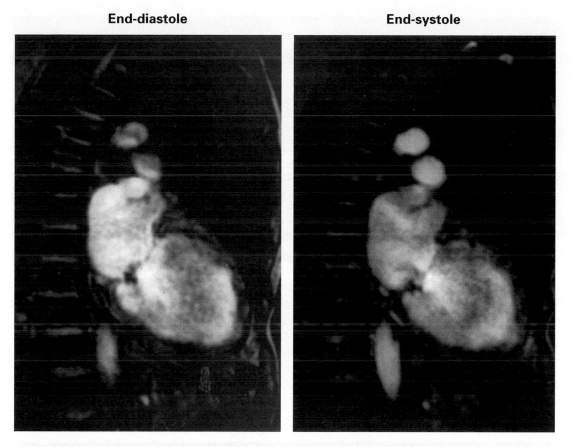

FIGURE 6-26 **A 52-year-old man with severe symptoms of heart failure.
End-diastolic and end-systolic frames from an RAO cine-MRI study show
that the left ventricle is dilated, with the very poor systolic function
characteristic of dilated cardiomyopathy. Calculated ejection fraction in
this patient was 17 percent, with an enlarged end-diastolic volume of 386 mL.**

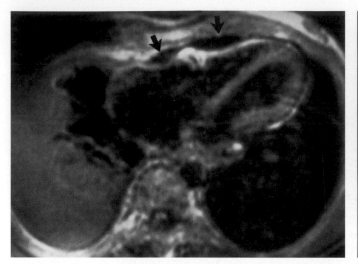

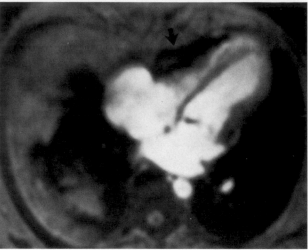

FIGURE 6-27   A 30-year-old man with progressive shortness of breath
and peripheral edema. Spin-echo *(left panel)* and gradient-echo *(right
panel)* images demonstrate classic MRI findings in constrictive pericardial
disease. There is marked thickening of the pericardium *(arrows)*. In
addition, distortion of the right ventricle, an enlarged right atrium, and
an associated pleural effusion are seen. The patient underwent successful
pericardiectomy with a return to normal functional status.

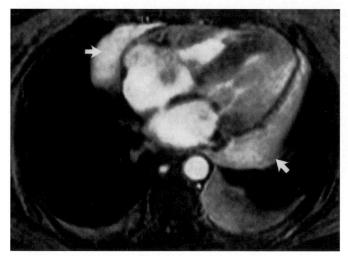

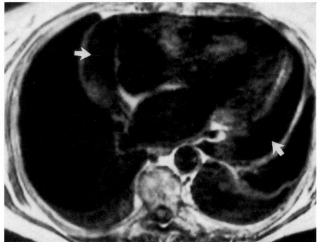

FIGURE 6-28   An 81-year-old woman with chronic renal insufficiency
and a large pericardial effusion. Gradient-echo *(left panel)* and spin-echo
(right panel) images identify freely mobile fluid around the posterolateral
right atrium and the posterior left ventricle *(arrows)*. Bilateral pleural
effusions are also identified. Transthoracic echocardiography is the
modality of choice for uncomplicated pericardial effusions. However,
MRI can provide useful information in patients with loculated effusions
and can help distinguish between pericardial and pleural effusions.

PARACARDIAC MASSES

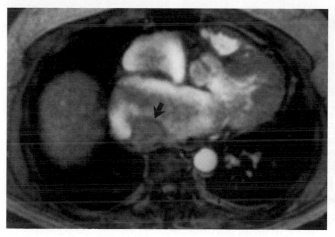
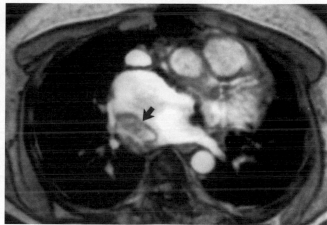

FIGURE 6-29 A 50-year-old patient several years after cardiac transplantation. Multislice axial gradient-echo images identify a left atrial mass *(arrows)* that is firmly adherent to the posterior left atrial wall. At surgery, this mass was found to be a large left atrial thrombus. Magnetic resonance imaging and transesophageal echocardiography are both useful for further investigation of mass lesions that are incompletely evaluated by transthoracic echocardiography.

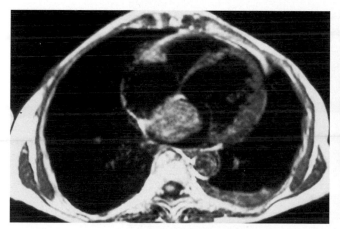
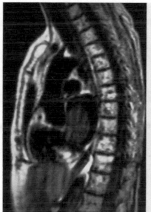
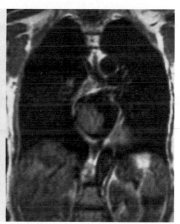

FIGURE 6-30 Left atrial myxoma. Transverse *(left panel)*, sagittal *(middle panel)*, and coronal *(right panel)* spin-echo images demonstrate a large left atrial myxoma. The three-dimensional characteristics of this intracardiac mass are well identified using MRI.

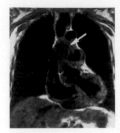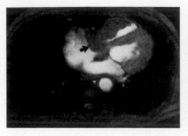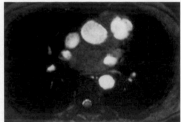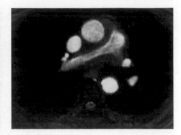

FIGURE 6-31 A 75-year-old man who presented with progessive shortness of breath. On physical examination, a low-pitched, soft diastolic rumble was audible at the lower sternal border, and chest x-ray showed a prominent mediastinum. Magnetic resonance imaging revealed an extensive mediastinal mass with encroachment into the right ventricle and functional tricuspid stenosis. The coronal spin-echo image demonstrates a homogeneous mass in the aortopulmonary window *(white arrow)*. Multislice axial gradial-echo images demonstrate encroachment of this lesion into the right atrium *(black arrow)* and encasement of the aorta and central pulmonary arteries. At surgery, this lesion was found to be an amyloidoma.

ADULT CONGENITAL HEART DISEASE

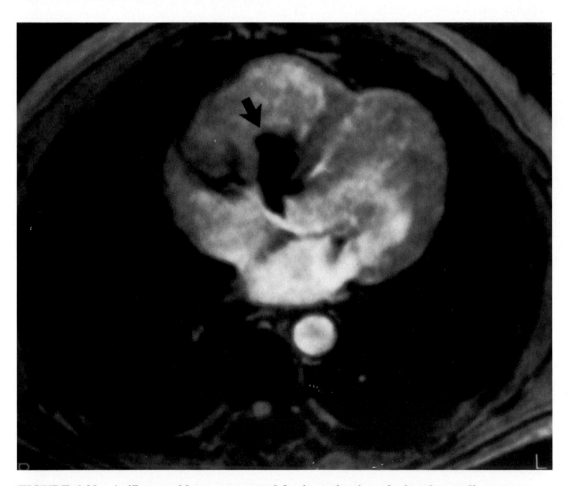

FIGURE 6-32 A 47-year-old-man presented for investigation of a harsh systolic murmur along the left sternal border. In this four-chamber gradient-echo image, the extensive black MRI signal void *(arrow)* represents shunt flow across a ventricular septal defect. The sensitivity of MRI signal to disturbed flow and the ability to obtain images from any desired tomographic plane makes MRI very useful in the identification of intracardiac shunts.

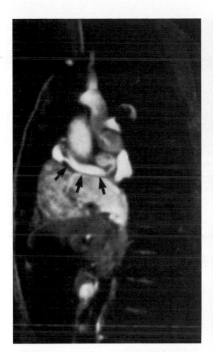 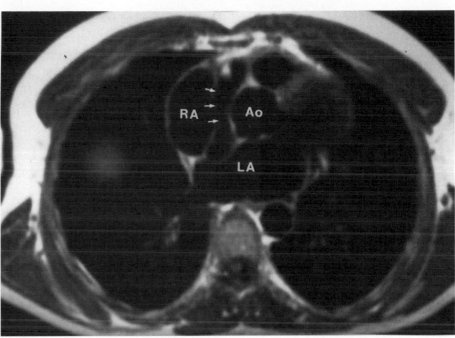

FIGURE 6-33 A 49-year-old man presented with symptoms of mild fatigue. Cardiac MRI demonstrates a coronary artery fistula. The left-hand panel is an angulated sagittal gradient-echo frame with arrows demarcating the fistula. In the axial spin-echo image *(right panel)*, the fistula can be clearly identified in its course between the aorta and the right atrium. Arrows indicate the coronary artery fistula. RA = right atrium; Ao = aorta; LA = left atrium.

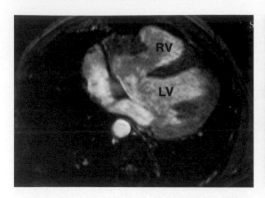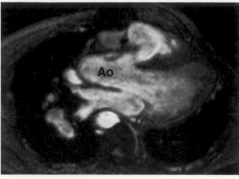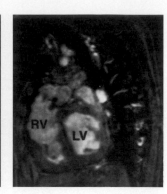

FIGURE 6-34   A 31-year-old man with tetralogy of Fallot. The left panel is an axial gradient-echo slice demonstrating a large ventricular septal defect. The middle slice is a left ventricular outflow tract view demonstrating the overriding aorta. The right panel is a right ventricular outflow-tract view demonstrating the relationship of the ventricular chambers and proximal portion of the pulmonary artery. RV = right ventricle; LV = left ventricle; AO = aorta.

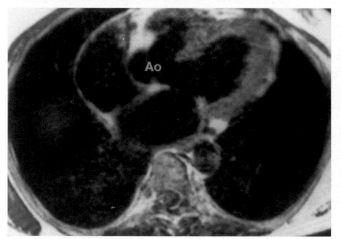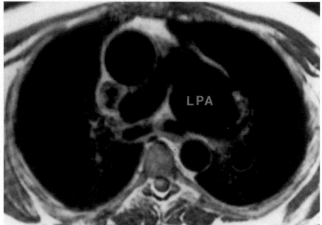

FIGURE 6-35   A 48-year-old male with aneurysmal dilatation of the central left pulmonary artery after a Blalock-Taussig shunt for tetralogy of Fallot. The axial spin-echo image on the left shows the aorta overriding the right ventricle; the right-hand panel shows dilatation of the central left pulmonary artery. Ao = aorta; LPA = left pulmonary artery.

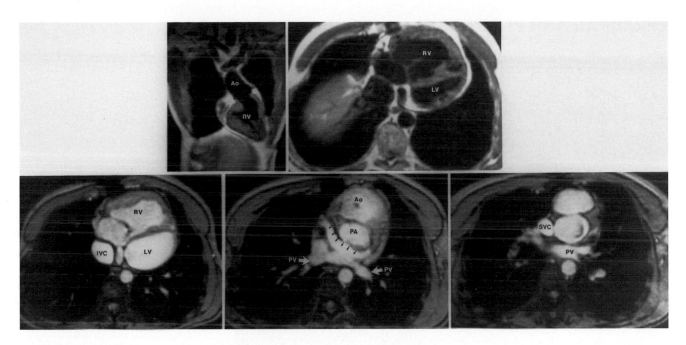

FIGURE 6-36 Surgically corrected transposition of the great arteries.
Top panels: coronal and transverse spin-echo images showing a
hypertrophied and enlarged morphologic right ventricle (RV), which gives
rise to the anteriorly located area (Ao). *Bottom panels*: tomographic slices
demonstrating ventricular morphology, relationships of the transposed
great arteries, and the course of systemic and pulmonary venous inflow in
this patient after an interatrial baffle procedure. RV = right ventricle;
LV = left ventricle; IVC = inferior vena cava; PV = pulmonary vein;
Ao = aorta; PA = pulmonary artery; SVC = superior vena cava;
small arrows = baffle.

CEREBRAL AND PERIPHERAL ANGIOGRAPHY

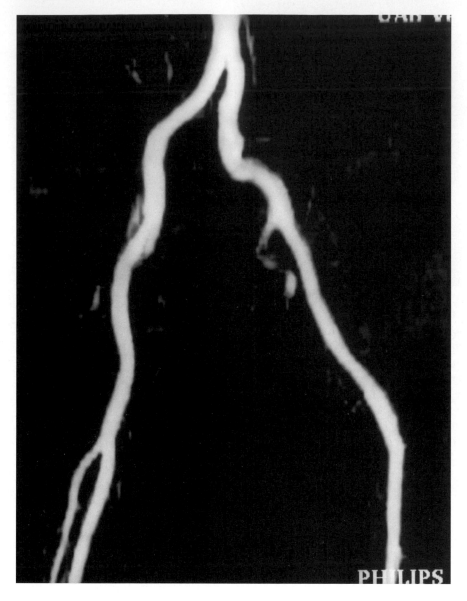

FIGURE 6-37   Normal iliofemoral MR angiogram.

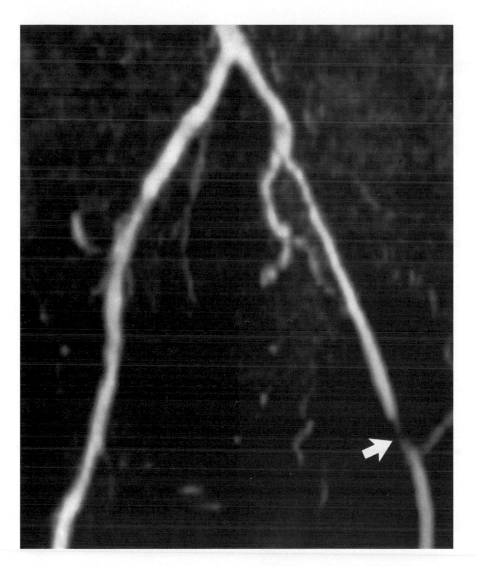

**FIGURE 6-38   A 67-year-old man with left leg claudication. An MR
angiogram of the distal abdominal aorta and iliofemoral arterial tree
demonstrates high-grade obstructive disease in the distal left system. Diffuse
nonobstructive disease is identified in the remainder of the arterial system.
Magnetic resonance angiograms have been shown to be useful in assessing
disease of both the major arterial channels as well as in identifying runoff
vessels in patients with severe lower-extremity peripheral vascular disease.**

MR Carotid Angiography

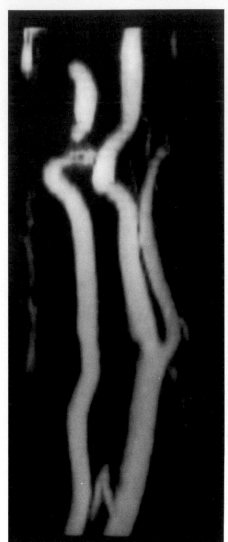 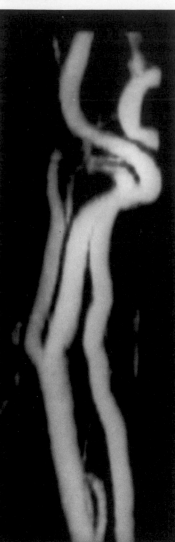

FIGURE 6-39   Normal MR angiogram of the extracranial cerebral vasculature. Excellent anatomic resolution is provided of the carotid and vertebral circulations without the need for intraarterial access or the use of contrast material.

Right   **Left**

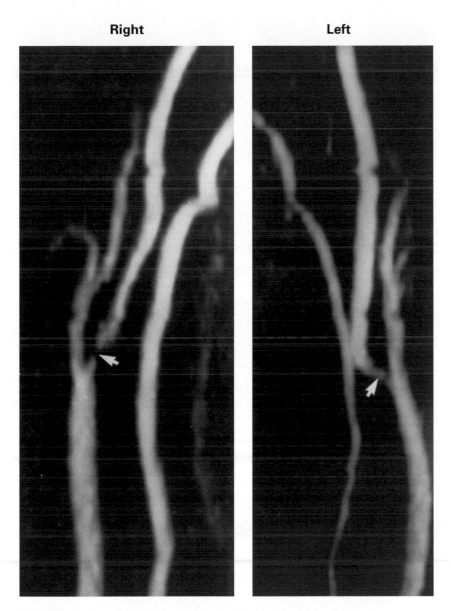

FIGURE 6-40 A 62-year-old man with bilateral carotid bruits. Magnetic resonance angiography reveals focal high-grade stenosis of the right internal carotid artery and mild disease of the left internal carotid artery. Some centers are gaining experience with surgical interventions guided by the combination of Doppler flow data and MR angiograms. The noninvasive diagnostic approach eliminates the morbidity associated with conventional four-vessel cerebral angiography.

REFERENCES

1. Blackwell GG, Pohost GM: The usefulness of cardiovascular magnetic resonance imaging. *Curr Probl Cardiol* 1994; 19:117–176.

2. Blackwell GG, Pohost GM: The evolving role of MRI in the assessment of coronary artery disease. *Am J Cardiol* 1995; 75:74D–78D.

3. Saini S, Frankel RB, Stark DD, Ferrucci JT: Magnetism: A primer and review. *AJR* 1988; 150:735–744.

4. Horowitz AL: *MRI Physics for Physicians.* New York: Springer-Verlag, 1989.

5. Mohiaddin RH, Longmore DB: Functional aspects of cardiovascular nuclear magnetic resonance imaging: Techniques and application. *Circulation* 1993; 88:264–281.

6. Pohost GM, Blackwell GG, Shellock F: Safety of patients with medical devices during application of magnetic resonance methods. *Ann NY Acad Sci* 1992; 649:302–312.

7. Blackwell GG: MRI assessment of paracardiac masses. In: Ezekowitz M (ed): *The Heart As a Source of Systemic Embolization.* New York, Marcel Dekker, 1993.

8. Owen RS, Carpenter JP, Baum RA, et al: Magnetic resonance imaging of angiographically occult runoff vessels in peripheral arterial occlusive disease. *N Engl J Med* 1992; 326:1577–1581.

9. Cranney GB, Lotan CS, Dean L, et al: Left ventricular volume measurement using cardiac axis NMR imaging—Validation by calibrated ventricular angiography. *Circulation* 1990; 82:154–163.

10. Lotan CS, Cranney GB, Bouchard A, et al: The value of cine NMR for assessing regional ventricular function. *J Am Coll Cardiol* 1989; 14:1721–1729.

11. Blackwell G, Cranney G, Pohost G, eds: *MRI: Cardiovascular System.* New York: Gower Medical Publishing, 1992.

CHAPTER 7

ELECTRON BEAM COMPUTED TOMOGRAPHY (EBCT) OF THE HEART AND BLOOD VESSELS

Bruce H. Brundage, M.D.

Song Shou Mao, M.D.

ULTRAFAST computed tomography (CT), or electron beam computed tomography (EBCT), recently the more popular designation, has been clinically available for more than 10 years, and yet the technique is not widely used. Most cardiologists have limited understanding of its diagnostic potential. The purpose of this chapter is to demonstrate the versatility of EBCT for evaluating virtually all types of cardiovascular disease. Space does not permit an encyclopedic depiction, but representative cases are presented to provide the reader with an appreciation of the diagnostic capability of this technology.

CORONARY ARTERY DISEASE

Over the past 35 years many studies have demonstrated a strong link between coronary calcium and atherosclerotic coronary artery disease. As detailed in recent reviews,[1,2] the detection and quantitation of coronary calcium by EBCT may prove to be the ideal method for screening asymptomatic people for subclinical coronary artery disease. In Fig. 7-1, dense calcification of the left coronary artery is seen. This amount of calcium is often associated with obstructive disease.

The EBCT technique can evaluate the impact of coronary artery disease on the left ventricle as well (Fig. 7-2). With the use of iodinated contrast medium, the cardiac chambers are well delineated. Images may be acquired as rapidly as every 58 ms so that cardiac wall motion can be assessed by displaying the scans in a cine loop.

The spatial resolution of EBCT is not yet sufficient to produce diagnostic coronary angiograms. However, in Fig. 7-3A and B, a left anterior descending coronary artery aneurysm is well demonstrated with currently available technology.

VALVULAR HEART DISEASE

Echocardiography and cardiac catheterization are the preferred imaging methods for evaluating valvular heart disease, but EBCT can provide useful adjunctive information in selected cases.[3] In Fig. 7-4A and B, the anatomic and hemodynamic effects of rheumatic heart disease are illustrated. Figure 7-5A and B are images of prosthetic mitral and aortic valves. Because cardiac motion is virtually eliminated with the high-speed imaging of EBCT, the streak artifacts common with conventional CT scanners are much less of a problem.

CONGENITAL HEART DISEASE

Magnetic resonance imaging (MRI) has received a great deal of attention as the ultimate tomographic method for evaluating congenital heart disease, and yet EBCT often rivals and sometimes surpasses the spatial resolution of MRI.[4] When routinely available, EBCT can be an effective method for defining the anatomy of complex congenital heart diseases (Fig. 7-6A through D). Moreover, EBCT can also determine the status of right and left ventricular function as well as detect and quantify any shunts that are present (Fig. 7-7).[5]

PERICARDIAL DISEASE

With the development of tomographic imaging techniques, the assessment of pericardial disease has been vastly improved.[6] The high spatial and temporal resolution of EBCT makes it possible to image normal pericardium (Fig. 7-8). The excellent density resolution of EBCT makes the technique ideal for detecting calcified pericardium (Fig. 7-9). With tomographic images at multiple levels, EBCT can evaluate the three-dimensional aspects of the heart and define the relationship of adjacent pathology (Fig. 7-10). Dynamic assessment of pericardial function and its impact on ventricular filling is also possible.[7]

CARDIAC TUMORS

Both primary and secondary tumors of the heart are well illustrated with contrast-enhanced EBCT. The high temporal resolution of the technique can be employed to define the dynamics of mobile tumors such as atrial myxomas (Fig. 7-11). Malignant tumors that spread to the heart are also well detected (Fig. 7-12).

AORTIC DISEASE

Conventional CT scanning has long been used to evaluate aortic aneurysms, particularly aortic dissection. Now EBCT, with its superior temporal resolution can provide exquisite detail of aortic dissection (Figs. 7-13 and 7-14); it is also effective for defining other types of thoracic aortic aneurysms.[9] Intraluminal and extraluminal thrombi are easily detected. Flow dynamics within true and false lumens can also be assessed. (See Chap. 10.)

PULMONARY ARTERY DISEASE

Pulmonary embolism is a common medical problem. Recently improvements in EBCT technology have led to preliminary studies indicating that this technique may be a powerful diagnostic tool for the diagnosis of acute pulmonary embolism.[10] The technique has been employed for some time to diagnose chronic pulmonary embolism[11] (Fig. 7-15). In addition, EBCT is useful for evaluating the effect of pulmonary hypertension on the heart (Fig. 7-16). It can, in fact, be used to image any type of lung pathology with superb resolution, as all motion artifact created by respiratory or vascular motion is eliminated (Fig. 7-17). (See Chap. 11.)

INFECTIOUS HEART DISEASE

Infective endocarditis is the most frequently encountered form of infectious heart disease in the United States. In other countries, particularly the developing ones, other forms of infectious heart disease are more common. The EBCT technique is a useful imaging modality in the evaluation of infectious heart disease. Myocardial abscess, complicating valvular endocarditis, may be detected when it is missed by other imaging techniques.[12] Unusual forms of myocardial infection may also be discovered (Figs. 7-18 and 7-19).

CONCLUSION

A diverse set of capabilities in the diagnosis and evaluation of heart disease is provided by EBCT. The examples presented here can only give the reader the "flavor" of the possibilities. Its dynamic capabilities, such as those used in the assessment of ventricular function, cannot be adequately represented in the still pictures of an atlas. Interested readers are referred to more detailed descriptions in comprehensive texts.[13–15]

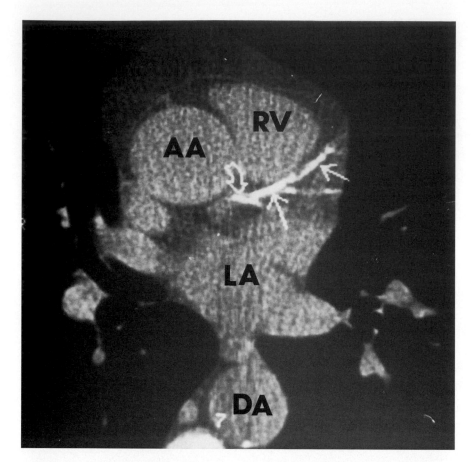

FIGURE 7-1   The entire proximal left coronary artery is calcified. The left main (*open arrow*) and left anterior descending coronary arteries (*stick arrows*) are well seen in this scan; also, the proximal circumflex and diagonal vessels are easily identified. AA = ascending aorta; DA = descending aorta; LA = left atrium; RV = right ventricular outflow tract.

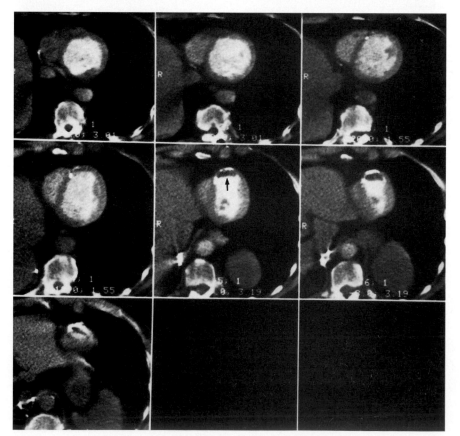

FIGURE 7-2   Seven adjacent 1-cm-thick scans of the left ventricle from midventricle to apex during contrast enhancement define an apical aneurysm with associated mural thrombus (*arrow*). Note the calcification of the aneurysm wall in scans 3 through 7.

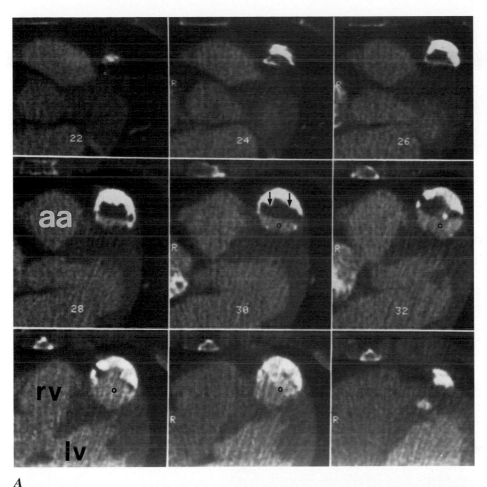

A

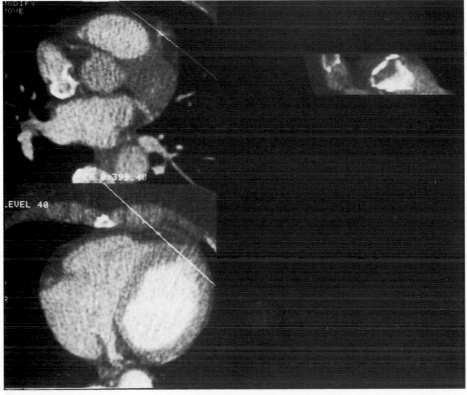

B

FIGURE 7-3   *A*. Nine adjacent 3-mm-thick contrast-enhanced scans of a calcified left anterior descending coronary artery aneurysm are shown. The anterior surface of the aneurysm is densely calcified. In the more cephalad scans (2 through 6), the anterior portion of the aneurysm is filled with thrombus (*arrows*); posteriorly, in the more caudad scans (4 through 8), the contrast-enhanced lumen is identified (°). aa = ascending aorta; lv = left ventricle; rv = right ventricle.   *B*. The 3-mm scans of the left anterior descending coronary artery aneurysm are "stacked" like coins and an off-axis plane is defined (white lines in the top and bottom scans). A longitudinal reformatting of the aneurysm is shown (right image). Again, note the calcified wall, thrombus, and contrast-enhanced lumen.

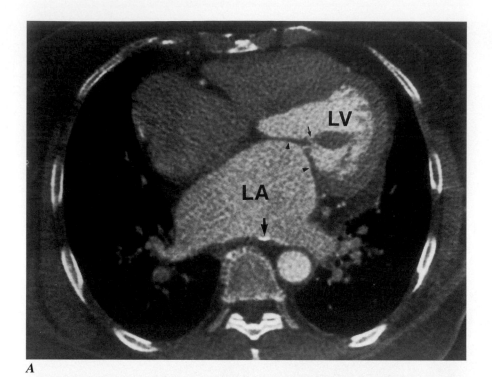

A

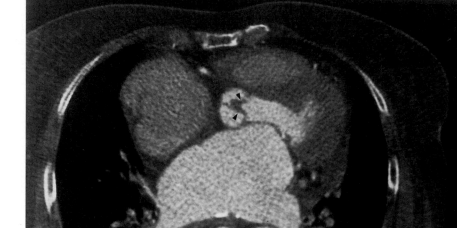

B

FIGURE 7-4 *A.* A contrast-enhanced scan at the level of the mitral valve depicts anterior and posterior valve thickening (*arrowheads*), chordal shortening (*small arrow*), and left atrial (LA) and pulmonary vein enlargement. Also note the calcification of the posterior left atrial wall (*large arrow*). LV = left ventricle. *B.* A contrast-enhanced scan of the same patient as in Fig. 7-4*A* a few cm more cephalad illustrates thickening of two aortic cusps (*arrowheads*).

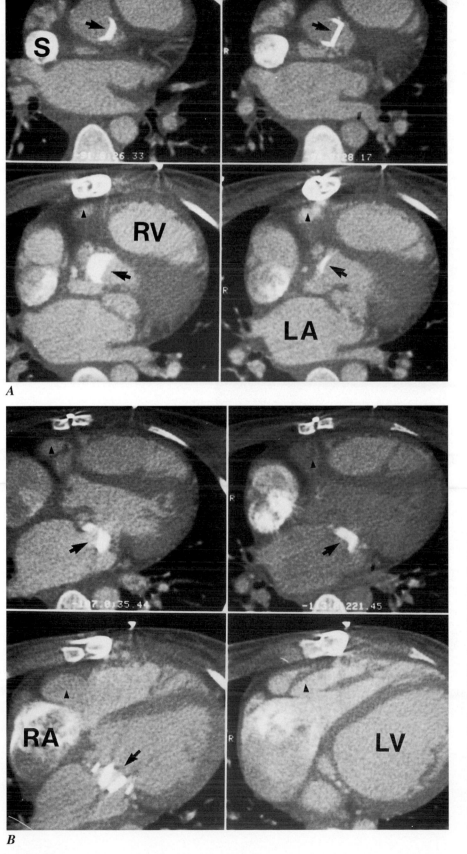

FIGURE 7-5 *A* and *B*. Selected contrast-enhanced images from the level of the right coronary artery to the mid left ventricle in a patient with St. Jude prosthetic aortic and mitral valves (*arrows*). The valves appear to be well seated and no thrombus or pannus is identified. This patient also had a right coronary artery to right ventricle fistula. The coronary artery can be tracked (*following arrowheads*) from the right sinus of Valsalva to entry into the right ventricle. LA = left atrium; LV = left ventricle; RA = right atrium; RV = right ventricle; S = superior vena cava.

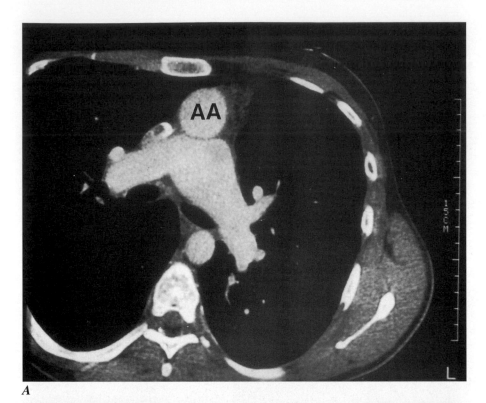

A

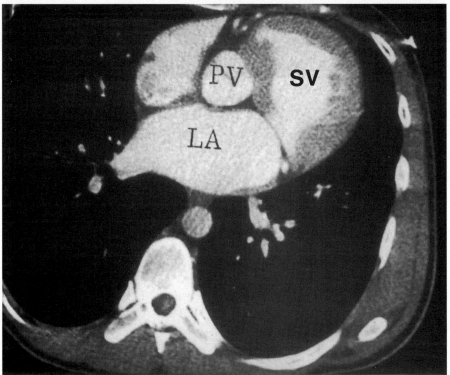

B

FIGURE 7-6   *A* through *D.*   In a patient with a complex form of corrected transposition, selected contrast-enhanced EBCT images define the salient anatomic abnormalities: the anterior position of the aorta (AA), the ventricular septal defect (*arrows*), and the superior-inferior relationship of the ventricles (scans *B* and *D*). PV = pulmonary valve; pulm vent = pulmonary ventricle; RA = right atrium; SV = systemic ventricle; LA = left atrium.

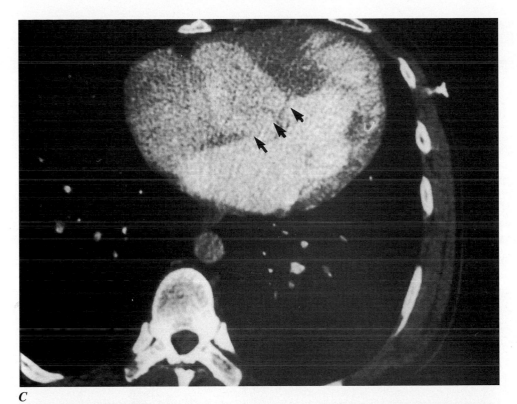

C

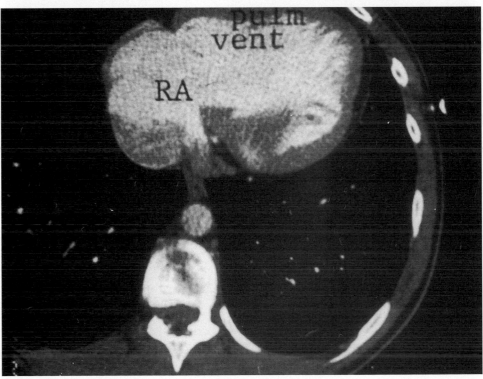

D

FIGURE 7-6 (*Continued*)

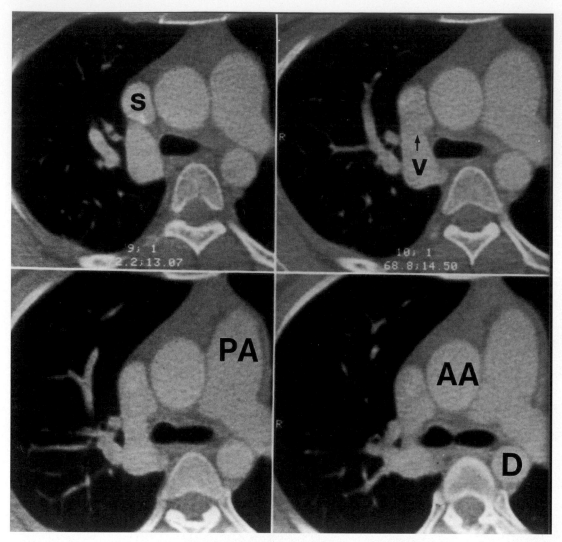

FIGURE 7-7   Four adjacent 3-mm-thick contrast-enhanced scans of the superior vena cava (s) define the presence of a sinus venosum defect (*arrow*) involving the right superior pulmonary vein (v), which drains into the superior vena cava. Note the enlarged main pulmonary artery (PA) from the left-to-right shunt. AA = ascending aorta; D = descending aorta.

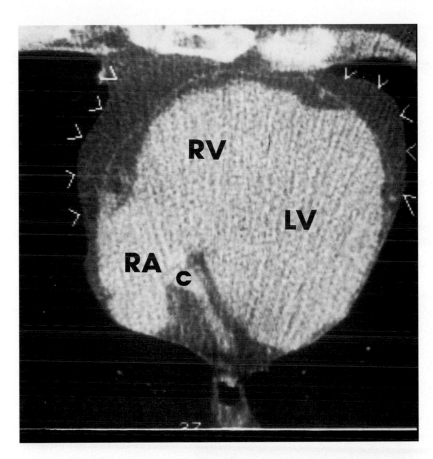

FIGURE 7-8 The fat that resides both inside and outside (*arrowheads*) the pericardium provides sufficient contrast to outline the normal pericardium, which is only 1 to 2 mm thick. Contrast enhancement with iodine agents is unnecessary. c = coronary sinus; LV = left ventricle; RA = right atrium; RV = right ventricle.

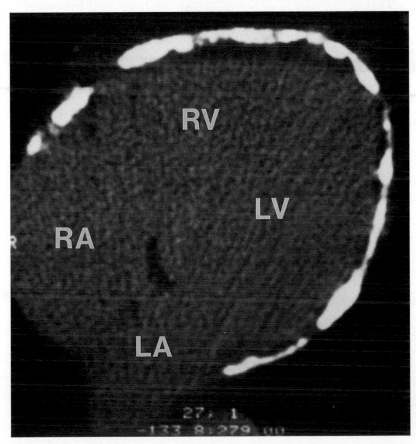

FIGURE 7-9 Densely calcified pericardium is easily identified in this scan of the mid-heart. LA = left atrium; LV = left ventricle; RA = right atrium; RV = right ventricle.

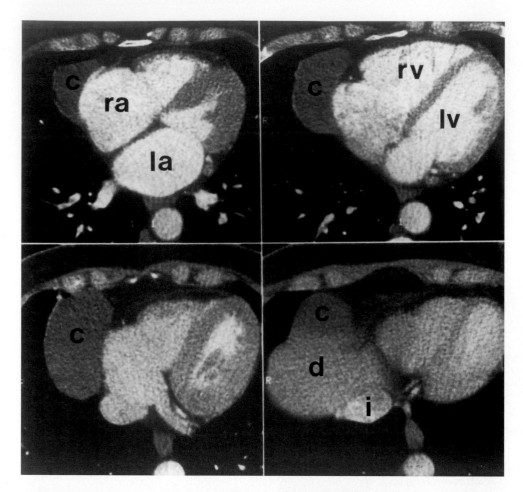

FIGURE 7-10
Four selected contrast-enhanced scans of the mid- to lower heart define the relationship of a pericardial cyst (c) to the right atrium (ra). d = diaphragm; i = inferior vena cava; la = left atrium; lv = left ventricle; rv = right ventricle.

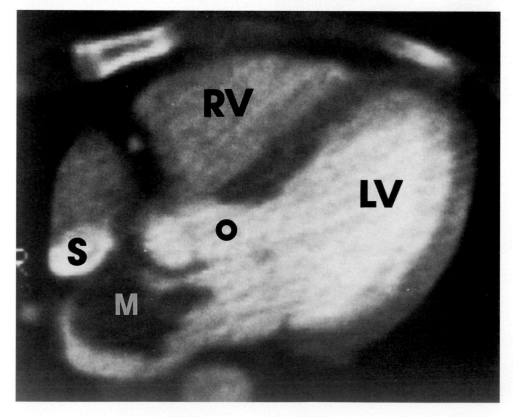

FIGURE 7-11   A single diastolic frame from a contrast-enhanced cine CT defines the left atrial septal attachment of a myxoma (M). The frond-like excrescences are characteristic of this tumor. LV = left ventricle; O = left ventricular outflow tract; RV = right ventricle; S = superior vena cava.

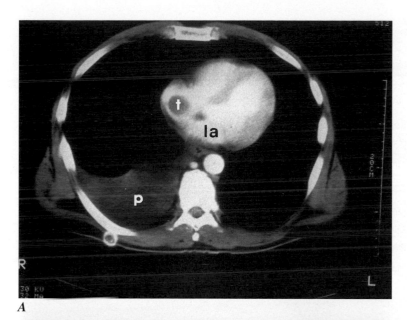

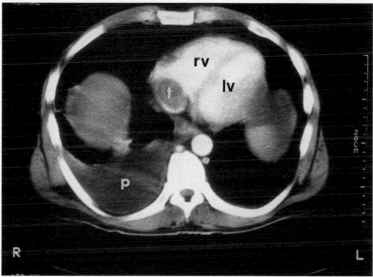

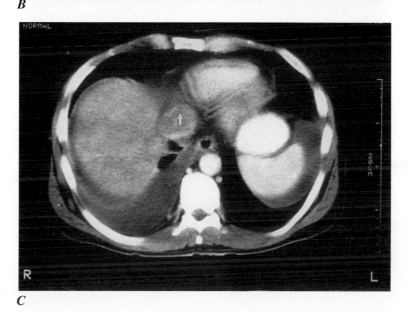

FIGURE 7-12   *A* through *C*. Selected contrast-enhanced scans demonstrated a filling defect (t) in the right atrium and inferior vena cava in a patient with a renal cell adenocarcinoma. The tumor could be tracked on more caudal scans to originate from the left kidney. la = left atrium; lv = left ventricle; p = pleural effusion; rv = right ventricle.

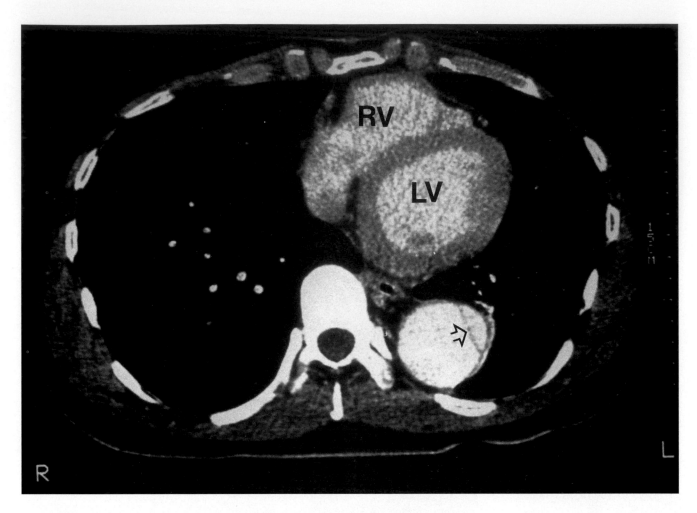

FIGURE 7-13 A typical type III aortic dissection is detected with contrast enhancement by the characteristic delineation of the intimal flap (*arrow*). LV = left ventricle; RV = right ventricle.

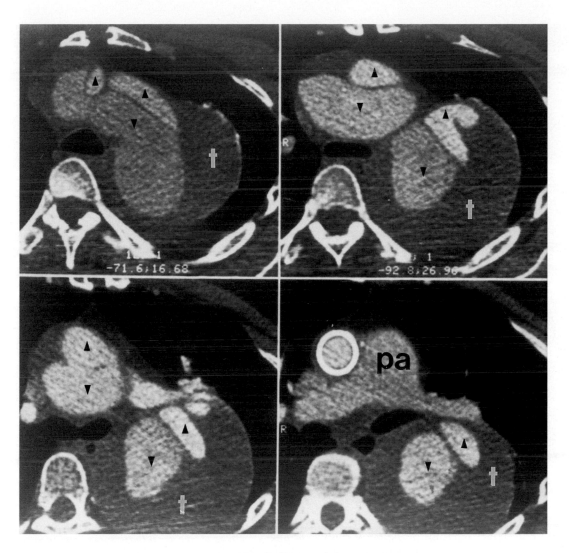

FIGURE 7-14 **Postoperative evaluation of a patient with Marfan syndrome by EBCT delineates the status of a type I dissection. Four selected contrast-enhanced scans of the ascending and descending aorta detail the anatomy of the true lumen (▲), false lumen (▼), and associated thrombus (t). The dense ring in the fourth panel is a graft conduit used to repair the ascending aorta. pa = pulmonary artery.**

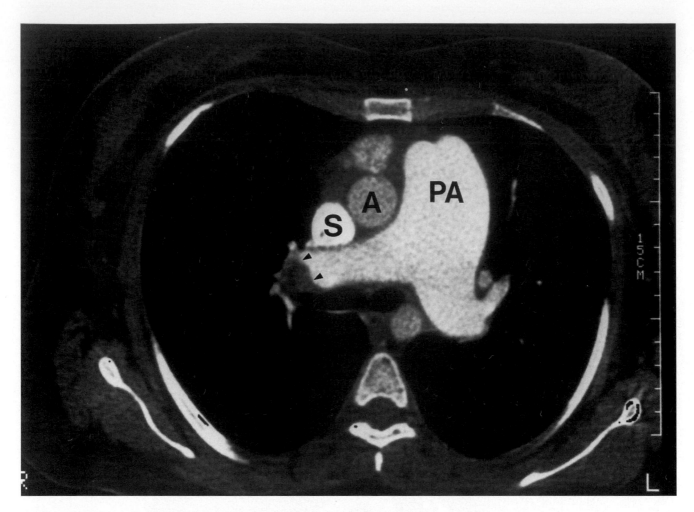

FIGURE 7-15   Contrast enhancement of the pulmonary artery (PA) defines a large chronic pulmonary embolus in the main right pulmonary artery (*arrowheads*). Note the marked enlargement of the main pulmonary artery compared to the ascending aorta (A), indicating severe pulmonary hypertension. S = superior vena cava.

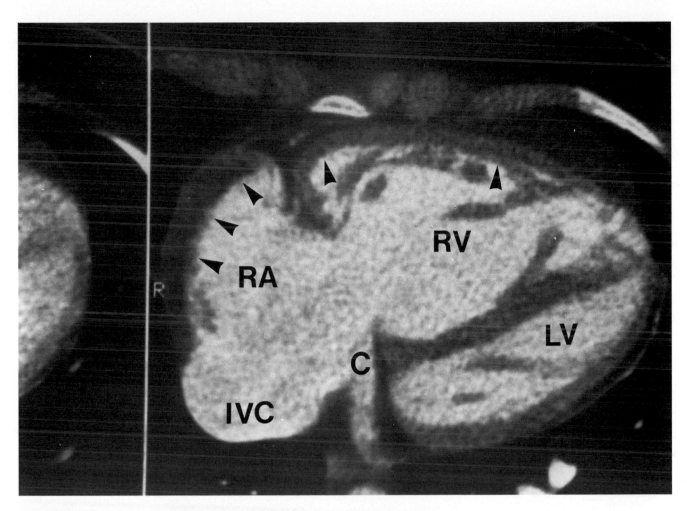

FIGURE 7-16   A contrast-enhanced scan of the mid-heart in the same patient as in Fig. 7-15 demonstrates the effects of severe pulmonary hypertension on the heart: right ventricular (RV) and atrial (RA) hypertrophy (*arrowheads*) and enlargement, leftward shift of the inter-ventricular septum, and reduced left ventricular volume (LV). C = coronary sinus ostium; IVC = inferior vena cava.

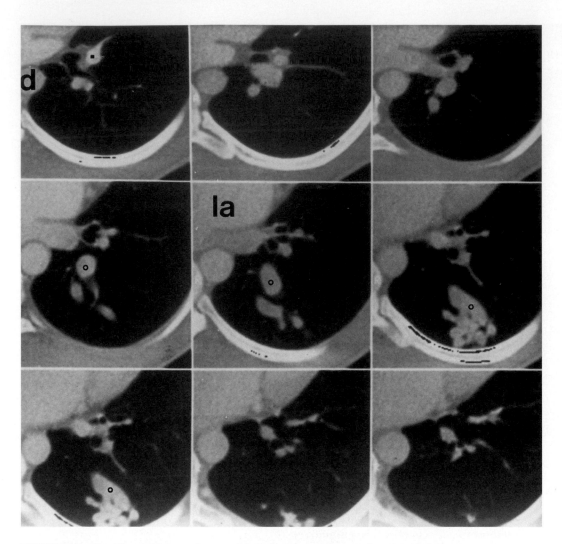

FIGURE 7-17   Nine adjacent 3-mm-thick contrast-enhanced scans of the left lung illustrate the presence of a large pulmonary arteriovenous fistula, with a large pulmonary vein (○) that drains toward the left atrium (la). ■ = pulmonary artery feeding the fistula; d = descending aorta. Other small pulmonary arteriovenous fistulas were also detected by EBCT. These were missed by conventional pulmonary angiography; the additional information guided the surgical management of this patient.

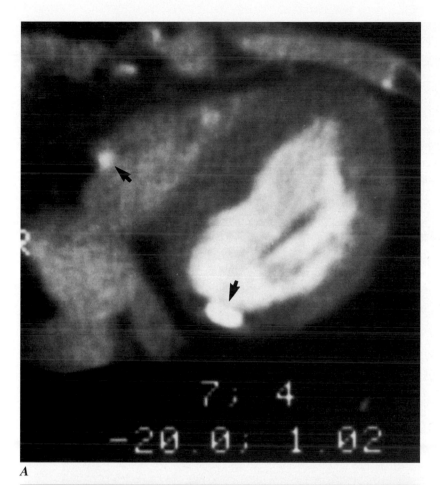

A

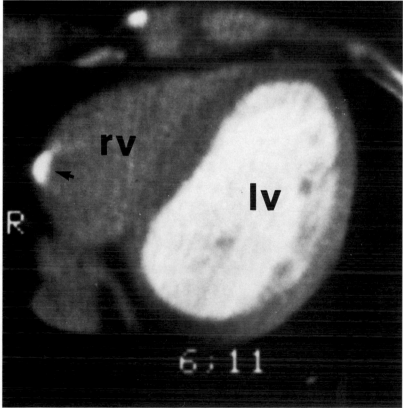

B

FIGURE 7-18 *A* and *B*. Systolic (*A*) and diastolic (*B*) images from a contrast-enhanced cine CT define intramyocardial calcifications (*arrows*) in a man with cysticercosis. The calcified cysts do not seem to impair either right ventricular (rv) or left ventricular (lv) function. The calcifications were noted during coronary angiography, but EBCT was required to define their exact location and etiology. Noncalcified intramyocardial cysts were also identified by EBCT, which was helpful in the surgical management of the man's atherosclerotic coronary artery disease.

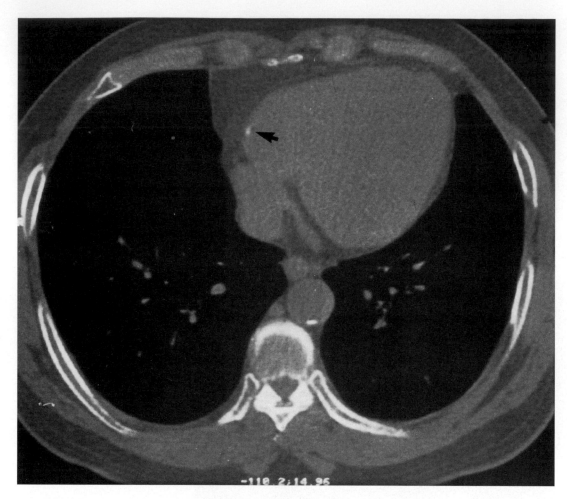

FIGURE 7-19   A nonenhanced 3-mm-thick scan of the mid-heart of the patient in Fig. 7-18 also identified the calcifications as intramyocardial (*arrow*). This simple technique could be used to screen populations at risk for infectious forms of heart disease that result in intramyocardial calcification.

REFERENCES

1. Brundage BH: Beyond perfusion. *Am J Cardiol* 1995; 75:69D–73D.

2. Brundage BH: The calcium story. *Am J Cardiol* 1995; in press.

3. Roig E, Chomka EV, Brundage BH: Evaluation of valvular heart disease by ultrafast computed tomography. In: Brundage BH (ed): *Comparative Cardiac Imaging—Function, Flow, Anatomy, Quantification.* Rockville, MD, Aspen Publishers, 1990:339–346.

4. Eldredge WJ: Comprehensive evaluation of congenital heart disease using ultrafast computed tomography. In: Marcus M, Schelbert H, Skorton D, Wolf G (eds): *Cardiac Imaging.* Philadelphia, Saunders, 1991:714–731.

5. Garrett JS, Jaschke W, Aherne T et al: Quantitation of intracardiac shunts by cine-CT. *J Comput Assist Tomogr* 1988; 12:82–85.

6. Oren RM, Grover-McKay M, Stanford W, et al: Accurate preoperative diagnosis of pericardial constriction using cine computed tomography. *J Am Coll Cardiol* 1993; 22:832–838.

7. Rumberger JA, Weiss RM, Feiring AJ, et al: Patterns of regional diastolic function in the normal human left ventricle: An ultrafast computed tomographic study. *J Am Coll Cardiol* 1989; 14:119–126.

8. Bertsch MJ, Chomka EV, Brundage BH: Imaging of cardiac tumors. In: BH Brundage (ed): *Comparative Cardiac Imagining—Function, Flow, Anatomy, Quantitation.* Rockville, MD, Aspen Publishers, 1990:505–514.

9. Thompson BH, Stanford W: Utility of ultrafast computed tomography in the detection of thoracic aortic aneurysms and dissections. *Semin Ultrasound CT MR* 1993; 14:117–128.

10. Tergin CL, Maus TP, Sheedy PF, et al: Pulmonary embolism: Diagnosis with electron beam CT. *Radiology* 1993; 188:839–845.

11. Rich S, Levitsky S, Brundage BH: Pulmonary hypertension from chronic pulmonary thromboembolism. *Ann Intern Med* 1988; 108:425–434.

12. Bleiweis MS, Milliken JC, Baumgartner FJ, et al: Application of ultrafast CT for diagnosis of perivalvular abscess: Surgical implications. *Chest* 1994; 106:629–632.

13. Brundage BH (ed): *Comparative Cardiac Imagining—Function, Flow, Anatomy, Quantitation.* Rockville, MD, Aspen Publishers, 1990.

14. Marcus M, Schelbert H, Skorton D, Wolf G (eds): *Cardiac Imaging.* Philadelphia, Saunders, 1991.

15. Stanford W, Rumberger J (eds): *Ultrafast Computed Tomography in Cardiac Imaging: Principles and Practice.* Mount Kisco, NY, Futura, 1992.

CHAPTER 8

CARDIAC POSITRON EMISSION TOMOGRAPHY IMAGING

Roxana Campisi, M.D.

Susanne Weismüller, M.D.

Heinrich R. Schelbert, M.D., Ph.D.

POSITRON emission tomography (PET) offers several advantages over conventional single photon emission computed tomography (SPECT). Foremost among these are (1) high spatial, temporal, and contrast resolution; (2) quantitative imaging capability as a result of correction for measured photon attenuation (which also eliminates or minimizes image artifacts) and, further, the relatively homogeneous spatial resolution; and (3) availability of a wide range of tracers of, for example, blood flow or substrate metabolism. Further, the combination of the quantitative imaging capability and high temporal spatial resolution of PET permits the measurement of regional tracer activity concentrations and their time-dependent changes. Thus, the principles of tracer kinetics, as widely employed throughout the biological sciences, can be applied in the noninvasive measurement of, for example, regional rates of myocardial blood flow and substrate metabolism.[1,2]

Clinically, PET has proved useful for detecting coronary artery disease, defining its extent and severity, and identifying myocardial viability. This chapter focuses on these clinical aspects of PET. It begins with a brief description of positron-emitting tracers used for cardiac imaging and their distribution in the left ventricular myocardium as it corresponds to the anatomy of the human heart. Following this, patterns of blood flow and metabolism in normal and diseased hearts are depicted, as are examples of coronary artery disease and myocardial viability. Finally, a series of case studies in patients with coronary artery disease is presented, showing how PET findings can influence the diagnostic and clinical decision-making process.

Detection of Coronary Artery Disease

Typically, each patient undergoes rest and stress myocardial blood-flow studies. Myocardial blood flow can be evaluated qualitatively with ^{82}Rb, ^{15}O water, and, as shown in this atlas, with ^{13}N ammonia. After the patient has rested and a myocardial blood-flow study has been acquired, he or she is given a stress test. This can be performed with bicycle or treadmill exercise. Most laboratories, however, employ pharmacologic stress testing with intravenous dipyridamole, intravenous adenosine, or, as proposed more recently, intravenous dobutamine.[3,4]

Assessment of Myocardial Viability

The evaluation of regional myocardial blood flow by using ^{13}N ammonia, ^{82}Rb, or ^{15}O water, and of metabolism, by assessing exogenous glucose utilization with ^{18}F deoxyglucose (FDG), serves as a highly accurate means for identifying "viable myocardium." Further, this approach affords the precise separation of viable from nonviable myocardium.

Viable myocardium is defined as myocardium with a potentially reversible impairment of contractile function. Such impairment may result from acute myocardial ischemia, "hibernation," myocardial stunning, or "repetitive stunning." It must be distinguished from an impairment or loss of contractile function that is irreversible and that, in most instances, results from myocardial necrosis and scar tissue formation. This latter state is defined as *nonviable myocardium.*

Positron emission tomography reveals three distinct patterns of myocardial blood flow and metabolism in regionally dysfunctional myocardium. Both blood flow and metabolism may be normal (pattern A) or blood flow may be decreased while FDG uptake is normal or increased (pattern B, defined by its operational term as *mismatch.*) These two patterns identify myocardium as viable. In contrast, concordant reductions in blood flow and FDG uptake (pattern C, defined as *match*) are consistent with nonviable myocardium.[5–8]

ACKNOWLEDGMENTS

The authors wish to thank Diane Martin and Melissa Sheldon for preparing the tables and figures and Eileen Rosenfeld for her skillful secretarial assistance. Dr. Roxana Campisi and Dr. Susanne Weismüller equally contributed in preparing this chapter.

ANATOMY OF THE HEART AND PET VIEWS

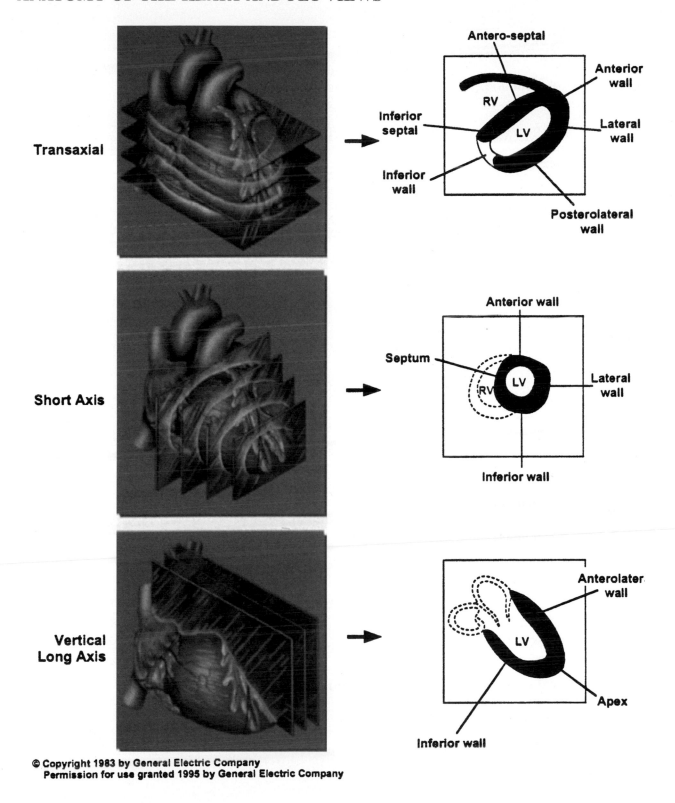

FIGURE 8-*A* Schematic illustrations of the orientation of the myocardial images of the left ventricular myocardium by PET.

RADIOPHARMACEUTICALS

TABLE 8-A

Positron-Emitting Tracers

Radionuclides	Production	Half-Life, min	Radio-pharmaceuticals	Cardiac Function
^{13}N	Cyclotron	9.96	NH_3	Blood flow
			Amino acids	Metabolism of amino acids
^{15}O	Cyclotron	2.07	H_2O	Blood flow
			CO_2	Blood flow
			CO	Blood volume
^{11}C	Cyclotron	20.4	Acetate	Oxidative metabolism
				Blood flow
			Palmitate	Fatty acid metabolism
			Glucose	Glucose metabolism
			Amino acids	Protein synthesis
			Hydroxyephedrine	Norepinephrine distribution
^{18}F	Cyclotron	109.7	Deoxyglucose	Glucose metabolism
^{82}Rb	Generator	1.26	RbCl	Blood flow
^{68}Ga	Generator	68	Microspheres	Blood flow

STRESS TESTING

TABLE 8-B

Stress Tests Used in Positron Emission Tomography

Pharmacologic stress tests	Exercise stress test	Others
Dipyridamole Adenosine Dobutamine	Supine bicycle exercise	Cold pressor test
Diagnosis and prognosis of coronary artery disease		Evaluation of coronary vasomotion

Transaxial

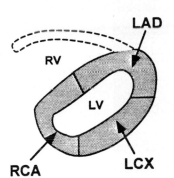

Short Axis

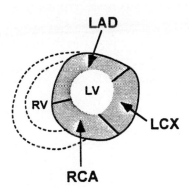

Long Axis

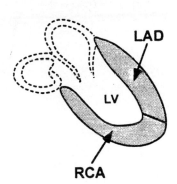

FIGURE 8-B   Estimated "normal" distribution of perfusion areas supplied by the three major epicardial arteries: left anterior descending (LAD), left circumflex artery (LCX), and right coronary artery (RCA).

TRACER DISTRIBUTION IN A NORMAL PET SCAN

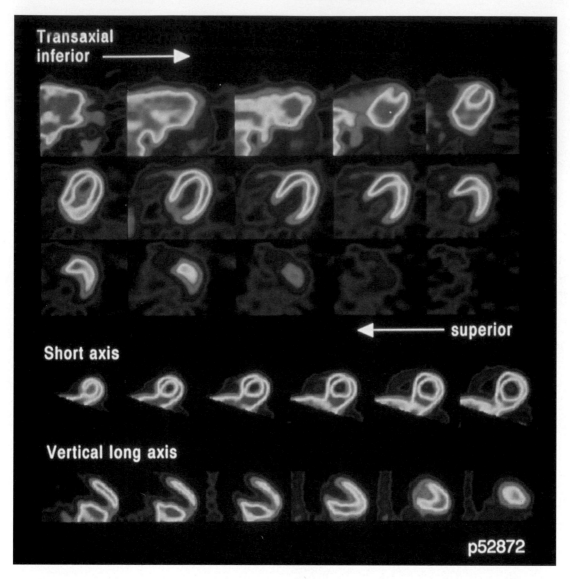

FIGURE 8-1   NORMAL VOLUNTEER. Set of 15 contiguous transaxial planes acquired after intravenous injection of ^{13}N ammonia. These images display the anterobasal, midventricular, and inferior diaphragmatic planes of the left ventricle and are viewed from the volunteer's feet. The right ventricular wall and papillary muscles are visualized. The tracer ^{13}N ammonia also accumulates in the liver, which is seen on the more inferior images. In normal volunteers, the tracer uptake of the left ventricular myocardium is homogeneous even though the postero-lateral and inferior walls sometimes show a slightly diminished uptake. The reason for this regional reduction has not been clarified but may be related to a regional alteration in amino acid or, more generally, substrate metabolism. After computer-processed reorientation, vertical long-axis and short-axis views are obtained. (*See color Plate 27.*)

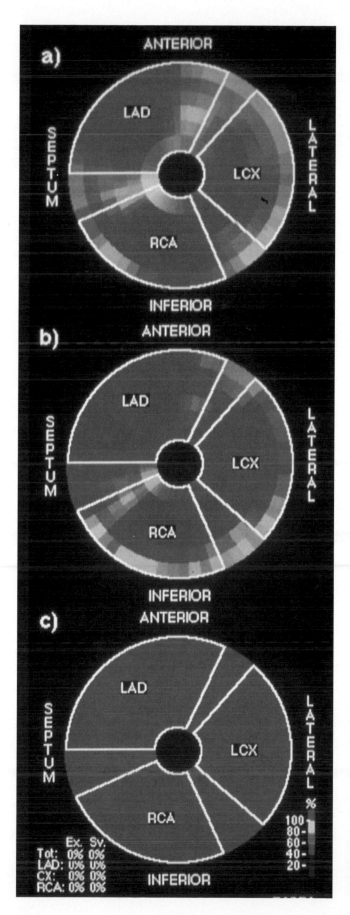

FIGURE 8-2   The three-dimensional distribution of tracer activity in the left ventricular myocardium can be displayed in the form of two-dimensional polar maps. These maps are generated from circumferential activity profiles of the six short-axis images (processing from the apex to the base of the left ventricle), shown in panel *a*. As depicted in panel *b*, regional tracer concentration is normalized to the top 5 percent of activity within the whole polar map. *Normal* is defined as a *pixel value within minus two standard deviations of the normal mean value* and is displayed in red. To identify abnormal myocardium in patients, polar maps are compared to a normal control group ("normal" database) using a color scale *c*. Normal myocardium is outlined in red, while a change in color to yellow, green, light blue, dark blue, and violet characterizes, stepwise, 20 percent reductions in tracer activity. To assess regional rather than global myocardial abnormalities, vascular territories can be defined on the polar maps, allowing estimation of the severity and the extent of a reduction in tracer uptake per vascular territory. The grade of severity describes the average reduction of activity relative to the normal myocardium, while the extent defines the fraction of abnormal myocardium in relation to the entire myocardium or to a myocardial territory related to a coronary artery. (*See color Plate 28.*)

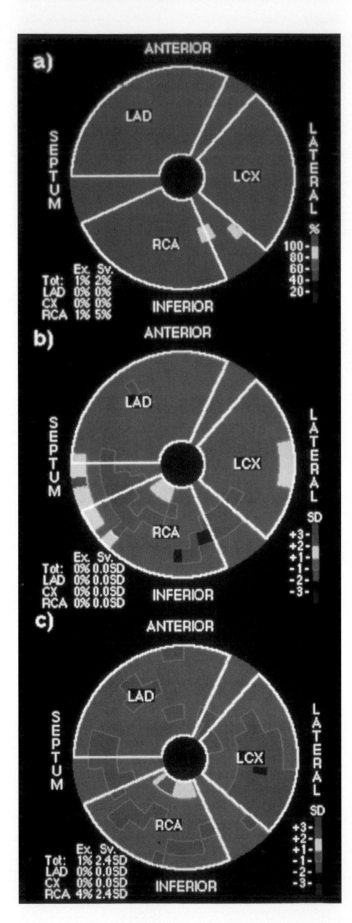

FIGURE 8-3   The normalized polar map (*a*), matched to a database of 11 healthy volunteers, presents a normal ¹³N ammonia blood pool study (as described in Fig. 8-4). The normalized polar map of glucose metabolism (*b*) displays normal ¹⁸F deoxyglucose (FDG) uptake in green, while yellow (uptake > 1 SD) and red (uptake > 2 SD) represent hypermetabolism and blue (uptake < 1 SD) and violet (uptake < 2 SD) hypometabolism. The difference polar map (*c*) compares the relative normalized ¹³N ammonia uptake (*a*) with the relative normalized FDG uptake (*b*) and displays the difference between glucose utilization and blood flow. Differences in regional tracer uptake within two standard deviations of the normal mean value are considered normal and are shown in red. Differences greater than two standard deviations of normal are considered abnormal and are depicted in green (2 to 3 SDs) and blue (more than three SDs). (*See color Plate 29.*)

PERFUSION ABNORMALITIES CORRESPONDING TO CORONARY ARTERY TERRITORIES

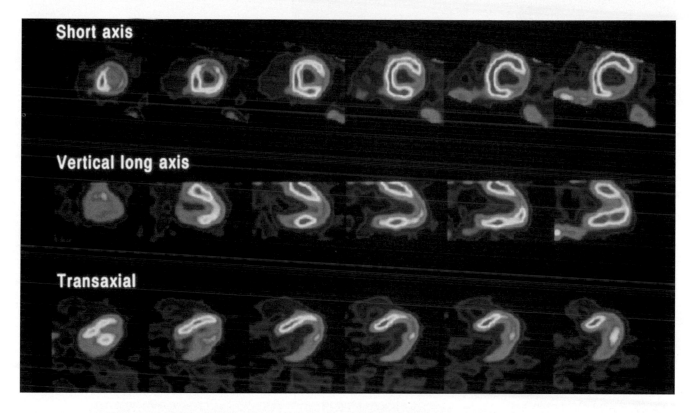

FIGURE 8-4   DISEASE OF THE LEFT ANTERIOR DESCENDING ARTERY. Short-axis, vertical long-axis, and transaxial views in a 61-year-old patient with coronary artery disease after intravenous injection of ^{13}N ammonia. Note the reduction in tracer uptake in the anterior wall, apex, and distal inferior wall, consistent with reduced myocardial blood flow in the LAD territory.

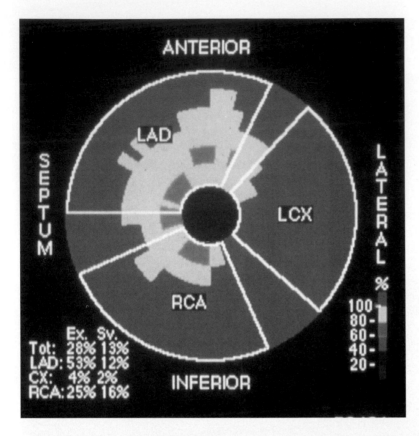

FIGURE 8-5 Comparison of the study shown in Fig. 8-4 to a database of normal demonstrates, on the polar map, a reduction in myocardial blood flow in the LAD territory, increasing in severity from base to apex. Additionally, the RCA territory shows a mild blood flow abnormality consistent with a flow defect in the distal inferior wall, which still might result from disease of the LAD. (*See color Plate 30.*)

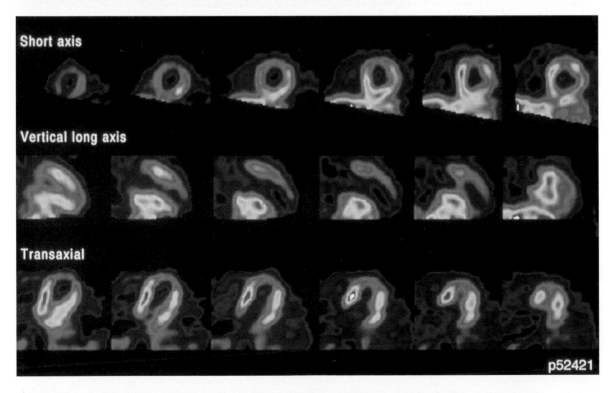

FIGURE 8-6 DISEASE OF THE LEFT CIRCUMFLEX ARTERY. Images acquired after intravenous administration of ^{13}N ammonia at rest. Note the reduced tracer uptake in the lateral and posterolateral walls, as seen best in the short-axis cuts. These findings are consistent with angiographically documented disease of the LCX.

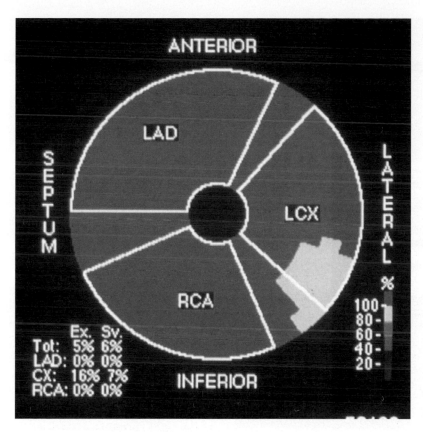

FIGURE 8-7   The semiquantitative polar map shows a moderate reduction in ^{13}N ammonia uptake in the lateral wall. The LAD and RCA territories are free of detectable abnormalities. This patient had angiographically documented disease of the LCX. (*See color Plate 31.*)

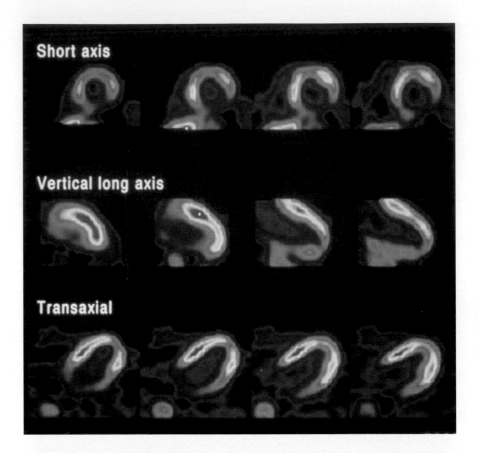

FIGURE 8-8 DISEASE OF THE RIGHT CORONARY ARTERY. Short-axis, vertical long-axis, and transaxial images of myocardial blood flow in a patient with coronary artery disease. Note the extensive flow defect in the inferior and inferolateral walls of the left ventricle, consistent with disease of the right coronary artery.

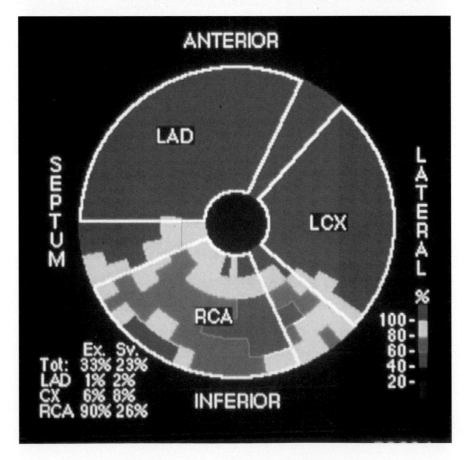

FIGURE 8-9 Polar map analysis confirms the severe reduction of tracer uptake in the inferior wall, whereas the LCX territory shows only a small abnormality. (*See color Plate 32.*)

MYOCARDIAL VIABILITY

Positron emission tomography is a diagnostic tool to assess myocardial viability by evaluating myocardial blood flow and metabolic activity. This is clinically important for deciding on the most appropriate treatment—as, for example, interventional revascularization, medical treatment, or cardiac transplantation.

Mismatch

Definition: Discordant uptake of the metabolic and blood-flow tracer in a myocardial region with impaired wall motion is defined as *blood-flow–metabolism mismatch* and indicates the presence of a reversible impairment of contractile function.

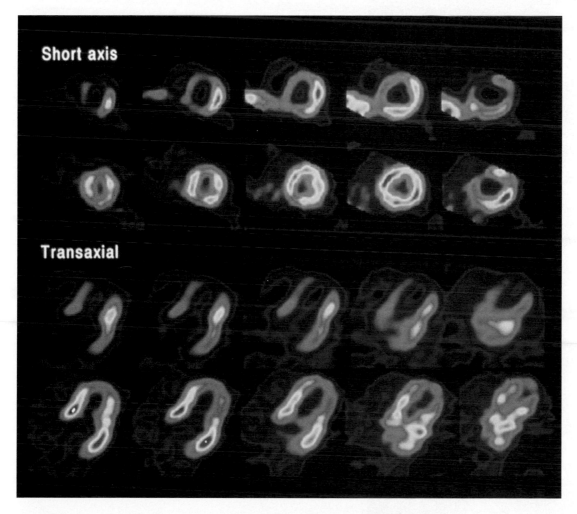

FIGURE 8-10   Short-axis and transaxial images of myocardial blood flow at rest (*upper row*) depict a reduction in tracer uptake in septum and anterior and inferior walls best seen in the short-axis views; yet exogenous glucose utilization (*lower row*) is maintained in these territories. This pattern represents a blood-flow–metabolism mismatch and indicates the presence of viable myocardium in the anterior wall and the interventricular septum.

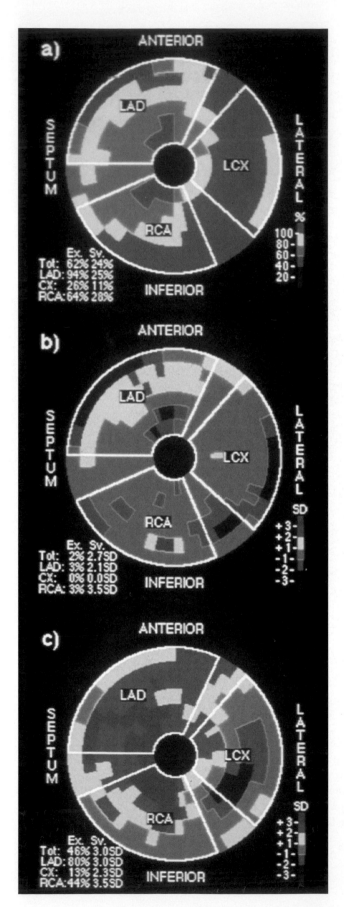

FIGURE 8-11   The normalized polar map of the myocardial blood flow (*a*) shows defects in the LAD and RCA territories, with increasing severity from the midventricular region to the apex; furthermore there is a mild defect in the LCX territory. The normalized FDG polar map (*b*) reveals an area of hypermetabolism in the LAD and RCA territories. The difference polar map (*c*) displays a mismatch pattern, confirming the presence of viable myocardium in this region. (*See color Plate 33.*)

Match

Definition: The operational term *blood-flow–metabolism match* describes a concordant decrease in myocardial blood flow and glucose utilization in regionally dysfunctional myocardium. It indicates the presence of a nonreversible impairment of contractile function resulting from scar tissue formation.

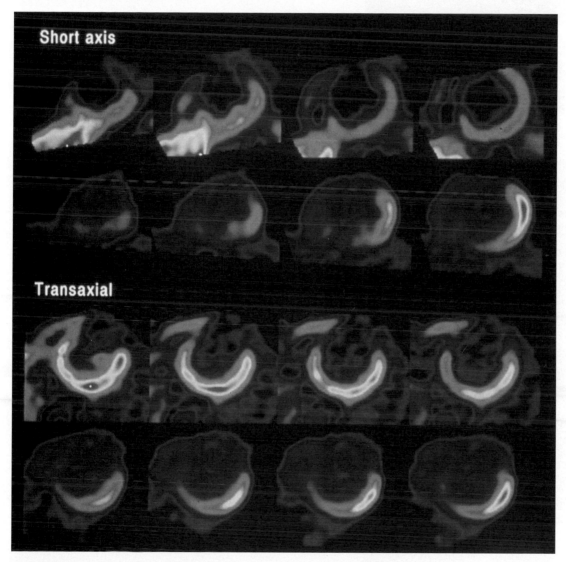

FIGURE 8-12   Short-axis and transaxial blood-flow images at rest (*upper row*) show a reduction in tracer uptake in the anterior and inferoseptal wall. The FDG images (*lower row*) demonstrate reduced glucose metabolism in the hypoperfused myocardium. The hypometabolism together with the reduced blood flow is consistent with a blood-flow–metabolism match.

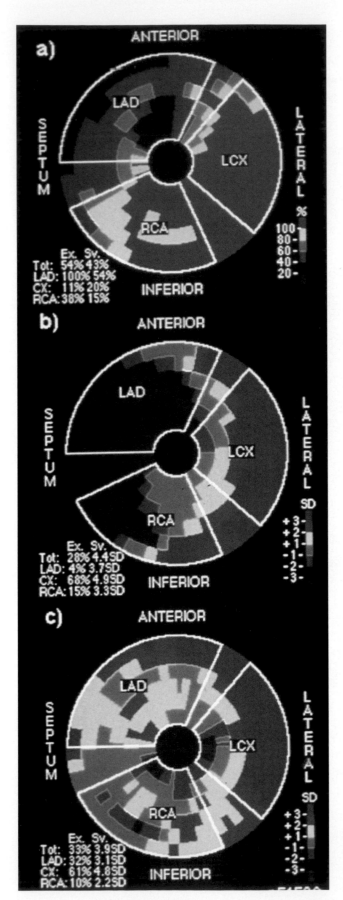

FIGURE 8-13 The polar map of myocardial blood flow (*a*) displays severe defect in the LAD territory, a moderate defect in the RCA territory, and a mild defect in LCX territory. The match pattern in the FDG polar map (*b*) supports the finding of nonviable myocardium in the LAD and RCA territories and is confirmed by the difference polar map (*c*). (*See color Plate 34.*)

CLINICAL CASE DEMONSTRATION

Ischemia and Infarction

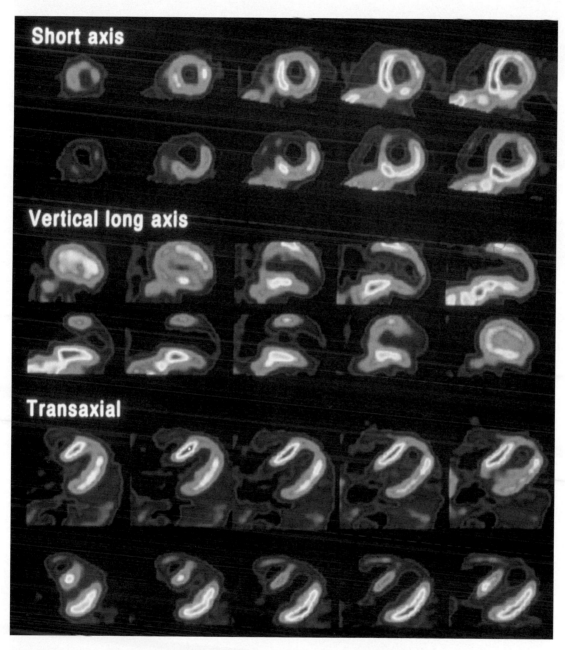

FIGURE 8-14 STRESS-INDUCED DEFECTS OF MYOCARDIAL BLOOD FLOW DUE
TO LAD DISEASE. **Short-axis, long-vertical-axis, and transaxial images at
rest (*upper row*) and after administration of 0.56 mg/kg dipyridamole
(*lower row*) in a patient with angiographically documented coronary artery
disease. At rest, small defects are seen in the distal anterior and inferior
walls and in the apex. Note the extensive flow defect in these territories
during stress.**

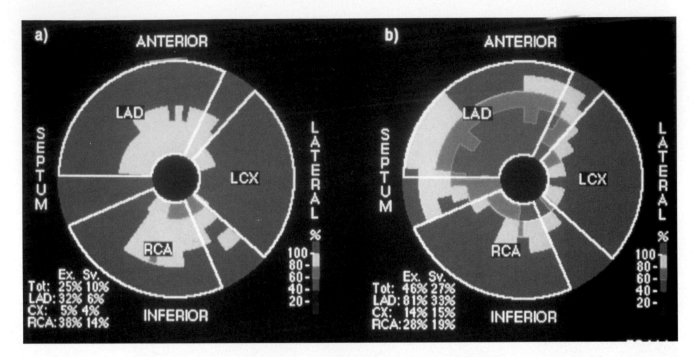

FIGURE 8-15   At rest (*a*) the semiquantitative analysis of the distribution of ^{13}N ammonia shows a mild defect in the anterior and distal inferior walls. During dipyridamole-induced hyperemia (*b*) the LAD territory demonstrates a severe perfusion defect consistent with disease of LAD, whereas the other vascular territories show only minor abnormalities. (*See color Plate 35.*)

Conclusion: Figure 8-15 represents a partially reversible stress-induced flow defect in the anterior wall, apex, and distal inferior wall. Because the defect involves the anterior septum, the hyperemic flow studies are consistent with a proximal LAD stenosis (proximal to the first septal perforator).

Note: Each plate is followed by a double-numbered figure in parentheses. The first digit refers to the chapter in which it is cited; the second digit indicates the figure within that chapter.

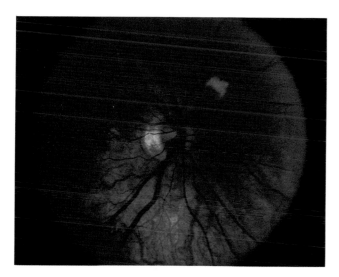

PLATE 1 (Fig. 2-1) Retinal cotton-wool spot. Cotton-wool spots are most frequently found close to the optic disk. Although they occur in acute uncontrolled systemic hypertension, the more common cause now, in younger patients, is infection with the human immunodeficiency virus. This normotensive 37-year-old man had no visual symptoms and no other retinopathy. There is a myopic crescent at the temporal disk edge, which is not abnormal. He died of complications related to the acquired immunodeficiency syndrome (AIDS) two years later.

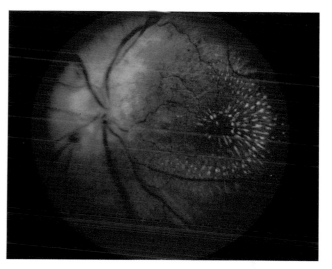

PLATE 2 (Fig. 2-2) Disk swelling and hard exudate in a macular "star" pattern. In this hypertensive patient with periarteritis nodosa, vascular leakage has led to the deposit of hard exudates around the fovea. Radial perifoveal connective tissue results in the star pattern of the exudate. Note also that the optic disk is edematous, with blurred margins, secondary to hypertension.

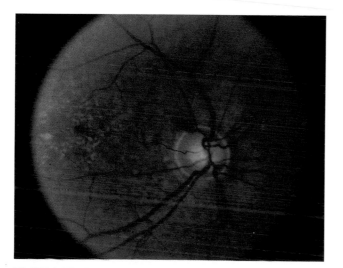

PLATE 3 (Fig. 2-3) Splinter or flame hemorrhage at the optic disk. Superficial hemorrhages such as this may be seen in hypertensive patients. Such hemorrhages may also be associated with glaucoma. In glaucoma, the hemorrhages usually overlie a portion of the disk as in this 61-year-old normotensive man. Note the temporal cupping of the disk, which is also a sign of glaucoma. Another very common condition of the elderly, macular degeneration, is also evident in this photograph. At the temporal edge of the field, pigment clumps can be seen in the macular area. Such retinal pigment disorganization is typical of the dry form of macular degeneration.

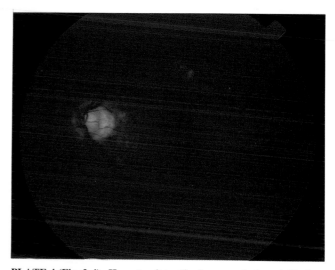

PLATE 4 (Fig. 2-4) Hypertensive retinal vaso-occlusion. *A.* Noting a spot in her vision, this previously healthy 63-year-old physician was found to have a small retinal venous occlusion with a patch of edematous retina superior to the left fovea. Hypertension and diabetes are associated with retinal vascular obstructions. After this lesion was discovered, brachial blood pressure was found to be 220/120.

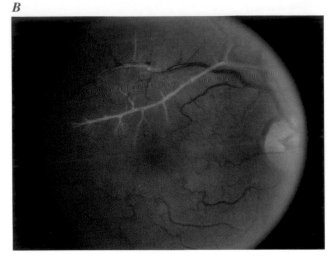

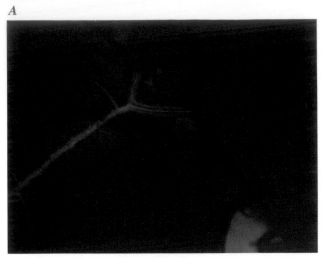

PLATE 5 (Fig. 2-5) *A.* Retinal arteriosclerosis. This 75-year-old hypertensive woman has marked arteriosclerosis of the upper temporal retinal arteriole and its branches. When the narrowed blood column can no longer be seen, the thickened wall produces the "silver-wire" appearance seen here. Where the arteriole crosses its associated vein, the course of the vein is altered, and its blood column cannot be seen. This venous "nicking" and "banking" is associated with impairment of outflow, and the affected veins become darker, larger, and more tortuous. *B.* Low-power view showing the silver-wire arteriole.

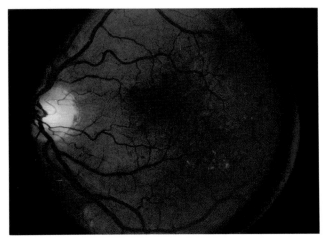

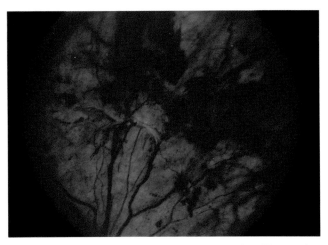

PLATE 6 (Fig. 2-6) Background diabetic retinopathy. Retinal microaneurysms, dot-and-blot hemorrhages, and a few fine upper temporal hard exudates are diagnostic of early diabetic retinopathy. The patient had no visual symptoms, but retinopathy of this magnitude can often be seen in patients with insulin-requiring diabetes of 15 or more years' duration.

PLATE 7 (Fig. 2-7) Proliferative diabetic retinopathy with preretinal hemorrhage. When neovascularization develops, preretinal and vitreous hemorrhages are much more likely to occur. Easily visible neovascularization either in the periphery of the retina, as in this diabetic patient, or at the disk is an indication for immediate panretinal laser photocoagulation.

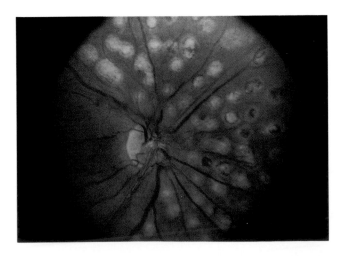

PLATE 8 (Fig. 2-8) Proliferative diabetic retinopathy treated with laser photocoagulation. The retina nasal to the optic disk has been treated with a panretinal pattern. Note the neovascularization at the disk, which is evidence of proliferative retinopathy and an indication for panretinal laser photocoagulation. Untreated, there is a high risk of blinding hemorrhage when neovascularization is present at the disk or in the periphery.

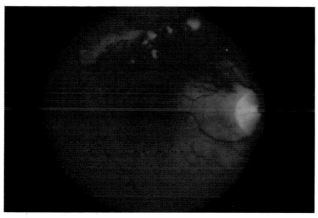

PLATE 9 (Fig. 2-9) Branch retinal vein obstruction. Thickening of the retinal arterial wall in diabetes and hypertension may compromise the lumen of the vein where they share a common adventitial sheath at an arteriovenous crossing. The resulting obstruction produces hemorrhagic retinopathy in the drainage area of the affected vein. Note here how the flame-shaped pattern of blood outlines the arcuate pattern of the nerve fibers as they run toward the optic disk.

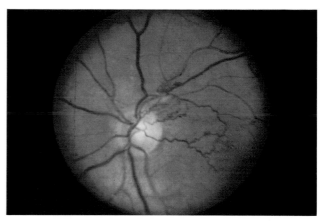

PLATE 10 (Fig. 2-10) Neovascularization after branch retinal vein obstruction. New vessels may develop late after obstruction of a branch of the central retinal vein. These most often serve to shunt flow around the obstructed vessel site and are thus not as exuberantly proliferative as those seen in diabetic retinopathy.

A

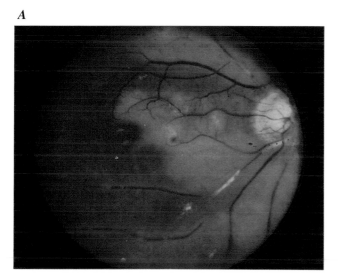

B

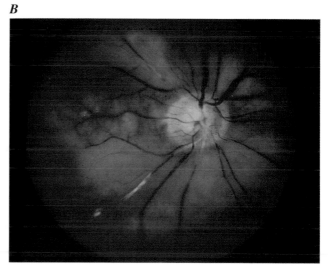

PLATE 11 (Fig. 2-11) Embolic retinal arterial obstruction (*A* and *B*). Cholesterol crystals may dislodge from the walls of the heart, aortic arch, or carotids. Carried into the retinal circulation as Hollenhorst plaques, they seldom completely obstruct the arterioles. Although amaurosis fugax is more common, the embolic burden may occasionally be so large as to produce retinal infarction. Note in the photograph of the macular area (*A*) that this patient's fovea remains red, while there is a pale, cloudy swelling nasal to it. This has produced a half "cherry-red" spot. With complete central retinal artery occlusion, the red foveal area is completely surrounded by pale swollen retina. Hollenhorst cholesterol plaques can be seen in both the upper and lower temporal retinal arteries. In *A*, the inferior temporal arteriole demonstrates "boxcar" segmentation of the blood column, indicative of very slow flow.

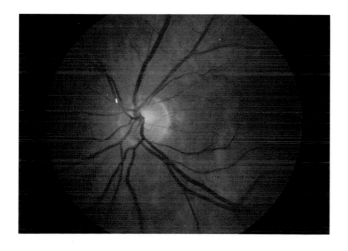

PLATE 12 (Fig. 2-12) Calcific retinal embolus associated with aortic valvular disease. Calcific aortic valvular disease and valve replacement surgery may result in retinal emboli. Like cholesterol emboli, these calcific flecks lodge at arterial bifurcations but seldom completely obstruct flow. They are white and glitter in the ophthalmoscope beam. Somewhat similar emboli may be seen after the intravenous injection of illicit drugs expanded with talc.

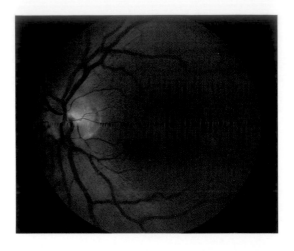

PLATE 13 (Fig. 2-13) Retinal hemorrhages after cardiac catheterization. Following cardiac catheterization, symptomatic and asymptomatic retinal hemorrhages may occur. The latter are more common. Presumably, these are the result of embolic events. Note, in this recently catheterized patient, the two oval hemorrhages and a small area of cloudy swelling just inferior and temporal to the fovea.

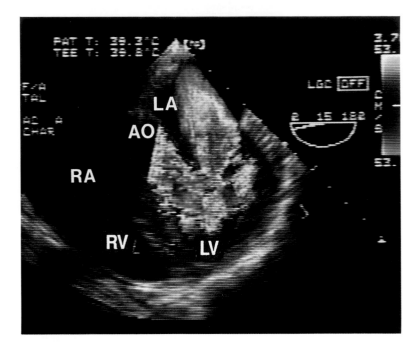

PLATE 14 (Fig. 4-14) Transesophageal echocardiography was performed in a patient with presumed severe aortic regurgitation to evaluate the structure and integrity of the aortic valve. This transesophageal echocardiogram, performed in the horizontal plane at 0° during diastole, reveals severe aortic regurgitation with significant diastolic mitral regurgitation in the left atrium (LA). The right atrium (RA), right ventricle (RV), and left ventricle (LV) are identified. Significant diastolic mitral regurgitation can occur in the setting of severe acute aortic regurgitation when left ventricular diastolic pressures exceed left atrial pressures.

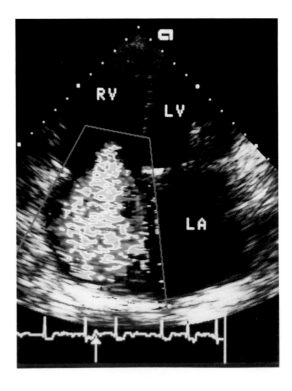

PLATE 15 (Fig. 4-15) A 46-year-old woman who had had multiple pulmonary emboli presented in the echocardiography lab for evaluation of the size, shape, and function of her right ventricle and/or the severity of tricuspid regurgitation. She had bounding neck veins and a pulsatile liver. This apical transthoracic echocardiogram was obtained, showing the right ventricle (RV), left ventricle (LV), and left atrium (LA). Severe tricuspid regurgitation is noted by the mosaic color. Continuous-wave Doppler interrogation of this jet showed a peak flow velocity of 4.5 m/s. This gave an estimated minimum right ventricular systolic pressure of 95 mmHg, which was nearly systemic. Continuous-wave Doppler has been shown to be useful in estimating right ventricular systolic pressure.

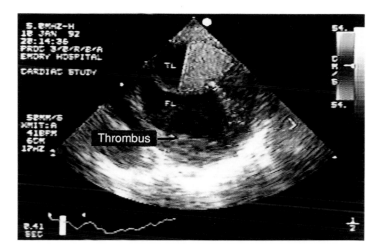

PLATE 16 (Fig. 4-20)   This transesophageal echocardiogram was obtained in a patient who was suspected of having a descending thoracic aneurysm and a possible dissection. These images show a type III dissection in the setting of a large dilated descending thoracic aorta. The true lumen is labeled (TL) and is easily distinguished from the false lumen (FL). Within the false lumen there is stagnant flow and thrombus. Communication between the true and false lumens is identified by the blue color Doppler. (See also Chap. 10.)

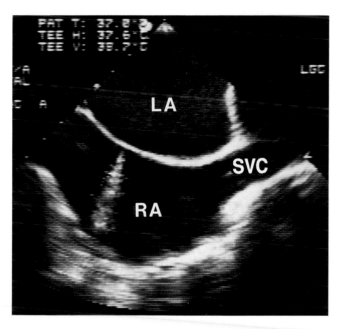

PLATE 17 (Fig. 4-22)   An 18-year-old woman was believed to have secundum atrial septal defect (ASD). Transthoracic echocardiography did not reveal substantial shunting; therefore transesophageal echocardiography was performed. These images reveal a vertical or 90° axis, showing what appears to be an intact interatrial septum between the left atrium (LA) and right atrium (RA). However, there is clearly a left-to-right shunt, noted by the blue jet of color Doppler. It is important to remember that while no defect in the interatrial septum is seen on this plane, advancing or retracting the transesophageal echocardiographic probe will interrogate different sections of the interatrial septum. When this was done, a small but definite ASD was noted. The patient had no signs of marked pulmonary hypertension, and she and her family elected to be followed despite advice that operative closure should be undertaken.

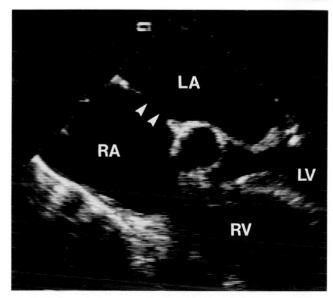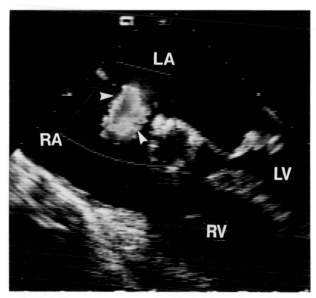

PLATE 18 (Fig. 4-23)   This patient, a 32-year-old woman, presented with atrial arrhythmias and increasing shortness of breath. Cardiovascular evaluation revealed a loud 2/6 systolic murmur with a wide and fixed split second heart sound. Transesophageal echocardiography was performed to look for an atrial septal defect. The left-hand image was obtained with a horizontal zero plane and shows a large ASD in the secundum septum *(white arrowheads)*. The left atrium (LA), right atrium (RA), right ventricle (RV), and left ventricle (LV) are identified. The right-hand panel shows obvious left-to-right shunting, as witnessed by the broad color Doppler jet. This jet measured 1.5 cm, compatible with a significant shunt. Transesophageal echocardiography is extremely useful in detecting the presence of an ASD, classifying its type, and locating the pulmonary veins. This patient had a simple secundum ASD and underwent successful surgical repair.

PLATE 19 (Fig. 4-33) A 51-year-old man with a previous myocardial infarction presented with atrial fibrillation. Two-dimensional transthoracic echocardiography, with the parasternal long axis *(A)* and apical two-chamber *(B)* views shown, was performed to determine left atrial size and left ventricular contractility. A color display communicating time and motion was used to facilitate the assessment of left ventricular (LV) regional wall motion. This technique provides better visualization of the extent and synchrony of endocardial contraction and expansion throughout the cardiac cycle. The arrows point to the endocardial wall segments that move in a direction opposite to their expected motion; i.e., they are dyskinetic, consistent with the past history of a myocardial infarction. A large left atrium (LA) is present. RV = right ventricle; Ao = aorta.

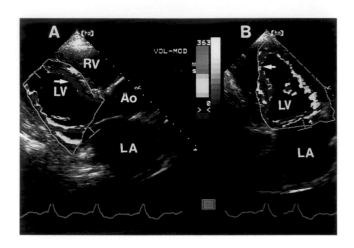

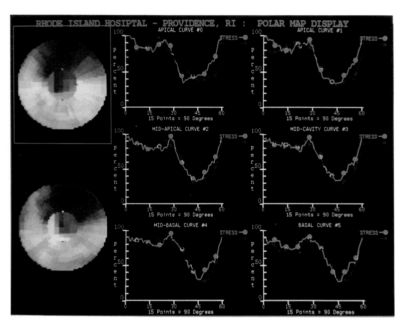

PLATE 20 (Fig. 5-6) Polar map display. The polar maps are created by telescoping the short-axis slices into a circular display in which the base is at the periphery of the circle and the apex in the center. Each map is scaled to the hottest pixel for that scan (either stress or rest). On the color display, the highest counts are represented as white and light yellow through shades of orange to brown and black (0 counts). The center of the polar map display is derived from count data from the apex of the midvertical long-axis slices. The polar map on the top is the stress map and the one below the rest map. Displayed to the right are six circumferential count profiles from representative short-axis slices from apex *(upper left corner)* to base *(bottom right corner)*. Zero degrees is at 3 o'clock, and the maps go clockwise. The blue curve is stress, the red curve redistribution. As can be seen in these displays, the inferior wall counts are high, while the anterior wall counts are profoundly reduced to between 30 and 35 percent of peak counts and do not change between stress and redistribution, consistent with scar in the distribution of the LAD.

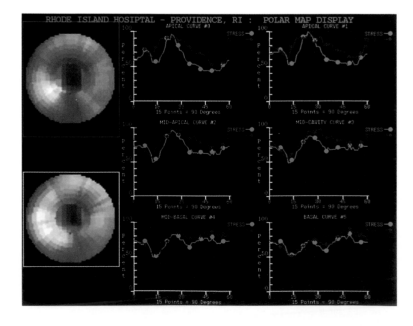

PLATE 21 (Fig. 5-15) The polar display shows redistribution in the inferior wall (distal), as well as anterior and anteroseptal walls (distal). The apex, which is not displayed, was reduced to 25 percent of peak counts and did not change. The quantitative data reveal extensive myocardial viability based on the presence of redistribution following a rest injection of thallium as well as count levels above 50 percent of peak counts in most of the heart except the apex.

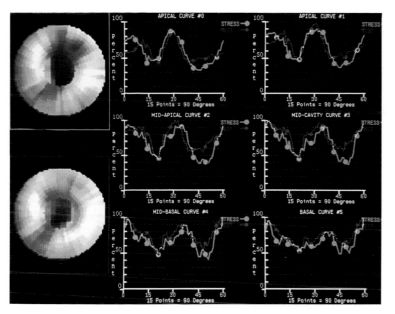

PLATE 22 (Fig. 5-20) Polar display from the same patient. The two defects are seen as the two dips in the curves, and the difference between the blue and red curves distally corresponds to the defect fill-in seen on the scans. Profiles from the apex are not included in this display. The apex shows the most severe count reduction, and the defect is fixed.

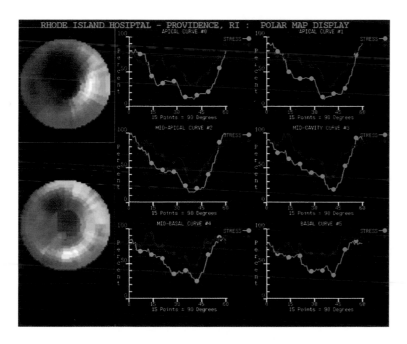

PLATE 23 (Fig. 5-24) Polar maps derived from scan data of the patient in Fig. 5-23.

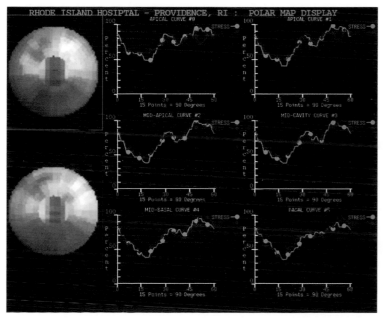

PLATE 24 (Fig. 5-27) Polar map showing fixed inferior wall defect.

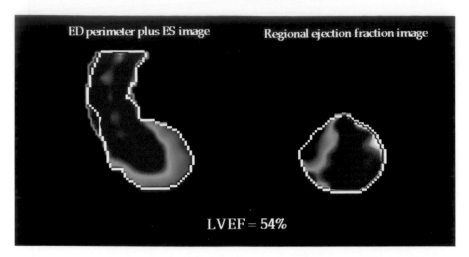

ED perimeter plus ES image   Regional ejection fraction image

LVEF = 54%

PLATE 25 (Fig. 5-28)   During the injection of the rest dose of sestamibi, a dynamic first-pass acquisition was performed for measurement of LVEF and evaluation of wall motion. This figure shows the first-pass study with low-normal LVEF and mild inferior hypokinesis seen on both the combined ED perimeter and ES image and on the regional ejection fraction image, in which regional ejection fractions in the LV region are color-coded with yellow, being the highest, through shades of red to purple, blue, green, and black. ED = end-diastolic; ES = end-systolic.

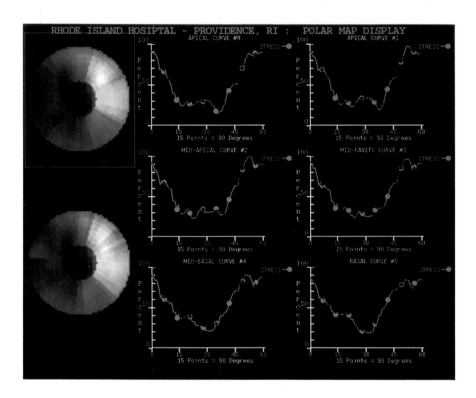

RHODE ISLAND HOSIPTAL - PROVIDENCE, RI : POLAR MAP DISPLAY

PLATE 26 (Fig. 5-30)   The polar map also demonstrates an extensive and severe fixed defect in the inferior wall and anteroseptum. The apical defect was also severe with 16 percent of peak activity.

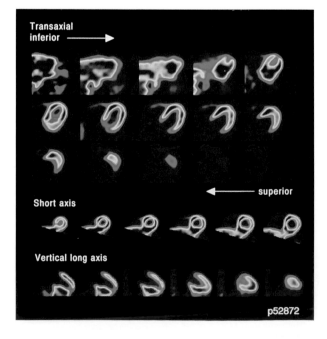

Transaxial inferior →

← superior

Short axis

Vertical long axis

p52872

PLATE 27 (Fig. 8-1)   NORMAL VOLUNTEER. Set of 15 contiguous transaxial planes acquired after intravenous injection of ^{13}N ammonia. These images display the anterobasal, midventricular, and inferior diaphragmatic planes of the left ventricle and are viewed from the volunteer's feet. The right ventricular wall and papillary muscles are visualized. The tracer ^{13}N ammonia also accumulates in the liver, which is seen on the more inferior images. In normal volunteers, the tracer uptake of the left ventricular myocardium is homogeneous even though the posterolateral and inferior walls sometimes show a slightly diminished uptake. The reason for this regional reduction has not been clarified but may be related to a regional alteration in amino acid or, more generally, substrate metabolism. After computer-processed reorientation, vertical long-axis and short-axis views are obtained.

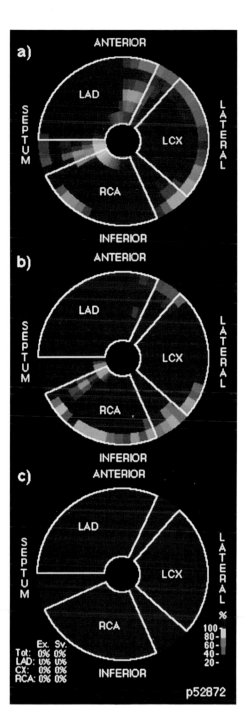

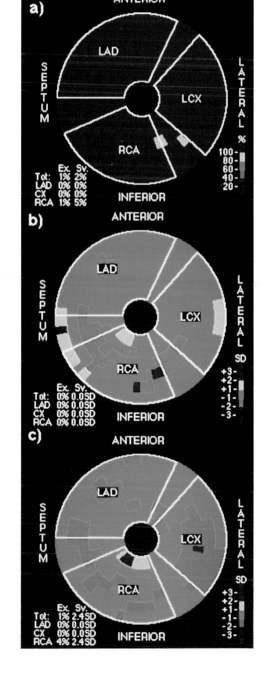

PLATE 28 (Fig. 8-2) The three-dimensional distribution of tracer activity in the left ventricular myocardium can be displayed in the form of two-dimensional polar maps. These maps are generated from circumferential activity profiles of the six short-axis images (processing from the apex to the base of the left ventricle), shown in panel *a*. As depicted in panel *b*, regional tracer concentration is normalized to the top 5 percent of activity within the whole polar map. *Normal* is defined as a *pixel value within plus/minus two standard deviations of the normal mean value* and is displayed in red. To identify abnormal myocardium in patients, polar maps are compared to a normal control group ("normal" database) using a color scale *c*. Normal myocardium is outlined in red, while a change in color to yellow, green, light blue, dark blue, and violet characterizes, stepwise, 20 percent reductions in tracer activity. To assess regional rather than global myocardial abnormalities, vascular territories can be defined on the polar maps, allowing to estimate the severity and the extent of a reduction in tracer uptake per vascular territory. The grade of severity describes the average reduction of activity relative to the normal myocardium, while the extent defines the fraction of abnormal myocardium in relation to the entire myocardium or to a myocardial territory related to a coronary artery.

PLATE 29 (Fig. 8-3) The normalized polar map (*a*), matched to a database of 11 healthy volunteers, presents a normal ^{13}N ammonia blood pool study (as described in Fig. 8-4). The normalized polar map of glucose metabolism (*b*) displays normal ^{18}F deoxyglucose (FDG) uptake in green, while yellow (uptake > 1 SD) and red (uptake > 2 SD) represent hypermetabolism and blue (uptake < 1 SD) and violet (uptake < 2 SD) hypometabolism. The difference polar map (*c*) compares the relative normalized ^{13}N ammonia uptake *a* with the relative normalized FDG uptake (*b*) and displays the difference between glucose utilization and blood flow. Differences in regional tracer uptake within two standard deviations of the normal mean value are considered normal and are shown in red. Differences greater than two standard deviations of normal are considered abnormal and are depicted in green (2 to 3 SDs) and blue (more than three SDs).

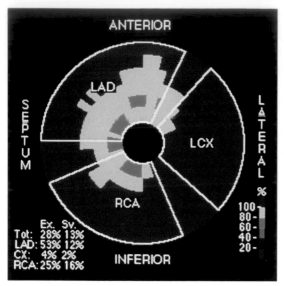

PLATE 30 (Fig. 8-5) Comparison of the study shown in Fig. 8-4 to a database of normal demonstrates, on the polar map, a reduction in myocardial blood flow in the LAD territory, increasing in severity from base to apex. Additionally, the RCA territory shows a mild blood-flow abnormality consistent with a flow defect in the distal inferior wall, which still might result from the disease of the LAD.

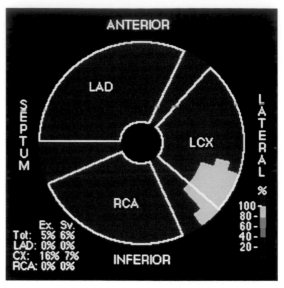

PLATE 31 (Fig. 8-7) The semiquantitative polar map shows a moderate reduction in ¹³N ammonia uptake in the lateral wall. The LAD and RCA territories are free of detectable abnormalities. This patient had angiographically documented disease of the LCX.

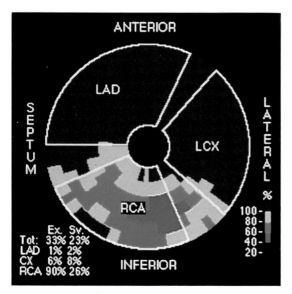

PLATE 32 (Fig. 8-9) Polar map analysis confirms the severe reduction of tracer uptake in the inferior wall, whereas the LCX territory shows only a small abnormality.

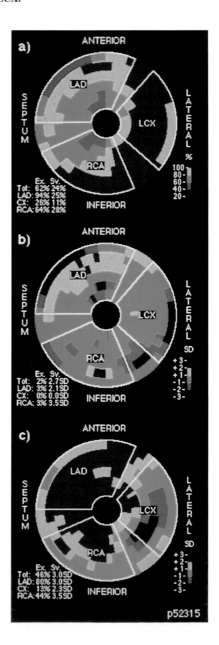

PLATE 33 (Fig. 8-11) The normalized polar map of the myocardial blood flow (*a*) shows defects in the LAD and RCA territories, with increasing severity from the midventricular region to the apex; furthermore there is a mild defect in the LCX territory. The normalized FDG polar map (*b*) reveals an area of hypermetabolism in the LAD and RCA territories. The difference polar map (*c*) displays a mismatch pattern, confirming the presence of viable myocardium in this region. ▶

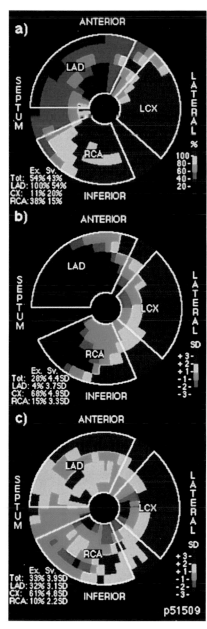

PLATE 34 (Fig. 8-13) The polar map of myocardial blood flow (*a*) displays severe defect in the LAD territory, a moderate defect in the RCA territory, and a mild defect in LCX territory. The match pattern in the FDG polar map (*b*) supports the finding of nonviable myocardium in the LAD and RCA territories and is confirmed by the difference polar map (*c*).

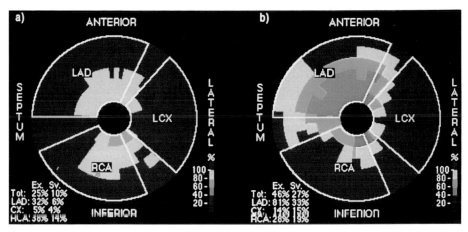

PLATE 35 (Fig. 8-15) At rest (*a*), the semiquantitative analysis of the distribution of ^{13}N ammonia shows a mild defect in the anterior and distal inferior walls. During dipyridamole-induced hyperemia (*b*), the LAD territory demonstrates a severe perfusion defect consistent with disease of LAD, whereas the other vascular territories show only minor abnormalities.

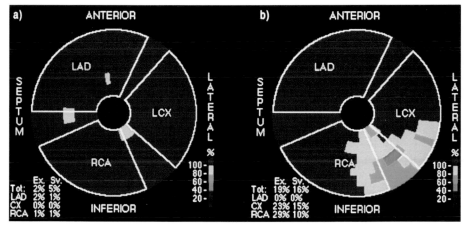

PLATE 36 (Fig. 8-17) Polar maps confirm the normal perfusion at rest (*a*). During stress (*b*), a moderate perfusion defect in the LCX territory is noted. A reduction of tracer uptake in the RCA, adjacent to the abnormality in the LCX territory, is seen.

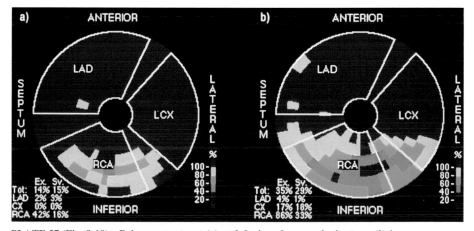

PLATE 37 (Fig. 8-19) Polar maps at rest (*a*) and during pharmacologic stress (*b*) in the same patient. The semiquantitative analysis of the myocardial coronary blood flow at rest reveals a moderate perfusion defect in the RCA territory. During pharmacologically induced hyperemia, note an increase in extent and severity of this abnormality. Furthermore, a moderate reduction in tracer uptake can be noted within the LCX territory.

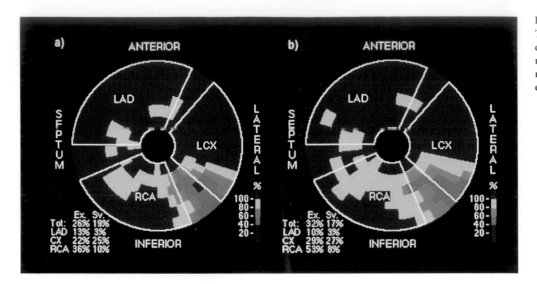

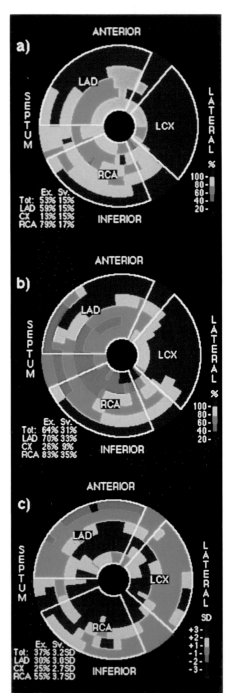

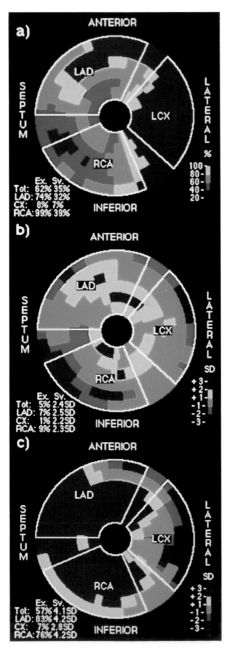

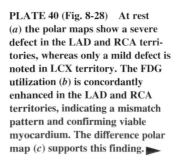

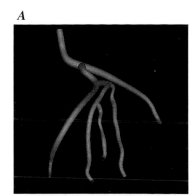

A

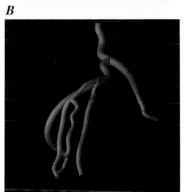

B

PLATE 41 (Fig. 12-9) Three-dimensional coronary trees. Three-dimensional visualization or quantitation of the vascular tree can be obtained with stereoscopic imaging.[24] As images are acquired, the x-ray source alternates between two positions separated by approximately 2 to 6 cm. When the two images are viewed together, with each eye looking at a different one of the two stereoscopic images, the eye-brain system can perceive the 3D relationships between the vessels. When the stereoscopic images are digitized, the vessels can be tracked and the centerline position of the vessels in the images determined.[25] From these positions and the known stereoscopic imaging geometry, the 3D positions of the vessel centerlines can be determined.[26] The 3D positions and the measured vessel sizes can then be used for rendering the 3D vasculature at arbitrary projection angles. The right anterior oblique (RAO) (*A*) and 45° from RAO (*B*) projections of the left coronary tree are generated by the computer after determination of the 3D positions by means of vessel tracking and correlation of the vessels in the tree and knowledge of the imaging geometry. In the second projection, the several vessels overlap, which can hinder diagnosis. With the 3D rendered tree, projections can be identified with minimal obscuring of the vessels of interest, and the gantry can be positioned for that acquisition geometry. Techniques have also been developed to determine 3D vascular positions from biplane views, from which 3D renderings can also be generated. In addition, methods have been developed to determine the "triple-orthogonal axis," i.e., the axis that is perpendicular to the vessel centerline in the two views.[27]

A

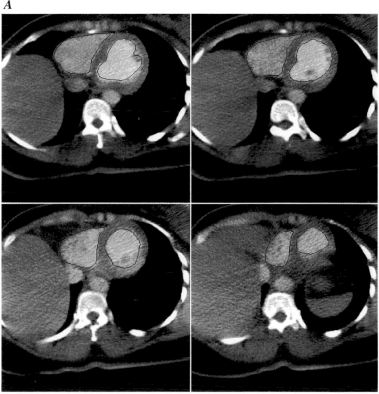

PLATE 42 (Fig. 12-12) Three-dimensional extraction and rendering of the ventricular surface. When cross-sectional images of the heart are obtained, the various levels of the heart can be inspected visually. Because CT and MRI are digital modalities, quantitative techniques can be applied. In particular, the ventricular regions can be identified using boundary-detection techniques. *A*. Individual contours (*red*) extracted semiautomatically from EBCT using an adaptive segmentation algorithm.[29,30] These contours can be stacked (*B*) and interpolated (*C*) or the surface can be shaded (*D*) to give a 3D perspective of the ventricular and aortic surfaces. *E*. When the boundaries of the epicardium are also obtained, volume-rendering techniques can be employed to render the cardiac structures for visualization. From such data, ventricular or myocardial volumes can be calculated by summing the areas of the individual regions and multiplying by the slice thickness (Simpson's rule). (From Chen SY, Carroll JD, Chen CT, et al: Three-dimensional ventricle reconstruction from serial cross sections. *Proc SPIE* 1993; 1905:93–99. Reproduced with permission from the publisher and authors.)

B

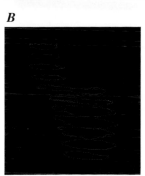

C

D

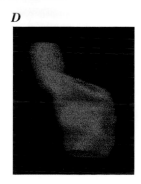

E

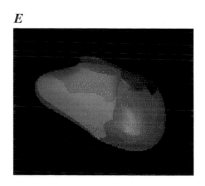

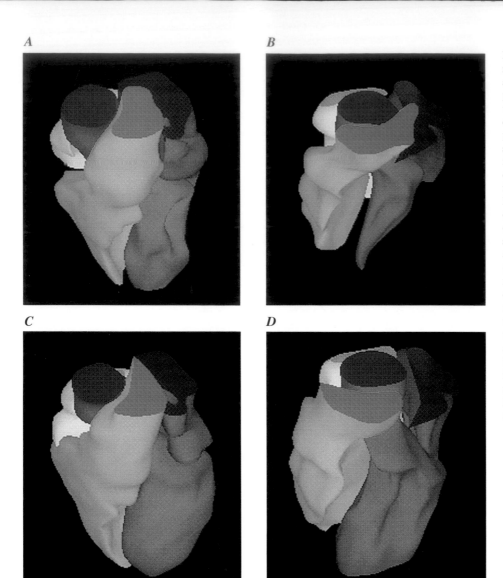

PLATE 43 (Fig. 12-13) Ventricular motion from EBCT. Cardiac images are usually obtained at various phases of the cardiac cycle. Thus, the ventricular or myocardial surfaces can be rendered for each of these phases and volumes calculated. The standard procedure is to analyze the images corresponding to systole and diastole and to calculate the ejection fraction or visualize ventricular or heart wall motion. The ventricles can be rendered from EBCT images obtained at end-diastole and end-systole. Illustrated are a normal heart at end-diastole (A) and end-systole (B), and a heart with dilated cardiomyopathy at end-diastole (C) and end-systole (D). With the 3D-rendered surfaces, the difference in the volume of the left ventricle of the two hearts at end-diastole is readily apparent. By comparing the changes between end-diastole and end-systole for the two hearts, the reduction of motion (or change of volume) for the heart with dilated cardiomyopathy is also apparent.

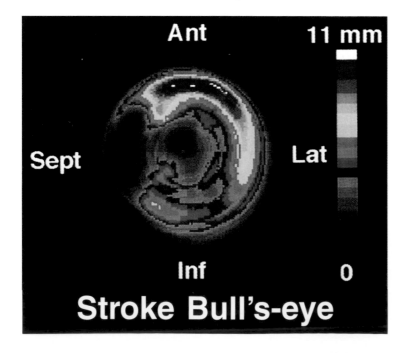

PLATE 44 (Fig. 12-15) Ventricular motion from PET. Methods have also been developed for measurement of wall motion from PET data. An ECG/seven-slice PET series was obtained using ^{15}O-carbon monoxide; the slice spacing was 14.2 mm, and the transaxial spatial resolution was 8.5 mm. By calculating the difference between the end-systolic data and end-diastolic data, "stroke" images were obtained. These data were then displayed using a polar bull's-eye display.[34,35] The results presented in this figure indicate that the patient had poor wall motion centered at the apex (center of the bull's-eye) and in the septal region, with good motion in the basal and lateral regions. Although PET studies do not have the spatial resolution of EBCT or MRI, PET can provide metabolic information (see Fig. 12-17) currently unavailable with the other modalities. (From Miller TR, Wallis JW, Landy BR, et al: Measurement of global and regional left ventricular function by cardiac PET. *J Nucl Med* 1994; 35:999–1005. Reproduced with permission from the publisher and authors.) (See also Chap. 8.)

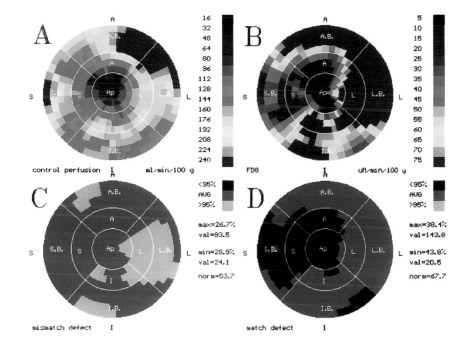

PLATE 45 (Fig.12-17) Perfusion, although providing information regarding ischemia, may not reflect the functional health of a region of the heart muscle. Studies with radio-isotope labeled [18]FDG (fluorodeoxyglucose) can provide information on glucose consumption and thereby metabolic function. Parametric polar maps of myocardial perfusion (*A*) and glucose consumption (*B*). The color scales pertinent to the maps are displayed to the right. In the bottom panel at left (*C*), the mismatch map is displayed as the ratio of *B* and *A*. In the map, the regions exceeding the 95 percent confidence interval are displayed in light green (increased [18]FDG uptake related to perfusion), the remainder in blue. At right, in the bottom panel (*D*), the match map is displayed. This is obtained by multiplying *A* and *B* and normalizing for mean flow. The match defect is the region below the 95 percent confidence interval (concomitant low perfusion and [18]FDG uptake) and displayed in black, the remainder in blue. In the right portion of *C* and *D*, the percentages of the myocardium that lie within, below, and above the 95 percent confidence interval are indicated along with their values. This example is from a patient with extensive myocardial infarction in the anteroseptal region and ischemia in the posterolateral and inferior regions. (From Blanksma PK, Willemsen ATM, Meeder JG, et al: Quantitative myocardial mapping of perfusion and metabolism using parametric polar map displays in cardiac PET. *J Nucl Med* 1995; 36:153–158. Reproduced with permission from the publisher and authors.)

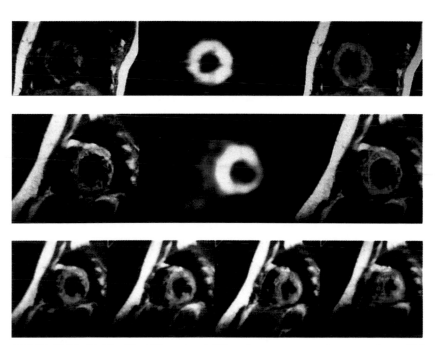

PLATE 46 (Fig 12-18) The different modalities often present complementary data, which must be integrated in the cardiologist's mind. Computational methods have been developed to facilitate this image integration when digital data are available. To integrate data, they are first registered (i.e., the corresponding regions in the two image sets must be made to overlap accurately). Registration can be performed with the individual planes of data. However, the different acquisitions are usually not obtained with the exact same imaging geometry; in addition, out-of-plane motion of the heart may further frustrate registration and thereby comparison of the image data. Thus, registration of the 3D data sets is required. Faber and colleagues[19] have developed techniques for registration of 3D single photon emission computed tomography (SPECT) and MR image sets of the heart. After registration, the information from the two modalities is combined by using the MRI to indicate anatomy as a gray scale image and the SPECT information as a color wash. The results are shown here. *Top*: One section of cardiac MR image is on the left, the corresponding section from the registered SPECT image is in the middle, and the fused image combining the MR and SPECT images is on the right. Note the uniformity of perfusion. These images are from a healthy subject. *Middle*: Registration and fusion of images from a subject with coronary artery disease. The MR image is on the left, the stress perfusion SPECT image is in the middle, and the fused image is on the right. Note the perfusion abnormality in the lateral wall, corresponding to an infarction. *Bottom*: Multiple frames of the rest study from the first subject. Fused short-axis sections from end diastole (*left*) to end systole (*right*). (From Faber TL, McColl RW, Opperman RM, et al: Spatial and temporal registration of cardiac SPECT and MR images: Methods and evaluation. *Radiology* 1991; 179:857–861. Reproduced with permission from the publisher and authors.)

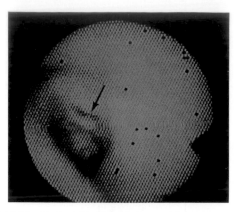

PLATE 47 (Fig. 13-6) This image is from a 72-year-old man with unstable angina who was unresponsive to medical therapy, which included aspirin, a beta blocker, and a calcium antagonist. Angiography revealed no thrombi or intimal disruption. Angioscopy, however, revealed a disrupted atheroma in the left anterior descending coronary artery. This disruption was undetectable in multiple angiographic views.

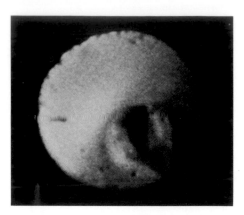

PLATE 48 (Fig. 13-7) A 74-year-old diabetic woman underwent an in situ femoral-popliteal bypass. This is an angioscopic image of a partially disrupted venous valve after initial valvotomy.

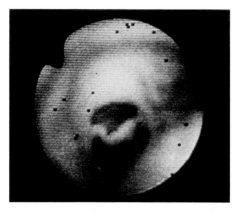

PLATE 49 (Fig.13-8) This image is from a 52-year-old man with severe stable angina who had acute closure during balloon angioplasty. Angiography revealed a long spiral dissection. By angioscopy, there is severe intimal change caused by the balloon angioplasty. The image shows the double lumen created by the dissection as well as subintimal hemorrhage.

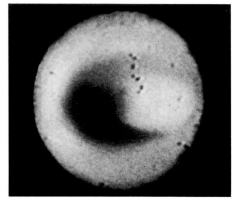

PLATE 50 (Fig. 13-9) This image is from the left anterior coronary artery of a 68-year-old woman with acute unstable angina pectoris at rest that was unresponsive to medical therapy. There is a crescent-shaped, fresh, partially occlusive coronary thrombosis. The surface of the clot undulated during routine flushing to clear blood from the imaging field. Coronary thrombi are typically adherent and do not dislodge during flushing.

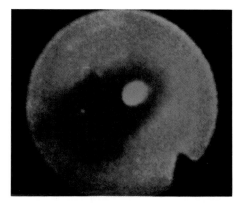

PLATE 51 (Fig. 13-10) A 70-year-old woman with known coronary artery disease presented with unrelenting chest pain of 4 h duration. Acute myocardial infarction was documented by electrocardiography and enzymes. Angioscopy revealed a completely occlusive coronary thrombosis in the left anterior descending coronary artery. The angioscope is very close to the thrombus. The vessel walls are outside the field of view. The central white spot is the angioscope's imaging light reflected back off the glistening thrombus.

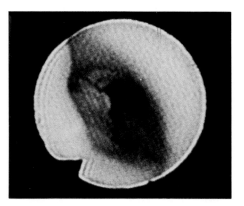

PLATE 52 (Fig. 13-11) A 56-year-old man was studied by angioscopy 2 weeks after transmural myocardial infarction. The image reveals an atheroma with residual disruption but without thrombosis. The patient had not been treated with a thrombolytic agent. Thus this is an example of spontaneous endogenous thrombolysis after presumed coronary occlusion.

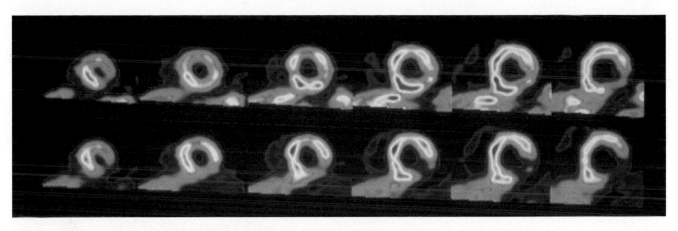

FIGURE 8-16 STRESS-INDUCED DEFECTS OF MYOCARDIAL BLOOD FLOW DUE TO LCX DISEASE.
Short-axis images of myocardial blood flow at rest (*upper row*) and during intravenous
dipyridamole-induced hyperemia (*lower row*) in a 57-year-old patient with a history of
multiple bypass graftings. Note the homogeneous tracer uptake throughout the left ventricular
myocardium at rest. A moderate defect in the inferolateral wall is seen during stress.
Quantitative image analysis confirmed the presence of this defect on the polar map, as
seen in Fig. 8-17.

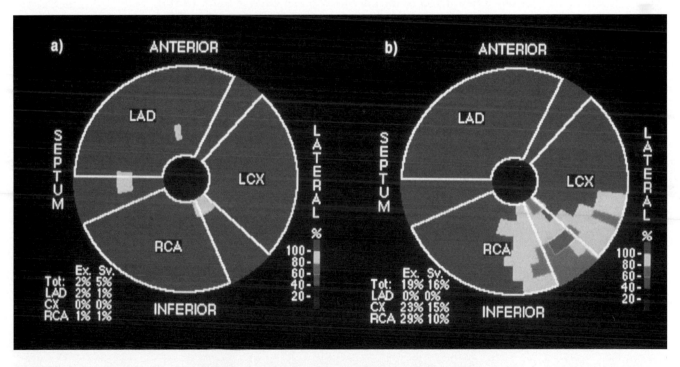

FIGURE 8-17   Polar maps confirm the normal perfusion at rest (*a*). During stress (*b*), a
moderate perfusion defect in the LCX territory is noted. A reduction of tracer uptake in the
RCA, adjacent to the abnormality in the LCX territory, is seen. (*See color Plate 36.*)

Conclusion: Stress-induced flow defect in the inferolateral wall consistent with
the patient's angiographically documented disease of the LCX.

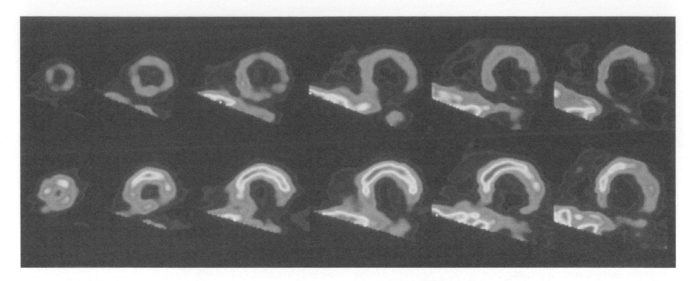

FIGURE 8-18   REVERSIBLE PERFUSION PATTERN—RIGHT CORONARY ARTERY. Short-axis ^{13}N ammonia images obtained at rest (*upper row*) and after intravenous administration of dipyridamole (*lower row*) in a 71-year-old patient with angiographically documented coronary artery disease. He had been treated unsuccessfully with angioplasty of the RCA. At rest, the images depict a moderate blood flow defect in the inferolateral and inferior walls. During stress, a moderate to severe reduction of tracer uptake is noted in the same segments. The defect spares the distal inferior wall, which was supplied by the LAD.

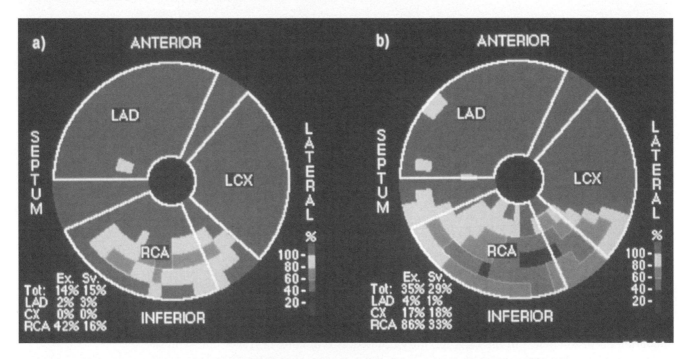

FIGURE 8-19   Polar maps at rest (*a*) and during pharmacologic stress (*b*) in the same patient. The semiquantitative analysis of the myocardial coronary blood flow at rest reveals a moderate perfusion defect in the RCA territory. During pharmacologically induced hyperemia, note an increase in extent and severity of this abnormality. Furthermore, a moderate reduction in tracer uptake can be noted within the LCX territory. (*See color Plate 37.*)

Conclusion: Partially reversible stress-induced blood-flow defect in the inferolateral and inferior walls, corresponding to RCA disease.

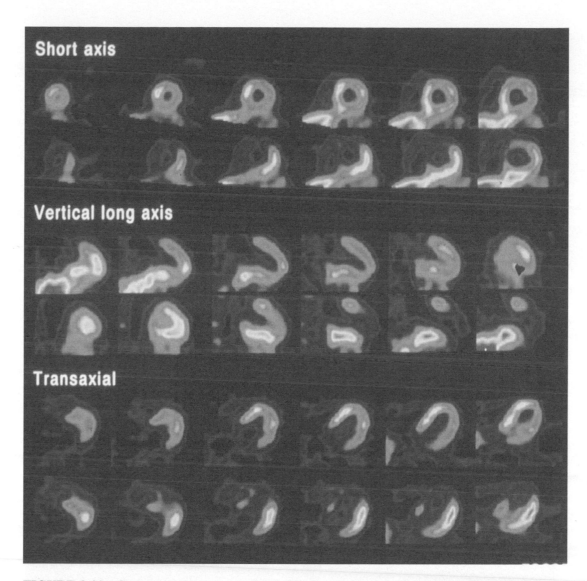

FIGURE 8-20   Severe disease of the **LAD.** Short-axis, long-vertical-axis, and transaxial images after intravenous injection of ^{13}N ammonia at rest (*upper row*) and after pharmacologic stress with dipyridamole (*lower row*). At rest, there is homogeneous tracer uptake. Note the reduction of tracer uptake in the septum and anterior wall during the stress study. There is also a transient left ventricular enlargement during stress, which is best seen in the short-axis cuts. Such chamber enlargement indicates extensive ischemia. Some decrease in tracer uptake is also noted in the posterior septum in the inferior wall, suggesting the presence of RCA disease.

Conclusion: The extensive stress-induced blood-flow defect involves the basal anterior wall and the anterior septum and extends into the apex and distal inferior wall. This is consistent with a proximal LAD stenosis, which affects the first septal perforator and causes the flow reduction in the anterior septum.

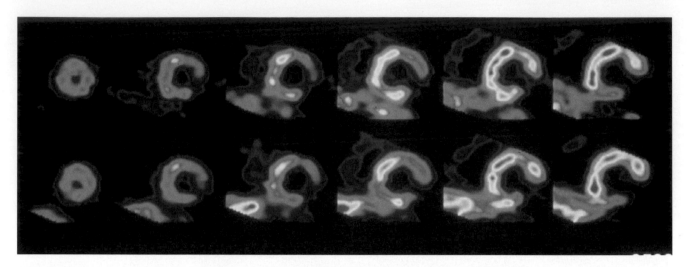

FIGURE 8-21 IRREVERSIBLE PERFUSION PATTERN. Short-axis cuts of myocardial blood flow at rest (*upper row*) and during pharmacologically induced stress (*lower row*) in a 63-year-old patient who had undergone coronary artery bypass grafting 7 years earlier. Six months prior to the PET study, the patient had suffered an inferolateral myocardial infarction and was treated by angioplasty. The rest and pharmacologic stress images reveal a severe flow defect in the inferolateral wall of the left ventricle.

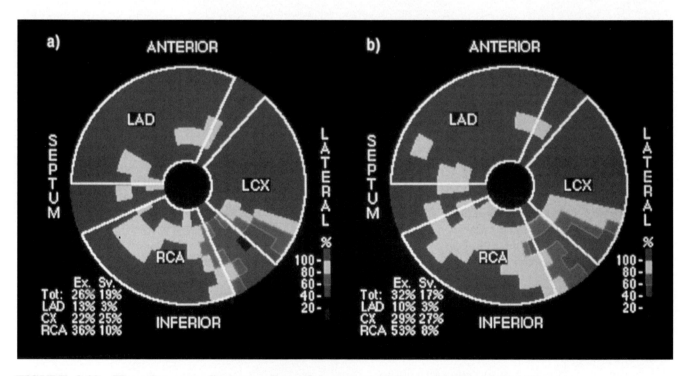

FIGURE 8-22 The polar maps display confirms the presence of the resting flow defect (*a*) but reveals some increase in its extent during dipyridamole (*b*). (*See color Plate 38.*)

Conclusion: Fixed flow defect (seen on the rest and hyperemic images) in the inferolateral wall is consistent with the patient's known previous myocardial infarction in the LCX territory.

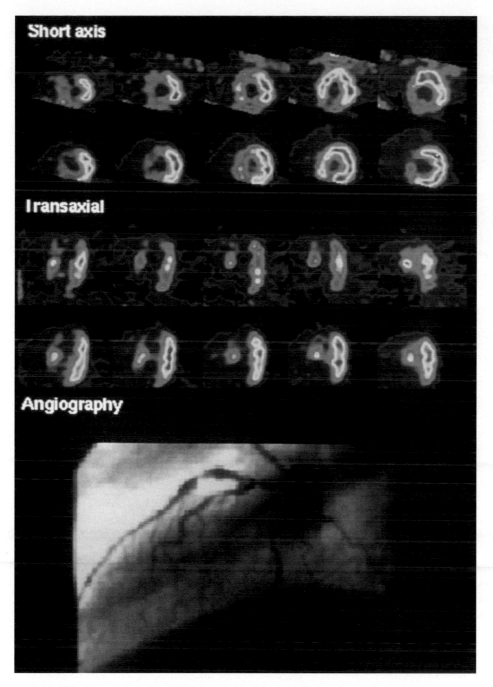

FIGURE 8-23 ACUTE MYOCARDIAL INFARCTION. Short-axis and transaxial perfusion images at rest (*upper row*) and during exogenous glucose utilization (*lower row*) from a 67-year-old male. The patient was admitted with an acute anteroseptal myocardial infarction; a PET scan was performed 4 days after the acute event. The patient had received thrombolytic therapy with evidence of reperfusion but developed postinfarction angina. This study was done to evaluate whether the thrombolysis had restored coronary blood flow adequately or whether additional revascularization was needed. The location and extent of the flow defect and the reduced FDG uptake are consistent with an extensive irreversible injury to the anterior and anteroseptal walls. The corresponding angiographic findings are depicted at the bottom of the figure and display two images showing sequential stenosis (70 to 80 percent) in the proximal LAD.

Conclusion: Since this study was performed early after myocardial infarction with akinesis of the anterior wall on echocardiography, the PET findings suggest the presence of nonviable or necrotic myocardium. Nevertheless, the patient underwent coronary angiography.

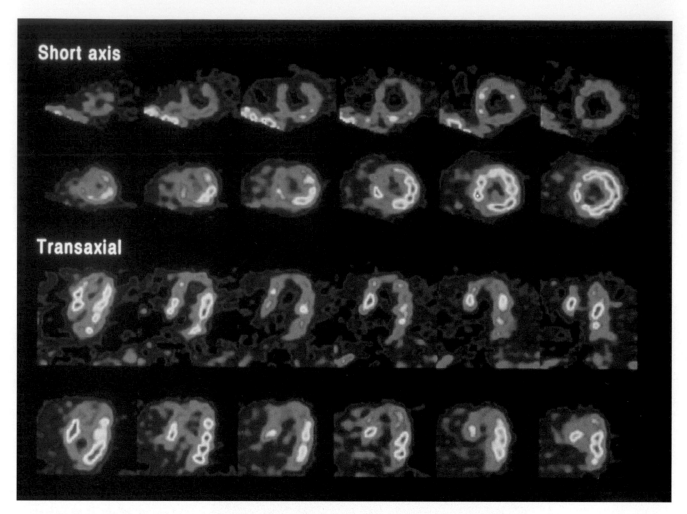

FIGURE 8-24   Myocardial infarction—follow-up. Short-axis and transaxial perfusion images at rest (*upper row*) and of FDG uptake (*lower row*), both at rest, were obtained 2 months after the acute myocardial infarction in the patient shown in Fig. 8-25. The purpose of this study was to assess possible changes in the regional blood-flow metabolism and to search for regional myocardial viability. In comparison with the previous PET study, the blood-flow study depicts a modest reduction in the extent of the anteroseptal wall defect. The FDG uptake images reveal a concordant reduction of tracer uptake, indicating nonviable myocardium.

Conclusion: A match pattern was found in the LAD territory consistent with necrosis and scar tissue formation in the "infarct territory," with low probability of an improvement in anterior wall motion.

ASSESSMENT OF MYOCARDIAL VIABILITY

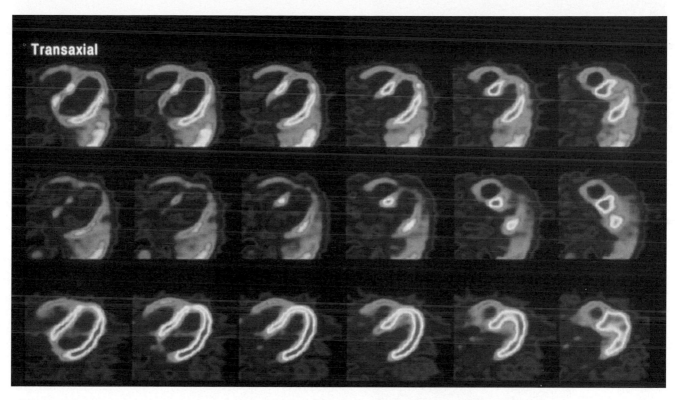

FIGURE 8-25 Transaxial images of blood flow at baseline (*upper row*), during dipyridamole-induced hyperemia (*middle row*) (both with ^{13}N ammonia), and of glucose utilization with FDG (*lower row*) in a 53-year-old man with type II diabetes. He had recently developed progressive shortness of breath and pulmonary edema. Echocardiography revealed poor left ventricular function (left ventricular diastolic dimension, 64 mm; systolic dimension, 47 mm; ejection fraction, 30 percent). Anteroseptal, apical, and inferior akinesis suggested previous anterior and inferior myocardial infarction. Coronary angiography revealed triple-vessel disease with proximal 95 percent LAD, 95 percent LCX, and 100 percent RCA stenosis. The objective of the PET study was to evaluate the presence and extent of ischemia as well as myocardial viability.

Note the enlargement of the right and left ventricles. At rest, there is substantially decreased perfusion in the proximal to distal inferoseptal, distal anteroseptal, and lateroapical walls. During dipyridamole-induced hyperemia, further widespread decreased perfusion in the mid- to distal anterolateral, lateral, inferolateral, and inferoseptal walls is seen. The FDG images show decreased uptake in the apex and proximal anterior and inferoseptal territories. Other than these findings, metabolic function was relatively well preserved.

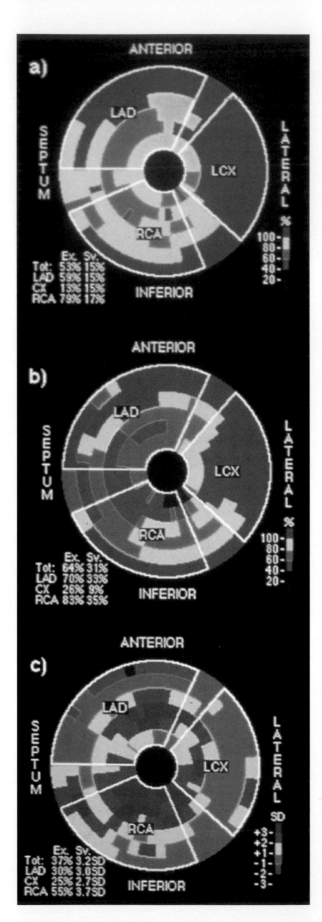

FIGURE 8-26 The semiquantitative analysis of polar maps at rest (*a*) reveals a reduced ^{13}N ammonia uptake mainly in the LAD and RCA territories, while only a moderate blood-flow defect was seen in the LCX territory. During stress (*b*) the extent of these defects increased. The difference polar map (*c*) confirms the presence of viable myocardium in all three territories. (*See color Plate 39.*)

Conclusion: Stress-induced ischemia in the LAD, LCX, and RCA territories. There is also a mismatch pattern in the LAD and RCA territories. This is consistent with viability in hypoperfused areas and is predictive of recovery of ventricular function following revascularization.

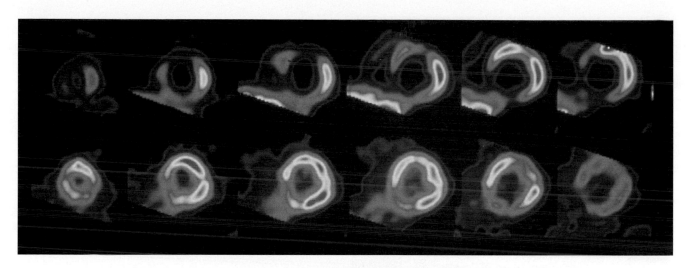

FIGURE 8-27   Short-axis images after intravenous ^{13}N ammonia matching (*upper row*) and of FDG (*lower row*) at rest in a 74-year-old male. The patient had a history of pulmonary edema. The ECG showed Q waves in the inferior leads. Echocardiography revealed a diffuse hypokinesis and poor left ventricular function (left ventricular ejection fraction, 27 percent). The objective of the PET study was to assess myocardial viability.

Note the enlargement of the left ventricle. In the resting study a moderate to severe decrease in tracer uptake is seen in the septum, anterior, inferior-septal, and inferior walls. The glucose utilization images show a marked increase in FDG uptake in the same hypoperfused territories.

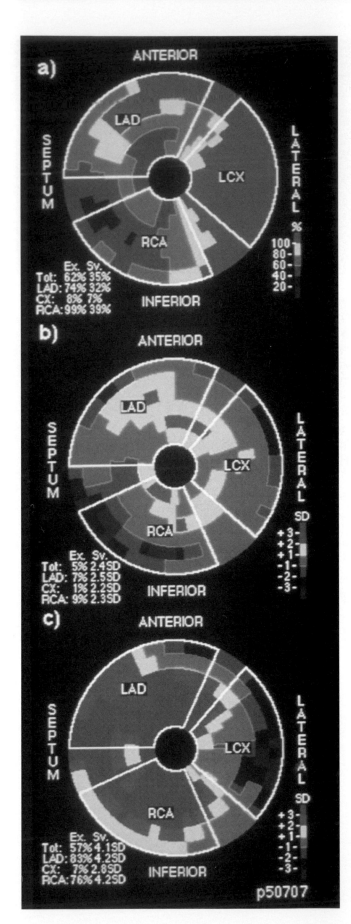

FIGURE 8-28 At rest (*a*) the polar maps show a severe defect in the LAD and RCA territories, whereas only a mild defect is noted in LCX territory. The FDG utilization (*b*) is concordantly enhanced in the LAD and RCA territories, indicating a mismatch pattern and confirming viable myocardium. The difference polar map (*c*) supports this finding. (*See color Plate 40.*)

Conclusion: Blood-flow metabolism mismatch in the LAD and RCA territories. The patient underwent coronary angiography, which confirmed an occlusion of the proximal LAD and RCA and a stenosis of the LCX (60 percent). Since PET revealed viable myocardium, the patient was treated successfully by coronary artery bypass grafting.

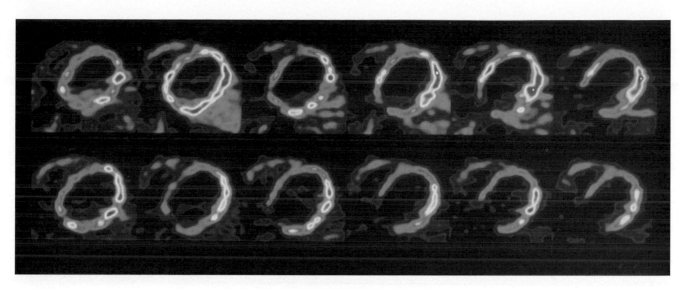

FIGURE 8-29 IDIOPATHIC CARDIOMYOPATHY. Transaxial images at rest (*upper row*) and after pharmacologic stress (*lower row*) in a 50-year-old patient with a history of idiopathic dilated cardiomyopathy (echocardiographic findings: left ventricular diastolic dimension, 80 mm; left ventricular systolic dimension, 69 mm; left ventricular ejection fraction, 18 percent.

The study was undertaken to investigate the etiology of the poor ventricular function. At rest and stress, the study shows a dilation of both chambers with a patchy distribution of tracer uptake. Note that the scattered blood-flow defects do not correspond to the distribution of the coronary vascular territories.

Conclusion: No stress-induced blood-flow defects. This scan is most commonly seen in patients with idiopathic cardiomyopathy. Positron emission tomography was critical in the decision to refer this patient for orthotopic heart transplantation.

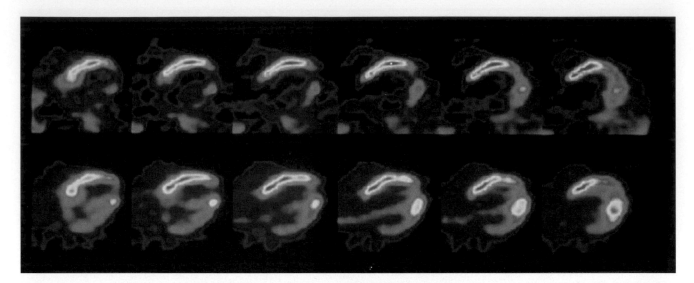

FIGURE 8-30   Contiguous transaxial images of ^{13}N ammonia uptake (*upper row*) and FDG uptake (*lower row*) in a 50-year-old man. He underwent coronary artery bypass grafting 10 years ago and is now presenting with chest pain and congestive heart failure. The PET study was performed to determine whether or not the patient had viable myocardium and would benefit from revascularization.

The PET studies showed a moderately enlarged left ventricle as well as a blood-flow metabolism mismatch in the mid- and distal anterior, anterolateral, inferolateral, and apical regions. This finding is consistent with hibernating myocardium in the mid-LAD and LCX territories. Blood-flow and metabolism matches are present throughout the inferior and inferoseptal segments of the RCA territory.

Conclusion: The PET scan offered convincing evidence of myocardial viability affecting a relatively large fraction of the ventricular myocardium. Accordingly, the patient underwent coronary angiography followed by coronary artery bypass grafting.

Severity of Angiographic Stenosis and PET Findings

The following examples depict a comparison of the noninvasively obtained images of myocardial blood flow at rest and during pharmacologic stress to the angiographically demonstrated luminal area stenosis. In these studies, myocardial blood flow was measured noninvasively at rest and during pharmacologic stress with intravenous ^{13}N ammonia, dynamic PET imaging, generation of time-activity curves, and use of a two-compartment tracer kinetic model.[1] Myocardial flow reserve represents the ratio of hyperemic to rest myocardial blood flow. The flow reserve declines progressively with increasingly severe coronary stenosis.

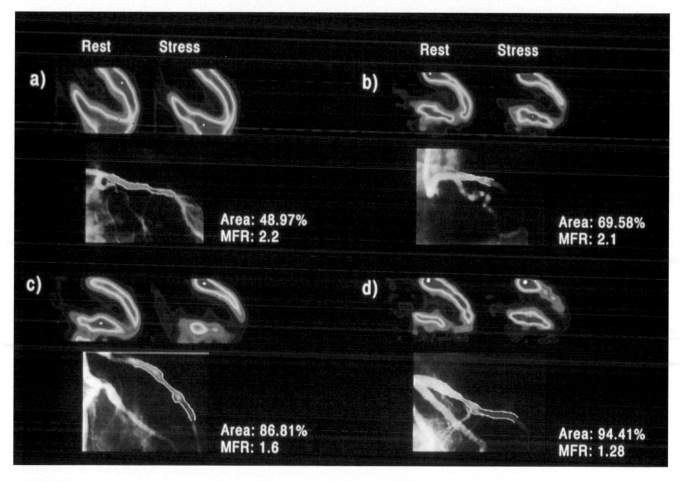

FIGURE 8-31 *a* through *d*   **These images demonstrate the progressive severity of stenosis in the LAD (48.97, 69.58, 86.81, and 94.41 percent) seen in the angiography. Note that in the corresponding PET scans, myocardial flow reserve declined (2.2, 2.1, 1.6, and 1.28).**

Conclusion: Positron emission tomography is a diagnostic method that can quantify the effects of coronary stenosis on blood flow in the dependent myocardium and, conversely, can serve as an indicator of stenosis severity.

REFERENCES

1. Porenta G: Positron emission tomography: Physics, instrumentation, and image analysis. *Wien Klin Wochenschr* 1994; 106/15:466–477.

2. Czernin J, Schelbert HR: Non-invasive quantification of myocardial blood flow and flow reserve using dynamic positron emission tomography. *Wien Klin Wochenschr* 1994; 106/15:478–486.

3. Go RT, Marwick TH, MacIntyre WJ, et al: A prospective comparison of rubidium-82 PET and thallium-201 SPECT myocardial perfusion imaging utilizing a single dipyridamole stress in the diagnosis of coronary artery disease. *J Nucl Med* 1990; 31:1899–1905.

4. Demer LL, Gould KL, Goldstein RA, et al: Assessment of coronary artery disease severity by positron emission tomography. Comparison with quantitative arteriography in 193 patients. *Circulation* 1989; 79:825–35.

5. Di Carli MF, Davidson M, Little R, et al: Value of metabolic imaging with positron emission tomography for evaluating prognosis in patients with coronary artery disease and left ventricular dysfunction. *Am J Cardiol* 1994; 73:527–533.

6. Tillisch J, Brunken R, Marshall R, et al: Reversibility of cardiac wall motion abnormalities predicted by positron tomography. *N Engl J Med* 1986; 314:884–888.

7. Tamaki N, Yonekura Y, Yamashita K, et al: Positron emission tomography using fluorine-18 deoxyglucose in evaluation of coronary artery bypass grafting. *Am J Cardiol* 1989; 64:860-865.

8. Porenta G, Kuhle W, Czernin J, et al: Semiquantitative assessment of myocardial blood flow and viability using polar map displays of cardiac PET images. *J Nucl Med* 1992; 33:1623–1631.

CHAPTER 9

CORONARY INTRAVASCULAR ULTRASOUND

Steven E. Nissen, M.D.

E. Murat Tuzcu, M.D.

Anthony De Franco, M.D.

FOR more than 35 years, contrast angiography has been the principal imaging modality used to assess the anatomic severity of coronary artery disease. Although angiography remains essential to diagnostic and interventional catheterization, coronary intravascular ultrasound provides the first practical alternative for clinical decision making.[1–11] The tomographic orientation of ultrasound visualizes lesions from a unique cross-sectional perspective. This alternative point of view provides incremental diagnostic information to confirm, deny, or supplement angiographic findings. Unlike angiography, ultrasound permits imaging of the soft tissues that comprise the vessel wall. Accordingly, intravascular imaging at the time of catheterization can characterize atheroma size, distribution, and composition. For percutaneous revascularization, ultrasound findings can be used to select interventional devices and assess the results of the procedure.

Catheter Features

Two dissimilar technical approaches to transducer design are currently employed—mechanically rotated devices and multielement electronic arrays.[1,2] Coronary intravascular imaging devices typically operate at ultrasound frequencies from 20 to 30 MHz. Recent technological progress has yielded a new generation of smaller devices,

2.9 to 3.5 Fr (0.96 to 1.17 mm) in diameter. Despite their small size, the most recent ultrasound transducers offer greatly improved image quality and improved mechanical properties. To facilitate subselective coronary cannulation, modern ultrasound catheters provide a lumen for a movable guide wire, usually a monorail design, to allow for easier catheter exchanges.

Artifacts and Limitations

Current intravascular ultrasound devices generate artifacts that may adversely affect image quality. Mechanical transducers may exhibit cyclical oscillations in rotational speed, known as nonuniform rotational distortion (NURD), which produces circumferential "stretching" of a portion of the image with compression of the contralateral vessel wall (Fig. 9-1). The severity of NURD has steadily decreased as manufacturers have improved the design of imaging catheters. All intravascular imaging systems are vulnerable to geometric distortion produced by oblique imaging, which can confound quantitative measurements. Ultrasound relies upon differences in the acoustic impedance of tissues to obtain imaging signals. Consequently, ultrasound can delineate the thickness and echogenicity of vessel wall structures but cannot provide actual histology.

Safety of Coronary Ultrasound

Although intravascular ultrasound requires intracoronary instrumentation, there are few serious untoward effects.[6] Transient spasm occurs in about 5 percent of patients but responds rapidly to administration of intracoronary nitroglycerin. The imaging transducer can occlude the coronary artery when it is advanced into tight stenoses or small vessels, but patients generally do not experience chest pain if the catheter is promptly withdrawn. Most experienced practitioners administer heparin (5000 to 10,000 U) prior to imaging; however, there are no prospective trials examining the necessity for anticoagulation. Despite the relative safety of intravascular ultrasound, any intracoronary instrumentation carries the risk of intimal injury or acute vessel dissection.

CORONARY MORPHOLOGY

Normal Anatomy

Studies report a distinctly laminar appearance to the normal vessel wall in many but not all normals[6,7] (Fig. 9-2). In some normal subjects, ultrasound reveals a discrete linear reflectance at the acoustic interface between the lumen and intima. However, other normal subjects exhibit an intimal leading edge that reflects ultrasound poorly, a phenomenon that leads to *dropout* of ultrasound signals. Thus, distinct laminations of the vessel wall are absent in about half of the normal coronary sites, particularly in younger normals (age below 30). In normal subjects with a distinct intimal leading edge, the maximum intimal thickness averages approximately 0.15 ± 0.07 mm, with most investigators considering an upper limit of normal as 0.25 to 0.30 mm.

Atherosclerotic Plaque Morphology

Coronary atherosclerotic plaques appear as variably echogenic intraluminal encroachments overlying a thin, sonolucent subintimal band representing the media[4–6] (Figs. 9-3 to 9-18). Atheromata less echogenic than the adventitia are commonly described as "soft" plaques because in vitro studies demonstrate a high lipid content. Soft atheromata range widely in echogenicity from plaques nearly as sonolucent as blood to more echogenic, highly textured lesions (Figs. 9-3 to 9-5). In tissues with a highly echogenic appearance, in vitro studies indicate the presence of significant fibrosis. Thus, plaques exhibiting more specular acoustic properties contain more fibrosis, whereas more sonolucent lesions contain greater lipid content. In the most extreme examples of plaque echogenicity, a dense lesion attenuates transmission of ultrasound, obscuring underlying structures (Fig. 9-6). Studies demonstrate that calcium is present in these lesions, which completely impedes the penetration of ultrasound. The lumen is primarily sonolucent, particularly when imaged using low-frequency intravascular devices (less than 20 MHz). Higher-frequency transducers (greater than 25 MHz) yield images with a distinctive faint, swirling pattern with finely textured echogenicity. The smokelike appearance of moving blood can prove invaluable in identifying vessel wall structures that communicate with the lumen.

DIAGNOSTIC APPLICATIONS

Angiographically Unrecognized Disease

In diagnostic or therapeutic catheterization, ultrasound commonly detects atherosclerotic abnormalities at angiographically normal sites, confirming the finding, previously noted in necropsy studies, that coronary disease is more extensive than apparent by radiography (Figs. 9-7 and 9-8). With the appearance of the first luminal irregularity, virtually the entirety of the coronary arterial tree exhibits abnormal intimal thickness by ultrasound. Several phenomena explain the greater sensitivity of ultrasound in the detection of atherosclerosis. Angiography relies upon luminal encroachment to identify diseased sites. However, in some cases, adventitial enlargement compensates for luminal encroachment by the atheroma, thus concealing the disease[12] (Fig. 9-8). Diffuse concentric atherosclerosis also represents a challenging problem for the angiographer because the entire vessel is reduced in caliber with no focal stenosis (Fig. 9-9). Patients with characteristic symptoms but "normal angiography" constitute a common and perplexing subgroup. Ultrasound will demonstrate coronary atherosclerosis in many of these patients, which can result in major alterations in therapy.

Assessment of Lesions of Uncertain Severity

Despite thorough radiographic imaging using multiple projections, angiographers commonly encounter lesions of uncertain severity in symptomatic patients. Other problematic coronary lesions include ostial stenoses of the right and left main coronaries, lesions at bifurcations, and stenoses visualized well in only a single angiographic projection. Intravascular ultrasound can frequently clarify the extent and severity of intermediate lesions, enabling quantitation of cross-sectional area independent of the radiographic projection.

Transplant Vasculopathy

Coronary vasculopathy remains the leading cause of late death following cardiac transplantation. Although most transplant programs perform annual arteriography, studies have documented a high prevalence of false-negative examinations. The inability to detect early transplant vasculopathy has impeded development of effective treatment strategies. Necropsy studies have emphasized that transplant recipients develop diffuse, concentric disease, involving both the proximal and distal vessels. The diffuse nature of vasculopathy confounds angiographic detection, because coronary segments contain no discrete luminal narrowing. Intravascular ultrasound, because of its tomographic orientation, enables early identification of intimal thickening in such patients. In the largest transplant centers, intravascular ultrasound has recently emerged as the "gold standard" for early detection of vasculopathy.[11]

INTERVENTIONAL APPLICATIONS

Quantitative Luminal Measurements

Many therapeutic decisions hinge upon assessment of coronary luminal dimensions. Studies have validated the accuracy of ultrasound luminal measurements in comparisons with quantitative angiography.[3,5,6] In normal vessels with a circular cross-sectional profile, ultrasound and angiographic measurements of lumen size correlate closely. In patients with atherosclerotic arteries, however, studies report only a moderate correlation between ultrasonic and angiographic dimensions, with the greatest disparities in atherosclerotic vessel segments with a noncircular lumen shape. The reduced correlation for diseased vessels almost certainly results from the inability of angiography to depict accurately the complex, irregular cross-sectional profile of atherosclerotic arteries.

The differences between ultrasound and angiography observed in eccentrically diseased coronaries have important implications for the assessment of lumen dimensions following angioplasty. Both ultrasound and necropsy studies illustrate that mechanical coronary revascularization, particularly balloon angioplasty, distorts the vessel wall, producing complex fractures or dissections within the intima, media, or adventitia. In this setting, measurements of the angiographic silhouette of the lumen predictably exhibit a relatively poor correlation with dimensions obtained by a tomographic method. In studies of residual stenosis after percutaneous transluminal coronary angioplasty, analysis of angiographic and ultrasonic measurements of diameter reveal a limited correlation, in the range of $r = .40$ to $.60$.

Morphology following Angioplasty

Intravascular ultrasound demonstrates a spectrum of morphologic findings following balloon angioplasty, including complex fractures or dissections in the vessel wall[5,6,8] (Figs. 9-10 to 9-13). The extreme distortion of lumen shape produced by balloon dilatation represents the most adverse environment for angiographic quantitation. Theoretically, extravasation of contrast through narrow dissection channels within the intima, media, or adventitia of the vessel can enhance the apparent angiographic diameter of the vessel (Figs. 9-10 and 9-11). In this setting, the angiographic appearance consists of a large but "hazy" lumen, in which intravascular ultrasound reveals minimal balloon augmentation of lumen size.

In some patients, intimal fracture constitutes the sole or principal mechanism responsible for luminal enlargement. The typical site of dissection occurs at the junction between hard and soft plaque elements. Ultrasound can readily determine the depth of the dissection, from superficial intimal disruption to extensive periadventitial tears (Fig. 9-10). In other cases, stretching of the vessel wall constitutes the sole mechanism responsible for the luminal gain (Fig. 9-12). Luminal enlargement can also result primarily from an apparent reduction in the cross-sectional area of the plaque (Fig. 9-13). Whether this phenomenon represents true plaque compression or simply axial redistribution of atheroma remains controversial. A potentially important morphologic feature, the presence or absence of thrombus, has thus far eluded accurate ultrasound characterization. The acoustic properties of intraluminal thrombus are similar to those of blood—a phenomenon that makes it difficult to identify thrombi with certainty. Several ongoing studies are examining the relationship between the mechanisms of luminal enlargement and long-term clinical outcome.

New Interventional Devices

The development of non-balloon revascularization devices has enhanced the clinical value of intracoronary ultrasound, particularly for the two widely used plaque removal techniques, directional atherectomy and rotablation[9] (Figs. 9-14 to 9-17). The reduced profile of catheters enables routine imaging of target lesions prior to treatment, which makes it possible to study the relationship between plaque morphology and clinical outcome. These examinations are enabling a novel interventional strategy in which plaque characteristics assist in the selection of the optimal type and size of revascularization device. Although this strategy has not yet withstood rigorous prospective clinical trials, the potential advantages of a lesion-specific approach are self-evident.

Directional Atherectomy

Most clinicians regard the location and distribution of the atheroma as important factors in the selection of patients for directional atherectomy. Initial angiographic studies suggested that eccentric plaque would represent the optimal target for atherectomy. Recent studies, however, have shown that the apparent distribution of the atheroma by angiography correlates poorly with plaque location by intravascular ultrasound (Fig. 9-14). Accordingly, lesions that appear concentric by angiography are often eccentric by ultrasound, and, conversely, angiographically eccentric lesions are frequently concentric by ultrasound. The poor correlation for plaque distribution probably reflects the disadvantages of a silhouette imaging method (angiography) as compared with a tomographic imaging technique (ultrasound).

In ultrasound-guided atherectomy, plaque distribution determines the device size and the orientation of atherectomy cuts (Fig. 9-15). Successful application of this approach, however, requires experience, patience, and careful planning. Although ultrasound provides an excellent view of the circumferential distribution of plaque, precise orientation of the image remains difficult. Experienced practitioners carefully examine the target segment prior to atherectomy to locate anatomic landmarks, particularly side branches to orient the intravascular image. For example, an eccentric plaque in the left anterior descending artery can be described as contralateral or ipsilateral to septal perforators. Using this information, the operator subsequently direct cuts toward the appropriate side of the vessel. Traditionally, significant fluoroscopic calcification has consituted a contraindication to atherectomy. Ultrasound, however, demonstrates calcification more frequently than fluoroscopy and can readily determine the circumferential location and depth of calcification. Vessels with extensive superficial calcification resist plaque removal by directional atherectomy, but arteries with extensive deep calcification can undergo successful atherectomy.

Rotational Ablation

Although experience remains limited, intravascular ultrasound can significantly benefit clinical application of the Rotoblator, a high-speed diamond-coated burr for percutaneous revascularization. This device is particularly effective at removing superficial intimal calcium, precisely the type of lesion least suitable for directional coronary atherectomy. Intravascular ultrasound determination of the location and extent of calcification enables differentiation of lesions most suitable for rotablation from vessels more suitable for directional atherectomy (Fig. 9-16). Precise vessel sizing provided by ultrasound facilitates selection of the appropraitely sized burr for rotablation.

Coronary Stenting

The importance of coronary stenting has increased following publication of data demonstrating a reduction in the risk of restenosis with this therapy. Studies show an increased risk of hemorrhagic complications following stenting, however, presumably secondary to the aggressive anticoagulation and large sheath sizes. Recent ultrasound studies have demonstrated failure to fully deploy coronary stents in a significant subset of patients when the procedure is guided solely by angiography (Fig. 9-17). Presumably, the porous nature of these stents results in the angiographic appearance of an enlarged lumen, although some stent struts are not fully apposed to the vessel wall. Several preliminary studies in which ultrasound was employed to assist stent deployment have reported a low stent thrombosis rate without vigorous anticoagulation. This approach will require careful testing through prospective randomized trials.

Future Directions

Industry engineers anticipate further reductions in the size of catheters and a 0.018-in. (0.457-mm) imaging guide wire is undergoing initial testing. A guide-wire-sized ultrasound probe would enable simultaneous imaging during many revascularization procedures. Several investigators have demonstrated three-dimensional reconstruction of ultrasound images, but artifacts and other limitations have precluded any practical application of this technique. Combination devices incorporating both diagnostic imaging and therapeutic capability are under development, and an angioplasty balloon incorporating an ultrasound transducer has been recently approved by the Food and Drug Administration.

SUMMARY

Recent advances in technology have permitted the development of miniaturized ultrasound devices capable of real-time intravascular imaging. This modality provides unique, detailed cross-sectional images of the arterial wall not previously obtainable in vivo by any other technique. Initial studies have successfully employed ultrasound to augment angiography in diagnostic and therapeutic catheterization. The cross-sectional perspective appears ideally suited for measurements of luminal dimensions. Ultrasound is more sensitive than angiography in the detection of atherosclerosis and may prove valuable in quantifying progression or regression.

For interventional applications, ultrasound analysis offers many potential advantages. Post-procedure, intravascular ultrasound often yields smaller luminal measurements than angiography. These differences probably reflect augmentation of the "apparent" angiographic diameter by extraluminal contrast within cracks, fissures, or dissection planes. New ultrasound instruments under development combine an imaging transducer with an interventional device, permitting on-line guidance during the procedure. The clinical value of routine ultrasound imaging following mechanical revascularization has not been tested by randomized trials. It seems likely, however, that the morphology following interventions will provide valuable insights into phenomena such as restenosis and abrupt occlusion (Fig. 9-18).

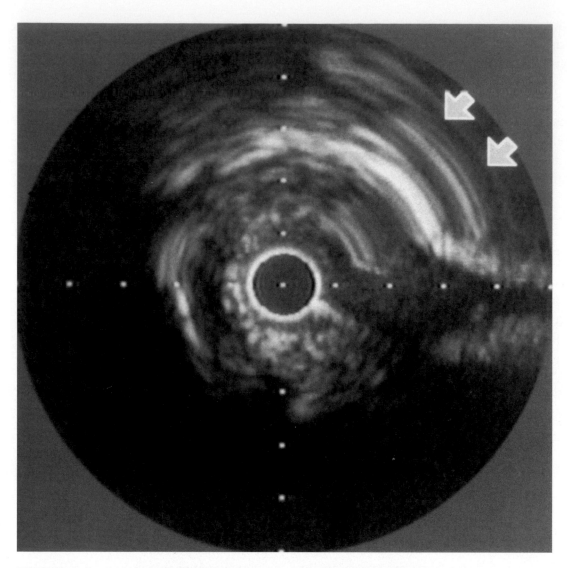

FIGURE 9-1   A common intravascular ultrasound artifact, nonuniform rotational distortion (NURD). This artifact is generated when the speed of a mechanical transducer varies excessively during rotation. This phenomenon causes a "stretching" of the image during a portion of the rotational cycle (*arrows*) with "compression" of the image in the contralateral side. Reducing the rotational speed of the transducer can often eliminate this artifact if it is clearly recognized.

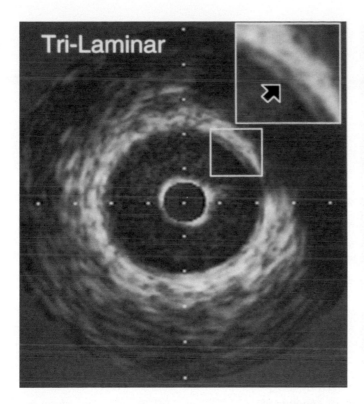
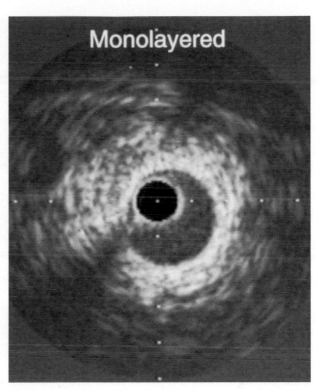

FIGURE 9-2 Two patterns of normal coronary anatomy as visualized by intravascular ultrasound. The left panel illustrates a normal coronary artery with a trilaminar structure and a portion of the wall enlarged to show structural detail. The arrow indicates a distinct intimal leading edge with a subintimal sonolucent zone. Available data indicate that the intimal leading edge echo represents the internal elastic lamina and the sonolucent zone the media of the vessel. In the right panel, a slightly different normal variant exhibits an intimal thickness and acoustic impedance that are sufficiently low that no distinct trilaminar structure is evident. Both examples represent typical normal vessels.

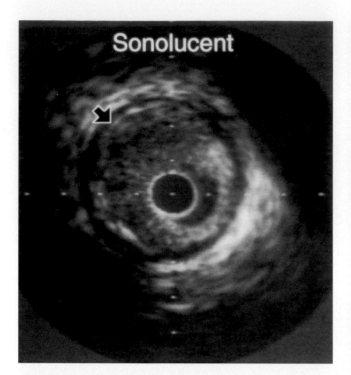 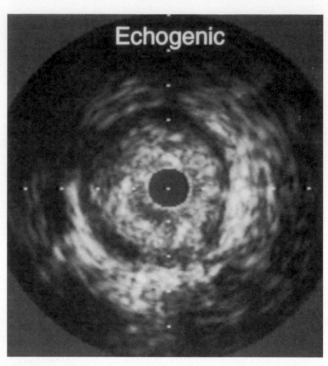

FIGURE 9-3   Two examples of atherosclerotic lesions imaged by intravascular ultrasound. In the left panel, the plaque is primarily sonolucent *(arrow),* which available data demonstrate to be lipid rich. The media is observed as a circumferential sonolucent band deep to the plaque. The lumen of this vessel is quite small, with the intravascular ultrasound catheter occupying about two-thirds of it. The right panel illustrates a more echogenic "hard" plaque, with an average acoustic intensity nearly equivalent to that of the adventitia. The lumen is severely reduced in size and entirely occupied by the intravascular ultrasound catheter.

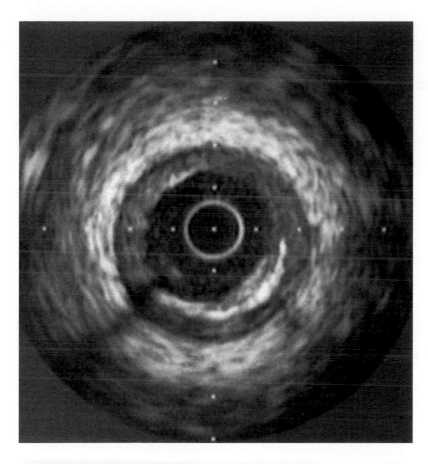

FIGURE 9-4 Mixed coronary plaque.
In this image, a circumferential plaque
distribution is evident with the intima
thickened to approximately 1 mm. There
is some variability in plaque echogenicity,
with a dense portion from 3 to 7 o'clock
and a sonolucent portion throughout the
rest of the circumference.

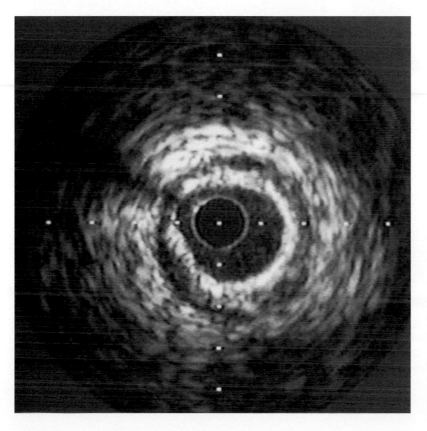

**FIGURE 9-5 Circumferential coronary
disease with a distinct fibrous cap.** In this
vessel, a highly echogenic intimal leading
edge is thickened to approximately 0.4 mm.
In vitro studies have demonstrated that
such structures represent well-formed
fibrous caps, in this case overlying a
relatively soft, sonolucent lesion. The
echo distinction between the media and
sonolucent plaque is indistinct in this case,
precluding definite indentification of each
layer.

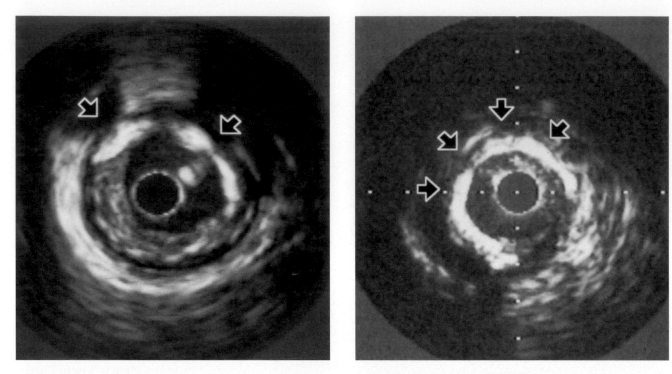

FIGURE 9-6   Calcified coronary atheromata. In both examples, the arrows indicate dense echogenic plaques that obstruct penetration of ultrasound, thus shadowing underlying structures.

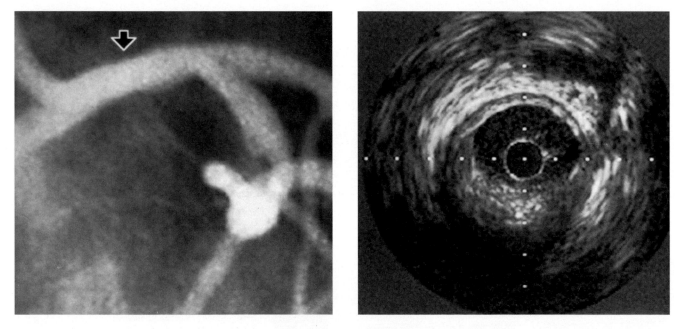

FIGURE 9-7   Angiographically unrecognized left main coronary artery disease. In the angiographic frame, the intravascular ultrasound imaging site is indicated by the arrow. The ultrasound shows a large crescent-shaped atheroma from 3 to 9 o'clock, which occupies between 40 and 50 percent of the lumen area. Such lesions are commonly observed at angiographically normal sites by intravascular ultrasound.

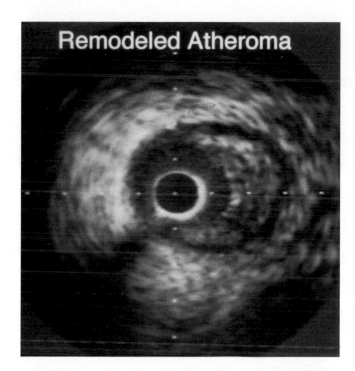
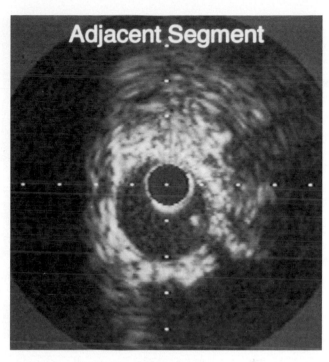

FIGURE 9-8   **The phenomenon of coronary remodeling. Originally described by Glagov et al.,[12] atherosclerosis commonly results in outward remodeling of the adventitia, which accommodates the atheroma, thus preserving lumen size. In the left frame, a large crescent-shaped atheroma is evident from 12 to 6 o'clock. However, in this remodeled artery, the adventitia has extended outward, preserving the lumen size. In the right panel, an adjacent segment is free from atherosclerotic disease. However, the lumen size for the adjacent segment is virtually identical to the atherosclerotic segment. Accordingly, the angiogram failed to reveal any narrowing.**

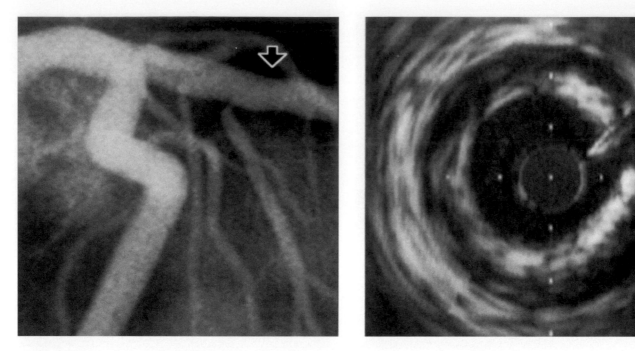

FIGURE 9-9   Circumferential coronary disease with a minimally abnormal angiogram. The intravascular ultrasound imaging site is indicated by the arrow. Despite a nearly normal angiogram, there is a concentric atheroma with a well-formed fibrous cap. The radial echogenic structure extending from the catheter at approximately 2 o'clock represents the shadow from a 0.014-in. guide wire.

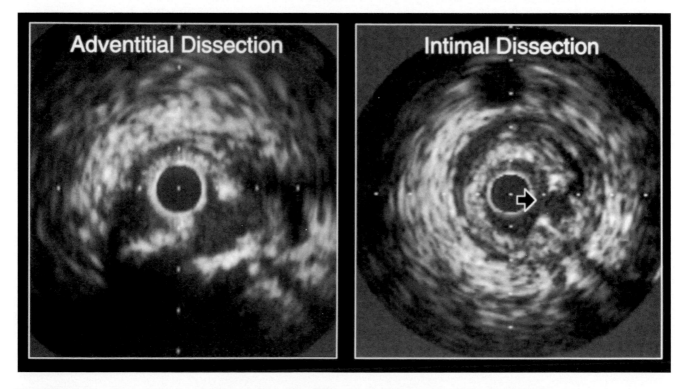

FIGURE 9-10   Two examples of arterial dissection following balloon angioplasty. In the left panel, a dissection (entry site at 3 o'clock) extends into the adventitia with a curving path. In the right panel, an intimal dissection *(arrow)* has split the plaque but does not extend to the level of the media.

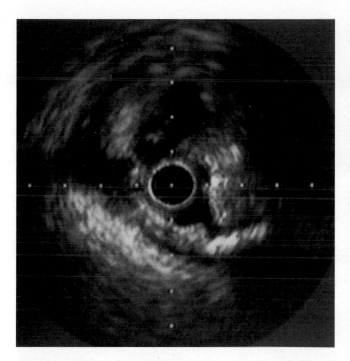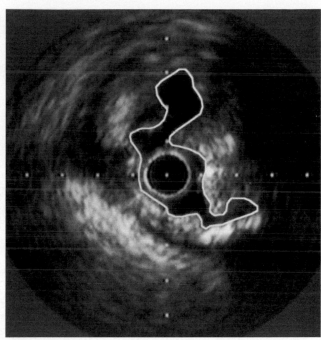

FIGURE 9-11   Complex coronary dissection following balloon angioplasty. There is a complex luminal shape following balloon angioplasty. In the right panel, the luminal border has been traced manually to illustrate the extraordinary irregularity of its shape.

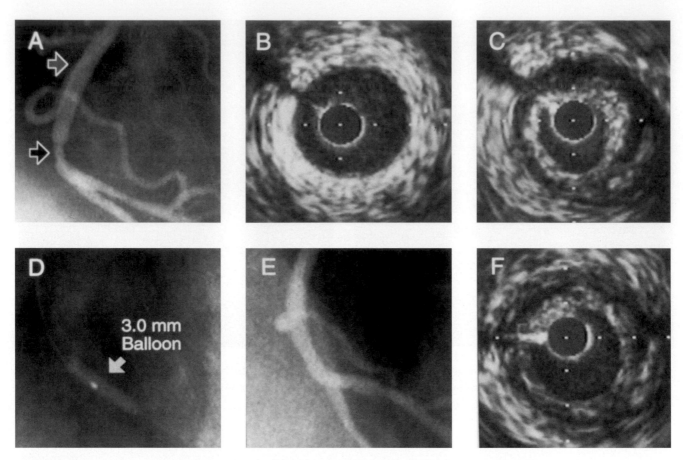

FIGURE 9-12   Balloon angioplasty where the mechanism of vessel enlargement is primarily stretching of the media/adventitia. Panel *A* shows the lesion by angiography prior to dilation. Ultrasound at the reference segment *(gray arrow)* is illustrated in panel *B* and shows no atherosclerosis. The target lesion *(black arrow* in panel *A)* is illustrated in panel *C*. This shows a circumferential plaque with a moderate degree of stenosis. In panel *D*, a 3.0-mm balloon is shown inflating, and in panel *E*, the final angiographic result is illustrated. In panel *F*, the postprocedure intravascular ultrasound shows moderate enlargement of the lumen, where the principal mechanism of luminal enlargement is stretching of the media-adventitia border. Preliminary data indicate that such methods of luminal enlargement may produce only transient benefit.

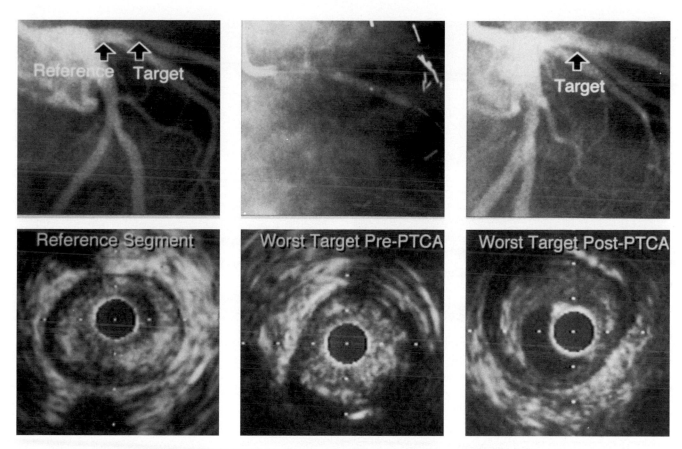

FIGURE 9-13   Angiography and intravascular ultrasound before and after balloon angioplasty. In the upper left frame, the angiogram shows the target lesion and an adjacent reference segment. Surprisingly, the ultrasound imaging within the reference segment *(bottom left)* shows extensive, severe atherosclerosis. In the bottom middle frame, ultrasound at the worst target lesion is illustrated, showing a severely obstructive lesion that is circumferential in distribution. At the upper right, the angiogram following the procedure shows an excellent result. In the bottom right panel, intravascular ultrasound after the procedure shows moderate luminal enlargement, but with significant residual plaque burden.

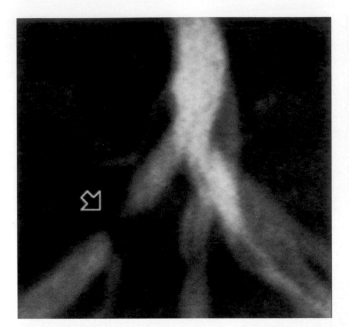
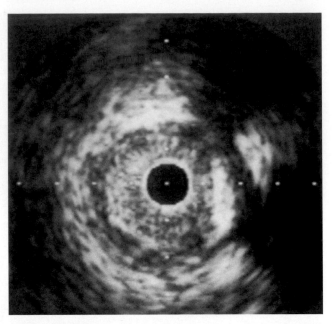

FIGURE 9-14 Differences between angiography and intravascular ultrasound in assessment of lesion eccentricity. In the left panel, the lesion *(arrow)* appears highly eccentric by angiography. In the right panel, intravascular ultrasound of the same site shows nearly circumferential plaque distribution. Systematic studies have revealed that intravascular ultrasound frequently disagrees with angiography in classifying plaque distribution.

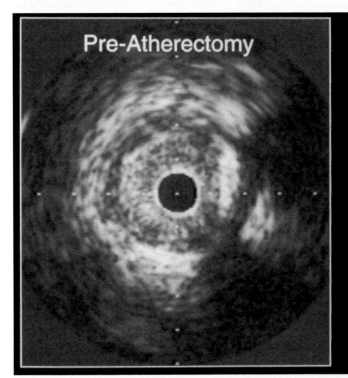
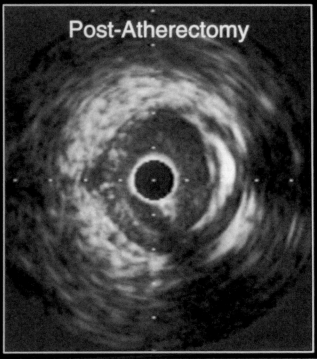

FIGURE 9-15 Intravascular ultrasound before and after directional coronary atherectomy in the same patient as illustrated in Fig. 9-14. Based upon the plaque distribution findings by intravascular ultrasound, the operator-directed atherectomy cuts around the 360° circumference of the vessel. This approach achieved excellent debulking of plaque, which is illustrated in the postatherectomy image *(right panel).*

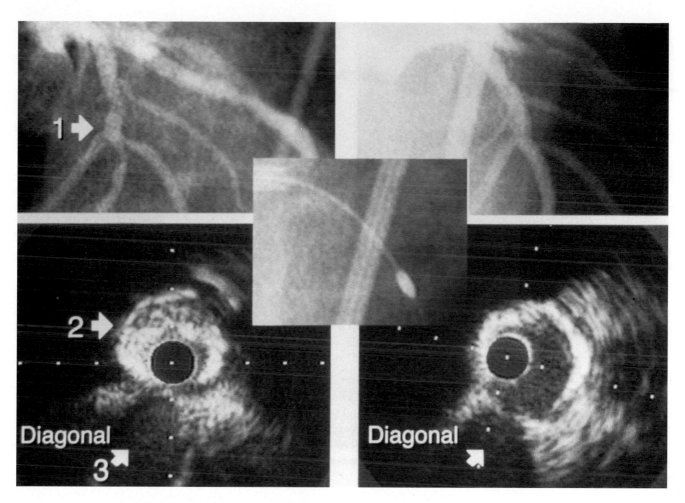

FIGURE 9-16   Angiography and intravascular ultrasound before and after rotational ablation. In the upper left panel (site 1), angiography reveals a moderate lesion involving the circumflex coronary artery. In the center image, angiography illustrates the use of the Rotoblator with a burr size of 2.25 mm. In the upper right panel, the angiographic image shows improvement following treatment. The lower left image shows a dense calcified lesion before intervention (site 2), with a lumen nearly completely occupied by the intravascular ultrasound catheter. A diagonal branch adjacent to the stenosis is identified (site 3). In the bottom right panel, after rotational ablation, a lumen approximately the size of the Rotoblator burr has been achieved, approximately 2.2 mm.

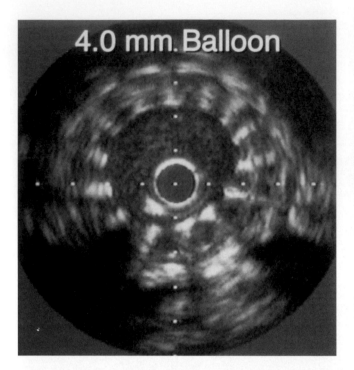
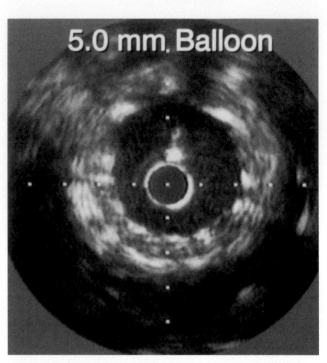

FIGURE 9-17   Intravascular ultrasound following deployment of a Palmaz-Schatz stent. In the left frame, following inflations with a 4.0-mm balloon, several struts (from 3 to 7 o'clock) are not fully apposed to the vessel wall. Although the angiogram showed apparently excellent results, the operator performed additional inflations with a 5.0-mm balloon, which yielded complete apposition of the stent struts to the vessel wall. Available data indicate that adequate deployment of stents is vital to achieving good long-term results without abrupt vessel occlusion due to thrombosis.

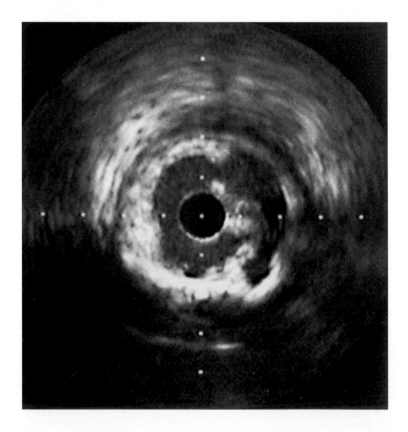

FIGURE 9-18   Example of atheroma morphology in a patient with an acute coronary syndrome. In this example, the patient presented with unstable angina and was treated for 5 to 7 days with aspirin/heparin and antianginal drug therapy. Subsequently, angiography showed an ulcerated coronary lesion. In the intravascular ultrasound image, the catheter is lying in the "true lumen." A secondary lumen from 12 to 5 o'clock is also evident. There is an opening connecting these two lumens at approximately 12 o'clock. Available evidence suggests that the secondary lumen from 1 to 5 o'clock represents a ruptured coronary plaque, which was subsequently recanalized after acute therapy.

REFERENCES

1. Bom N, Lancee CT, Van Egmond FC: An ultrasonic intracardiac scanner. *Ultrasonics* 1972; 10:72–76.
2. Yock PC, Johnson EL, Linker DT: Intravascular ultrasound: Development and clinical potential. *Am J Cardiac Imaging* 1988; 2:185–193.
3. Nissen SE, Grines CL, Gurley JC, et al: Application of a new phased-array ultrasound imaging catheter in the assessment of vascular dimensions: In vivo comparison to cineangiography. *Circulation* 1990; 81:660–666.
4. Hodgson J, Graham SP, Savakus AD, et al: Clinical percutaneous imaging of coronary anatomy using an over-the-wire ultrasound catheter system. *Int J Cardiac Imaging* 1989; 4:187–193.
5. Tobis JM, Mallery J, Mahon D, et al: Intravascular ultrasound imaging of human coronary arteries in vivo: Analysis of tissue characterizations with comparison to in vitro histological specimens. *Circulation* 1991; 83: 913–926.
6. Nissen SE, Gurley JC, Grines CL, et al: Intravascular ultrasound assessment of lumen size and wall morphology in normal subjects and coronary artery disease patients. *Circulation* 1991; 84:1087–1099.
7. St. Goar FG, Pinto FJ, Alderman EL, et al: Detection of coronary atherosclerosis in young adult hearts using intravascular ultrasound. *Circulation* 1992; 86:757–763.
8. Potkin BN, Keren G, Mintz GS, et al: Arterial responses to balloon coronary angioplasty: An intravascular ultrasound study. *J Am Coll Cardiol* 1992; 20: 942–951.
9. Suarez de Lezo J, Romero M, Medina A, et al: Intracoronary ultrasound assessment of directional coronary atherectomy: Immediate and follow-up findings. *J Am Coll Cardiol* 1993: 21:298–307.
10. Fitzgerald PJ, St. Goar FG, Connolly AJ, et al: Intravascular ultrasound imaging of coronary arteries: Is three layers the norm? *Circulation* 1992; 86: 154–158,
11. Tuzcu EM, Hobbs RE, Rincon G, et al: Occult and frequent transmission of atherosclerotic coronary disease with cardiac transplantation. *Circulation* 1995; 91:1706–1713.
12. Glagov S, Weisenberg E, Zarins CK, et al: Compensatory enlargement of human coronary arteries. *N Engl J Med* 1987; 316:1371–1375.

CHAPTER 10

DISEASES OF THE AORTA

Joseph Lindsay, Jr., M.D.

Steven A. Goldstein, M.D.

Bart L. Dolmatch, M.D.

"[WE limit] our pictures of nature to the kinds that can be understood by our minds. As we cannot draw one perfect picture, we make two imperfect pictures and turn to one or the other according as we want one property or the other to be accurately delineated. Our observations tell us which is the right picture to use for each particular purpose. . . ."[1]

Until very recently images of the aorta were provided only by standard radiographs and contrast aortography. The former provides sometimes important but limited information. The silhouette of the aorta may be seen in areas in which it abuts lung, and calcium deposits in its wall may be identified. Aortography provides a "luminogram" of the interior of the aorta. Although frequently important for diagnosis, the procedure is invasive and carries attendant risks. Further, it is a static image and provides little or no information regarding the aortic wall. Finally, details may be obscured by the column of contrast agent.

The development of computed tomography (CT) provided an important advance. With this technique, the radiologist may manipulate the relative contrast of the x-ray image and can reformat the images into tomographic slices. Far less invasive than aortography and far more informative than plain films, CT is, nevertheless, also limited. It provides little information about the aortic wall and produces only static images (see also "Electron Beam Computed Tomography (EBCT)," Chap. 7).

The two newest imaging modalities to be directed at aortic disease, transesophageal echocardiography (TEE) and magnetic resonance imaging (MRI), overcome many of the shortcomings of the three x-ray techniques. They add information that extends our knowledge of the appearance and pathogenesis of aortic disease. Both are noninvasive.

Now that an ultrasound transducer can be placed on an endoscope and positioned in the esophagus in proximity to the heart and descending aorta, many of the shortcomings of ultrasound for aortic imaging have been overcome. The TEE technique is safe, convenient, and reliable in even the sickest patient. Indeed, there are few contraindications to TEE. It can be employed in the operating room, in the emergency department, or in the intensive care unit. It has several additional advantages for imaging the aorta: it provides pictures of the aortic wall and its luminal surface and can demonstrate motion. Color-flow Doppler imaging indicates the direction and relative velocity of blood flow in the lumen or in connecting structures.

In addition to providing images of the aortic lumen with astonishing clarity, MRI provides quite detailed information about the composition of the aortic wall. With appropriate techniques, the flow of blood can be delineated as cine techniques become ever more useful. Currently, MRI has limited applicability in very ill patients, since examinations can only be conducted in the "magnet," not at the bedside. Moreover, during the somewhat extended time required for the examination, the very ill patient may not be readily accessible for monitoring and nursing attention.

Using the principle attributed to Jeans in the lead paragraph of the introduction to *Diseases of the Aorta*,[1] the interested physician can now combine the insights of these two new techniques with conventional radiography, angiography, and CT to diagnose his or her patients' illnesses and to learn more about the disease states with which they are afflicted.

The illustrations included in this chapter were chosen to be examples of the application of all these techniques. We particularly chose those that make a special teaching point or provide insight into the pathologic anatomy of aortic disease. For example, two newly described variations on the theme of aortic dissection, not addressed in the eighth edition of *Hurst's The Heart*, are included. The interested reader will find a more complete discussion of the imaging of aortic disease in a recent book[1–3] authored by two of us.

AORTIC DISSECTION

Longitudinal cleavage of the elastic lamina of the aortic media by a column of blood is the defining abnormality of aortic dissection. The "false channel" created by the dissecting hematoma communicates through one or more intimal tears with the "true" aortic lumen (Figs. 10-1 through 10-4). One of these tears is almost always located near the proximal limit of the false channel. Studies with TEE and MRI have recently identified hematomas (Fig. 10-5) that split the aortic media, as do aortic dissections, but which—unlike dissections—lack intimal tears.[4,5]

AORTIC ATHEROSCLEROSIS

Atherosclerosis of the aorta accompanies aging in most individuals in the western world, but it varies in severity from subject to subject. It is accelerated by diabetes, hypercholesterolemia, hypertension, and smoking. Most severe in the infrarenal segment, aortic atherosclerosis has been most often recognized clinically by aneurysm (Fig. 10-6) or obstruction (Fig. 10-7) of that segment. Recent evidence suggests that it is too simplistic to consider atherosclerosis as the sole cause of aneurysm of the abdominal aorta.[6] Moreover, aortic atherosclerosis is—far more often than has been thought—the origin of embolic material[7] (Fig. 10-8). Recently the "penetrating" atherosclerotic plaque has been recognized as a source of medial dissection and external rupture[8] (Fig. 10-9). Such atherosclerotic damage to the aortic media may allow saccular aneurysms as well (Fig. 10-10).

MEDIAL DEGENERATION

Like atherosclerosis, medial degeneration also accompanies aging. As a consequence, the aorta becomes elongated, tortuous, and inelastic in older individuals. Severe and premature medial degeneration is the cardiovascular hallmark of Marfan's syndrome. In that disorder, aneurysmal dilatation of the proximal aorta, including the sinuses of Valsalva, is characteristic (Fig. 10-11). The resulting bulb-shaped aortic root has been termed *anuloaortic ectasia*. While characteristic of Marfan's syndrome, these aneurysms are encountered more frequently in subjects with no other manifestations of that genetic disorder. Medial degeneration may be severe enough to produce clinical disease in individuals with coarctation of the aorta, bicuspid aortic valve, polycystic kidneys, and Turner's syndrome.

AORTITIS

Nonspecific aortitis, often associated with evidence of an "autoimmune" process, has been termed *Takayasu's aortitis* (Fig. 10-12). Temporal (giant-cell) arteritis, a disorder with similar clinical and pathologic characteristics, not infrequently affects the aorta (Fig. 10-13).

Bacterial aortitis may result from direct extension of aortic valve infection to the adjacent wall (Fig. 10-14) and, less often, from spread of infection in periaortic soft tissue. Although the intact aortic intima is resistant to blood-borne infection, areas damaged by atherosclerosis or other disease may be invaded by pathogens from the bloodstream (Fig. 10-15).

CONGENITAL AORTIC MALFORMATIONS

Common congenital anomalies encountered after early childhood include aortic coarctation (Fig. 10-16) and sinus of Valsalva aneurysm (Fig. 10-17). A congenitally bicuspid aortic valve is associated with dilatation, sometimes substantial, of the proximal aorta (Fig. 10-18).

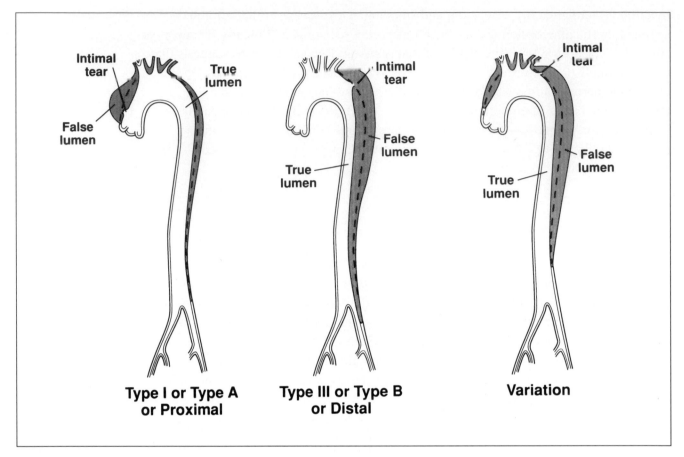

FIGURE 10-1 Artist's depiction of the three major anatomic patterns of aortic dissection. The left panel illustrates the most common variety, in which the intimal tear is located just above the aortic valve and the medial cleavage plane extends in the long axis for varying distances, often to the iliac bifurcation. The center panel illustrates the second most frequent variety. The intimal tear is located just beyond the left subclavian artery and the medial dissection extends distally. The right panel illustrates an important but relatively uncommon variation. From an intimal tear just distal to the left subclavian artery, the medial dissection extends both retrograde into the ascending segment and antegrade down the thoracic aorta. (From Lindsay J: Aortic dissection. *Heart Dis Stroke* 1992; 1:69. Reproduced with permission from the publisher and author.)

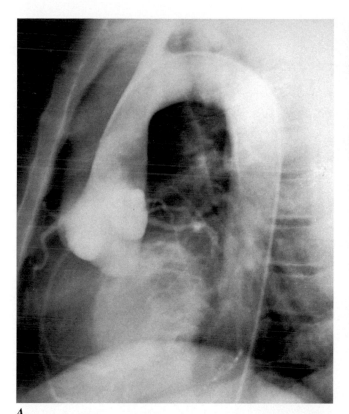

A

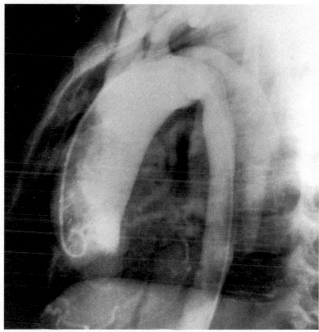

B

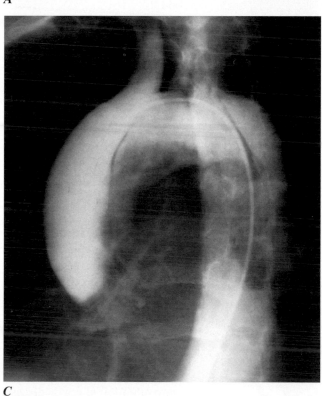

C

FIGURE 10-2   The appearance of the major varieties of aortic dissection as they appear on aortography. *A*. Dissection originates in the ascending aorta, as in the left panel of Fig. 10-1. Note the proximity of the dissection to the right coronary artery and the aortic regurgitation that results from the loss of support of the aortic valve. *B*. Dissection originates distal to the left subclavian artery, as in the center panel of Fig. 10-1. The laterally placed false channel is less well opacified than the true lumen. (From Lindsay J: Aortic dissection. *Heart Dis Stroke* 1992; 1:69. Reproduced with permission from the publisher and author.) *C*. This dissection involves both the ascending and descending aortic segments as well as the intervening arch. At surgery, the intimal tear was found to be located just distal to the left subclavian artery. This variety is represented by the right panel in Fig. 10-1. (From Lindsay J: Aortic dissection. In: Lindsay J (ed): *Diseases of the Aorta*. Philadelphia, Lea & Febiger, 1994. Reproduced with permission from the publisher and author.)

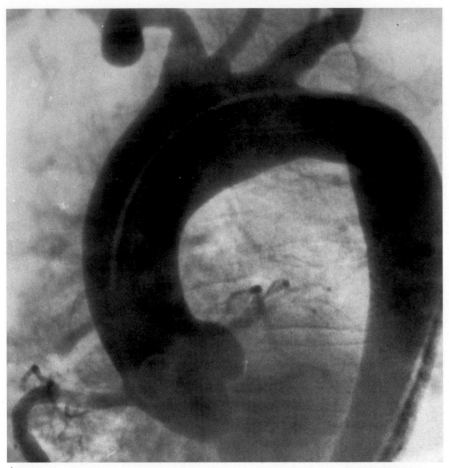

A

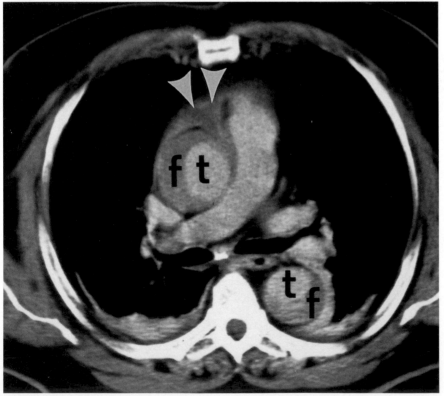

B

FIGURE 10-3   Aortography is not infallible in aortic dissection. *A.* A nondiagnostic aortogram in a patient with dissection demonstrated by CT *(B).* Arrowheads identify a small mediastinal hematoma. f = false lumen; t = true lumen. (From Dolmatch BL, Horton KM, Gray RJ, Rundback JH: Diagnostic imaging in the evaluation of aortic disease. In: Lindsay J (ed): *Diseases of the Aorta*, Philadelphia, Lea & Febiger, 1994. Reproduced with permission from the publisher and authors.) (See also Chap. 7.)

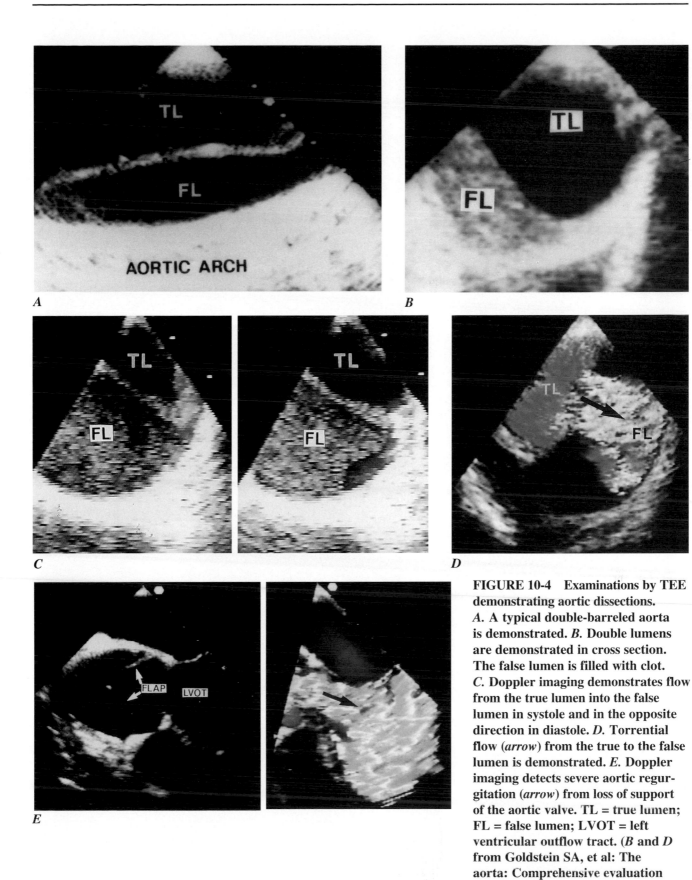

FIGURE 10-4 Examinations by TEE demonstrating aortic dissections. *A.* **A typical double-barreled aorta is demonstrated.** *B.* **Double lumens are demonstrated in cross section. The false lumen is filled with clot.** *C.* **Doppler imaging demonstrates flow from the true lumen into the false lumen in systole and in the opposite direction in diastole.** *D.* **Torrential flow (*arrow*) from the true to the false lumen is demonstrated.** *E.* **Doppler imaging detects severe aortic regurgitation (*arrow*) from loss of support of the aortic valve. TL = true lumen; FL = false lumen; LVOT = left ventricular outflow tract. (*B* and *D* from Goldstein SA, et al: The aorta: Comprehensive evaluation by echocardiography.** *J Am Soc Echocardiogr* **1993; 6:634. Reproduced with permission from the publisher and authors.)**

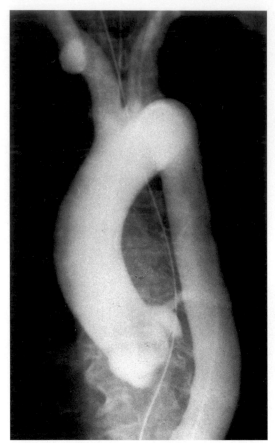

A

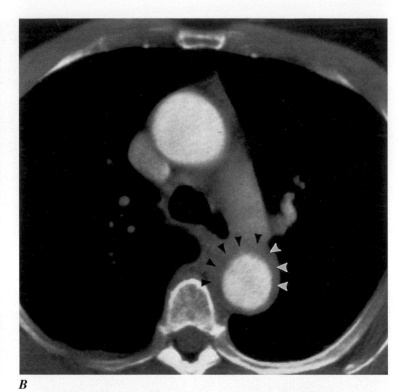

B

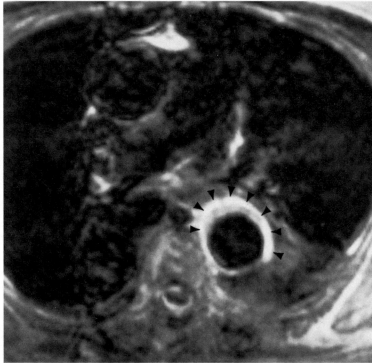

C

FIGURE 10-5   Imaging studies obtained in a patient admitted with severe back pain typical of aortic dissection. Her aortogram (*A*) was nondiagnostic. The anteromedial aortic wall was thickened (*arrowheads*) on CT (*B*), and MRI (*C*) demonstrated a high signal crescent in the medial, anterior, and lateral walls of the aorta (*arrowheads*). These findings are typical of intramural hematoma.[4,5] (From Dolmatch BL, Horton KM, Gray RJ, Rundback JH: Diagnostic imaging in the evaluation of aortic disease. In: Lindsay J (ed): *Diseases of the Aorta*. Philadelphia, Lea & Febiger, 1994. Reproduced with permission from the publisher and authors.)

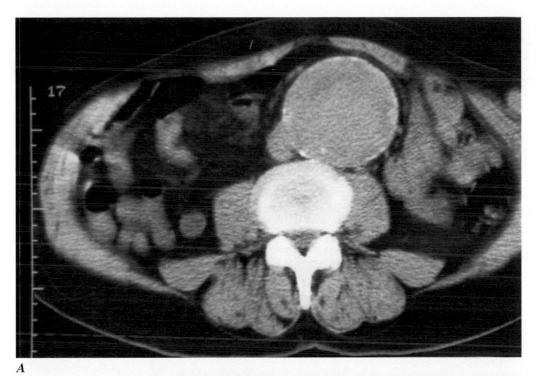

A

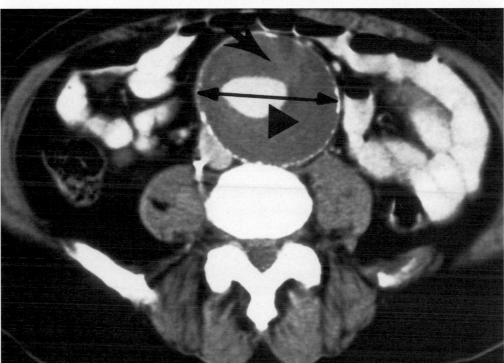

B

FIGURE 10-6   Computed tomography of the abdominal aorta demonstrates
a large (7-cm) aneurysm (*A*). Another large aneurysm (*B*) is filled with
organized thrombus, as are many of these. The arrowhead indicates the lumen,
and the double-headed arrow shows the true diameter of the aneurysm.
The organized thrombus is indicated by the arrow. (*B.* from Dolmatch BL,
Horton KM, Gray RJ, Rundbach JH: Diagnostic imaging in the evaluation of
aortic disease. In: Lindsay J (ed): *Diseases of the Aorta.* Philadelphia, Lea &
Febiger, 1994. Reproduced with permission from the publisher and authors.)
(See also Chap. 7.)

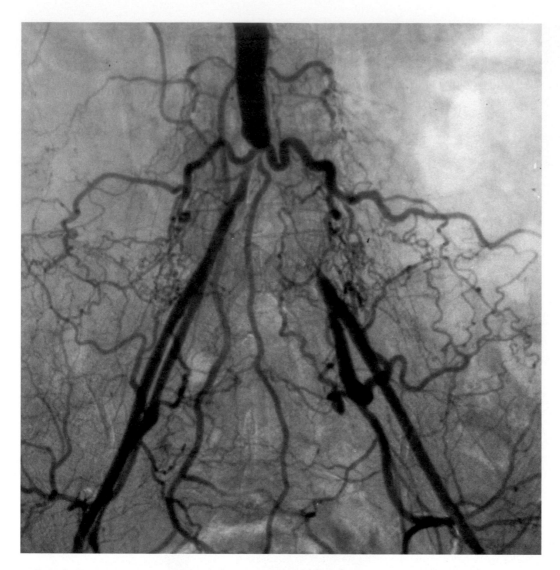

FIGURE 10-7 Arteriogram depicting severe obstruction of the terminal aorta and both iliac arteries. This represents the underlying pathoanatomy of the Leriche syndrome. (From Dolmatch BL, Horton KM, Gray RJ, Rundbach JH: Diagnostic imaging in the evaluation of aortic disease. In: Lindsay J (ed): *Diseases of the Aorta*. Philadelphia, Lea & Febiger, 1994. Reproduced with permission from the publisher and authors.)

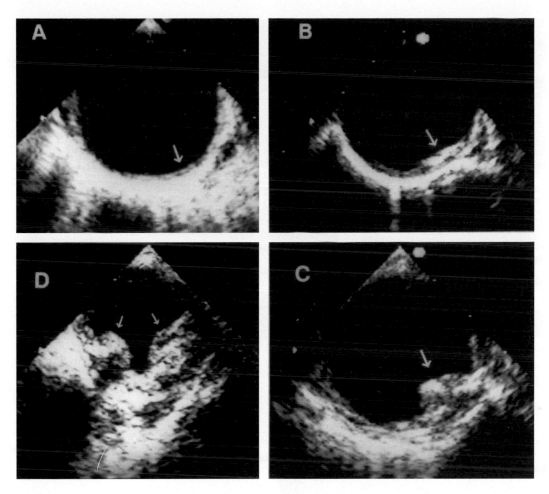

FIGURE 10-8   A TEE view of the aortas of four patients with varying degrees of atherosclerosis. The severity of the process varies from minimal (*A*; *upper left*) to severe and protruding (*D; lower left*). It has recently been recognized that such lesions represent a source of emboli to the brain and elsewhere.[7] Arrows indicate the atherosclerotic plaques.

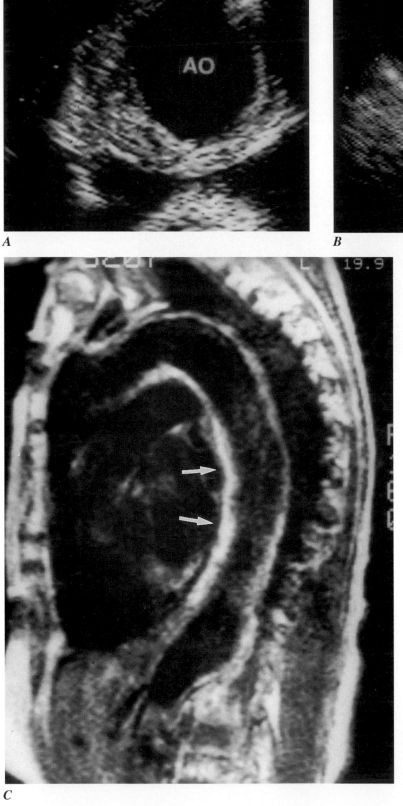

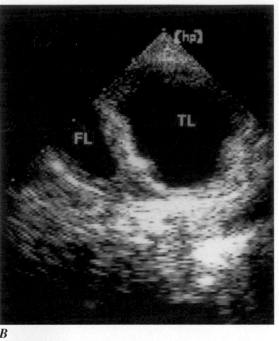

A

B

C

FIGURE 10-9 An elderly woman presented with back pain consistent with aortic dissection. An aortogram did not reveal a dissection; however, on TEE, severe atherosclerosis (*A*) and a double lumen (*B*) were demonstrated. On MRI, there was high signal density in the anterior, medial, and lateral walls of the descending thoracic aorta (*arrows*) (*C* and *D*). Necropsy examination revealed a penetrating atherosclerotic ulcer[8] (*E*, *upper left*), providing communication from the aortic lumen to a medial hematoma (*E*; *upper right and below*). AO = aortic lumen; TR = true lumen; FL = false lumen.

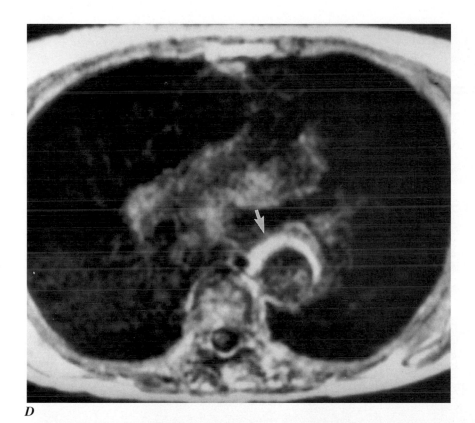

D

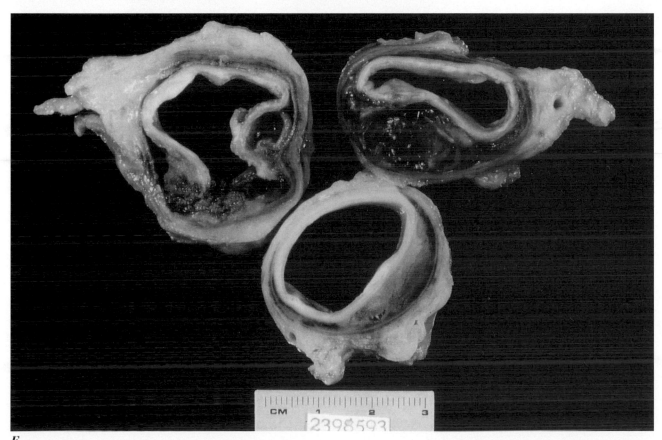

E

FIGURE 10-9 *(Continued)*

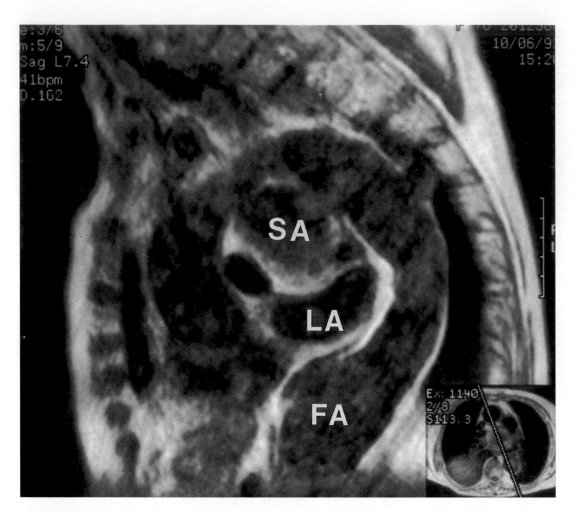

FIGURE 10-10 Magnetic resonance imaging demonstrates a saccular aneurysm (SA), which has protruded from the inferior aspect of the aortic arch and compressed the left atrium (LA). Also demonstrated is a fusiform aneurysm (FA) of the descending thoracic aorta.

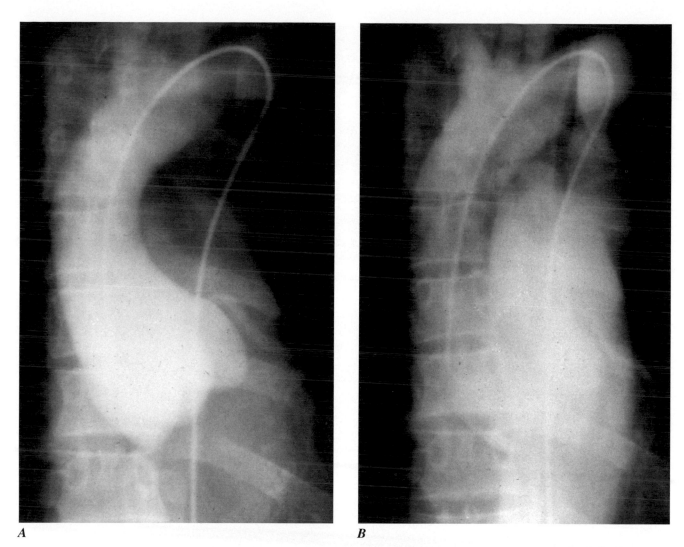

A   B

FIGURE 10-11   Two frames from an aortogram of a young man with
Marfan's syndrome. *A.* Dilatation of the sinuses of Valsalva and the proximal
ascending aorta is demonstrated. The amount of dilatation is modest
compared to that in many patients with this disorder. *B.* The opacification
of the descending thoracic aorta is depicted. An aneurysm is seen, probably
resulting from "healed dissection." (From Lindsay J: Atherosclerosis and
medial degeneration. In: Lindsay J (ed): *Diseases of the Aorta.* Philadelphia,
Lea & Febiger, 1994. Reproduced with permission from the publisher and
author.)

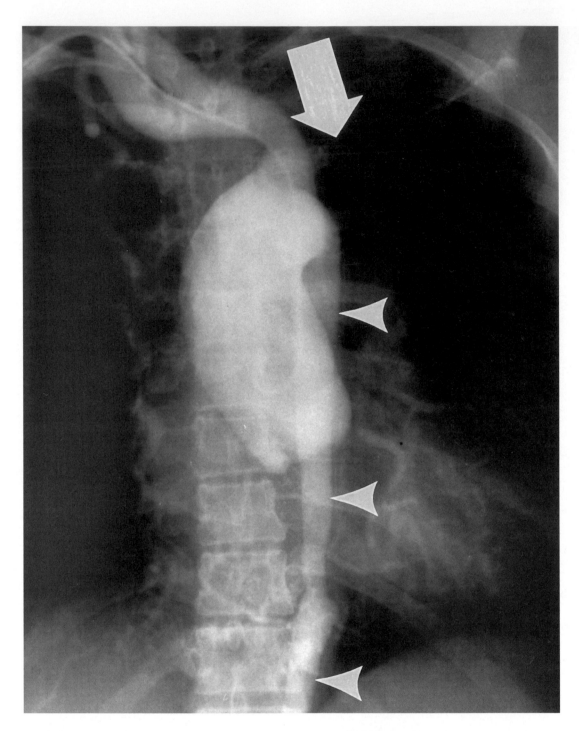

FIGURE 10-12 An aortogram from a young woman with Takayasu's arteritis. The left subclavian artery is occluded (*large arrow*). The descending thoracic and abdominal aortas are narrowed by the process (*arrowheads*). (From Dolmatch BL, Horton KM, Gray RJ, Rundback JH: Diagnostic imaging in the evaluation of aortic disease. In: Lindsay J (ed): *Diseases of the Aorta*, Philadelphia, Lea & Febiger, 1994. Reproduced with permission from the publisher and authors.)

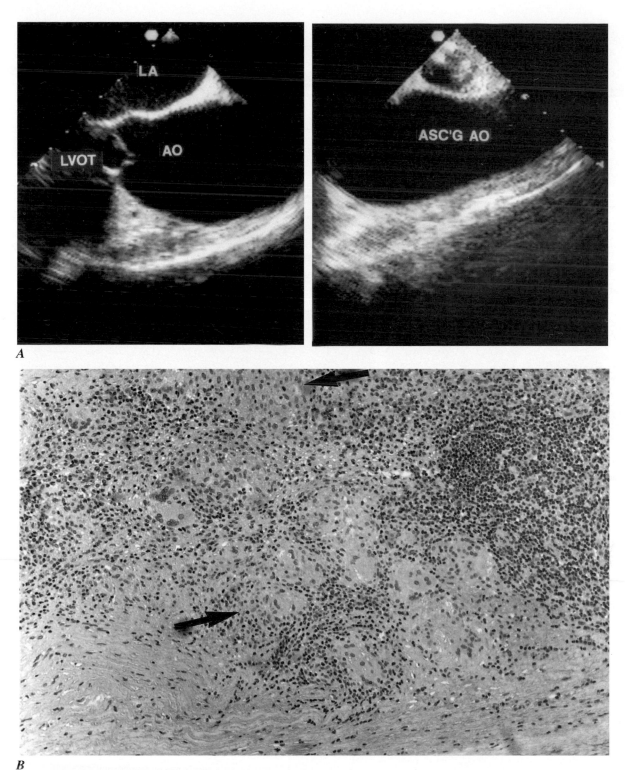

A

B

FIGURE 10-13   A 67-year-old woman who presented with severe congestive heart failure because of acute aortic regurgitation underwent successful aortic valve replacement. *A*. Her thickened, dilated aortic root is seen as demonstrated by TEE. *B*. A high-power photomicrograph of the aortic wall biopsy taken at operation. The normal constituents are replaced by granulation tissue containing numerous lymphocytes and giant cells (*arrows*). The histologic findings are characteristic of giant cell aortitis. LA = left atrium; AO = aorta; LVOT = left ventricular outflow tract; ASC'G AO = ascending aorta. (From Dollar AL: Aortitis. In: Lindsay J (ed): *Diseases of the Aorta*. Philadelphia, Lea & Febiger, 1994. Reproduced with permission from the publisher and author.)

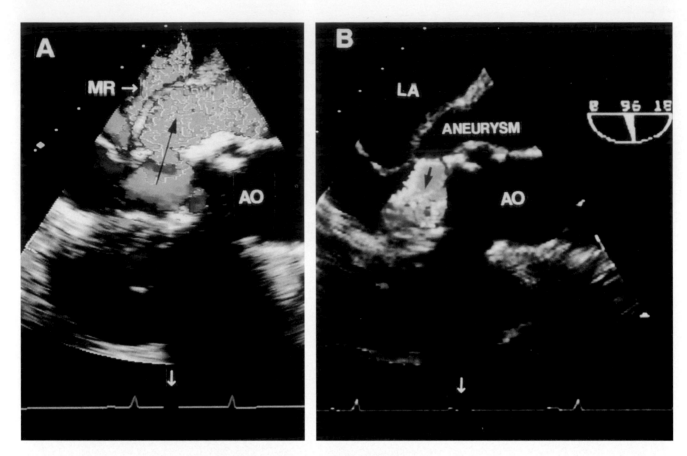

FIGURE 10-14 A TEE study of a patient with a perivalvular abscess (aneurysm) resulting from extension of aortic valve endocarditis into the narrow wedge of soft tissue between the aorta and the left atrium and rupturing into the left ventricular outflow tract. *A.* Systolic ejection from the left ventricle into the aneurysm (*arrow*). *B.* Return flow in diastole (*arrow*). No communication between the aorta and the abscess was discernible at operation. (See also Chap. 4.)

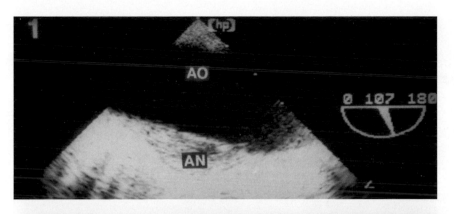

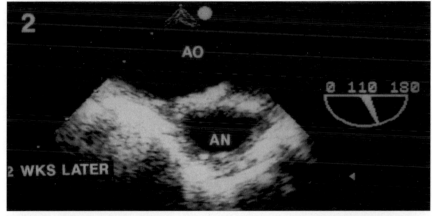

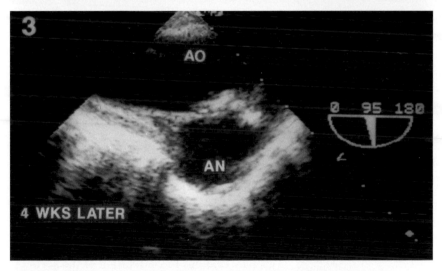

FIGURE 10-15   Bacterial infection of the aortic wall may complicate infective endocarditis. The growth of a "mycotic" aneurysm of the aortic arch is demonstrated in three TEE examinations of a patient with staphylococcal endocarditis. In the top panel, a study obtained shortly after admission demonstrated localized thickening in the aortic wall (AN) with "texture" suggestive of an abscess. The middle panel, from a study obtained 2 weeks later at the time of aortic valve replacement, depicts a definite aneurysm. The bottom panel, obtained 4 weeks later at planned operation for the aneurysm, demonstrates further enlargement. AO = aorta; AN = aneurysm. (From Goldstein SA, Lindsay J: Thoracic aortic aneurysms: Role of echocardiography. *Echocardiography* (in press, March 1996). Reproduced with permission from the publisher and authors.) (See also Chap. 4.)

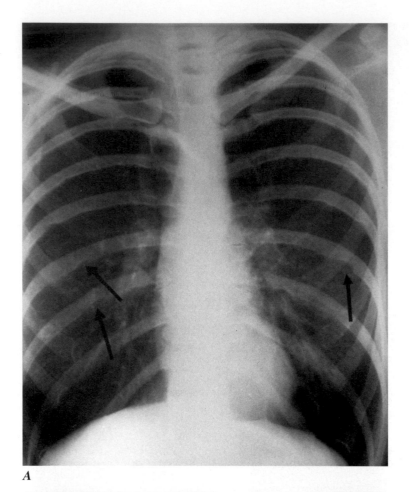

A

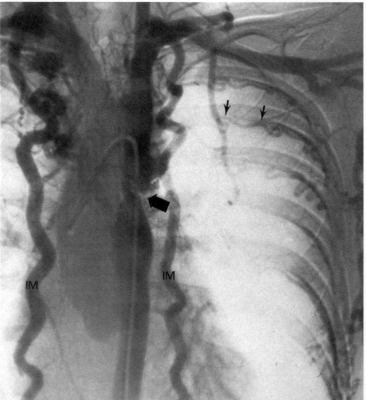

B

FIGURE 10-16   Typical plain film and aortographic findings in coarctation of the aorta. *A.* Notching of the underside of the ribs (*arrows*) is illustrated. *B.* An aortogram demonstrates the typical narrowing (*large arrow*) and the collateral circulation consisting of the dilated intercostal (*small arrows*) and internal mammary arteries (IM). (*B* from Dolmatch BL, Horton KM, Gray RJ, Rundback JH: *Diagnostic imaging in the evaluation of aortic disease. In: Lindsay J (ed): *Diseases of the Aorta*, Philadelphia, Lea & Febiger, 1994. Reproduced with permission from the publisher and authors.) (See also Chap. 3.)

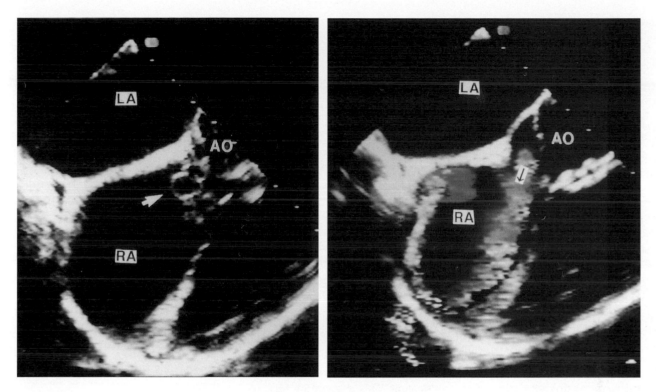

FIGURE 10-17   Imaging by TEE of a young man with a ruptured sinus of Valsalva aneurysm (*left panel, arrow*) and a resulting fistula into the right atrium (*right panel*). (From Lindsay J: Diseases of the aortic root. *Heart Dis Stroke* 1994; 3:377. Reproduced with permission from the publisher and author.)

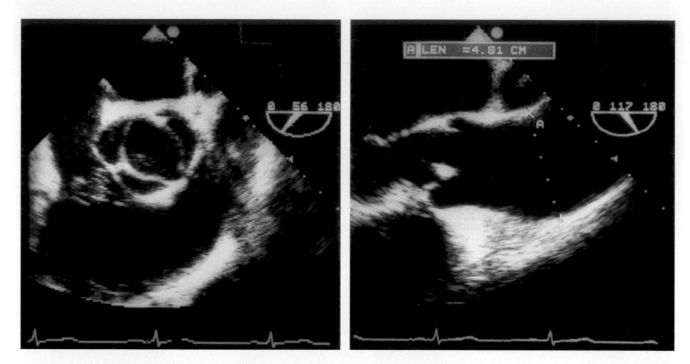

FIGURE 10-18 TEE study of a patient with a bicuspid aortic valve (*left panel*) demonstrating dilatation of the aortic root. This association has recently been recognized.[9,10] (From Lindsay J: Diseases of the aortic root. *Heart Dis Stroke* 1994; 3:377. Reproduced with permission from the publisher and author.)

REFERENCES

1. Dolmatch BL, Horton KM, Gray RJ, Rundback JH: Imaging studies used for aortic evaluation. In: Lindsay J Jr (Ed): *Diseases of the Aorta.* Philadelphia, Lea & Febiger, 1994; pp 179–195.

2. Dolmatch BL, Horton KM, Gray RJ, Rundback JH: Diagnostic imaging in the evaluation of aortic disease. In: Lindsay J Jr (Ed): *Diseases of the Aorta.* Philadelphia, Lea & Febiger, 1994; pp 197–250.

3. Goldstein SA: Ultrasound in the diagnosis of aortic disease. In: Lindsay J Jr (Ed): *Diseases of the Aorta.* Philadelphia, Lea & Febiger, 1994; pp 251–284.

4. Mohr-Kahaly S, Erbel R, Kearney P, et al: Aortic intramural hemorrhage visualized by transesophageal echocardiography: Findings and prognostic implications. *J Am Coll Cardiol* 1994; 23:658–664.

5. Robbins RC, McManus RP, Mitchell RS, et al: Management of patients with intramural hematoma of the thoracic aorta. *Circulation* 1993; 88II:II-1–II-10.

6. Tilson MD: Aortic aneurysms and atherosclerosis. *Circulation* 1992; 85:378–379.

7. Tunick PA, Perez JL, Kronzon I: Protruding atheromas in the thoracic aorta and systemic embolization. *Ann Intern Med* 1991; 115:423–427.

8. Movsowitz HD, Lampert C, Jacobs LE, Kotler MN: Penetrating atherosclerotic aortic ulcers. *Am Heart J* 1994; 128:1210–1217.

9. Hahn RT, Roman MJ, Mogtader AH, Devereux RB: Association of aortic dilatation with regurgitant, stenotic, and functionally normal bicuspid aortic valves. *J Am Coll Cardiol* 1992; 19:283–288.

10. Pachulski RT, Weinberg AL, Chan K-L: Aortic aneurysm in patients with functionally normal or minimally stenotic bicuspid aortic valve. *Am J Cardiol* 1991; 67:781–782.

CHAPTER 11

PULMONARY ARTERY IMAGING

Jeffrey A. Leef, M.D.

Martin J. Lipton, M.D.

A VARIETY of imaging techniques are available for evaluating the pulmonary circulation. Diseases of the left and right heart as well as lung disease may change the normal appearance of the pulmonary vasculature and provide critical diagnostic information. The two major radiographic patterns of disease are those reflecting pulmonary venous hypertension and pulmonary arterial hypertension. This chapter focuses on state-of-the-art techniques including computed tomography (CT) and magnetic resonance imaging (MRI), which are now playing an increasing role in the diagnosis of pulmonary disease. However, the basic chest roentgenogram remains one of the simplest, least expensive, and most indispensable noninvasive techniques.[1] Since it is usually the first imaging study obtained, it should always be evaluated prior to the performance of more sophisticated and expensive investigations (see also Chap. 3).

Pulmonary venous hypertension is a very familiar picture to cardiologists; the major causes producing this physiology are listed in Table 11-1.[1]

PULMONARY ARTERIAL HYPERTENSION

The clinical feature of pulmonary arterial hypertension is enlargement of the main and central pulmonary arteries. Figure 11-1 shows a typical example. Dilatation of these vessels is most pronounced in patients with atrial septal and Eisenmenger's syndrome. In advanced cases of pulmonary hypertension, calcification in the main or hilar

TABLE 11-1

Pulmonary Venous Hypertension—Sites of Lesions

1. *Pulmonary veins*
   Pulmonary venocclusive disease
   Anomalous pulmonary venous return
   Extrinsic compression by tumor
2. *Left atrium*
   Tumor—myxoma, lipoma, sarcoma, thrombus, cortriatriatum
3. *Mitral valve*
   Mitral stenosis—congenital or acquired
   Mitral regurgitation
4. *Left ventricle*
   LV failure—myocardial infarction
      Cardiomyopathy
      Valvular heart disease
      Hypertensive heart disease

pulmonary arteries may occur in atherosclerotic plaques and can be detected on the chest roentgenogram. Additionally, tortuousity of the pulmonary arteries is also indicative of very high pulmonary artery pressure (see also Chap. 3).

In pulmonary hypertension caused by hyperkinetic blood flow, the peripheral pulmonary arteries increase in size and number. The heart may also be enlarged in proportion to the size of the left-to-right shunt. With the onset of the Eisenmenger's syndrome, the peripheral pulmonary vascularity is reduced and central pulmonary artery enlargement occurs. The important causes of pulmonary arterial hypertension are listed in Table 11-2.

TABLE 11-2

Common Causes of Pulmonary Arterial Hypertension

Mitral valve stenosis
Pulmonary embolism
Destructive lung disease
Intracardiac shunts—congenital or iatrogenic
Extracardiac shunts (e.g., arteriovenous fistulas)
Constrictive pericarditis
Idiopathic

PULMONARY EMBOLISM

Pulmonary embolism may be acute or chronic.[2] Figure 11-2*A* and *B* illustrates a ventilation/perfusion lung scan obtained in a 45-year-old patient presenting with acute chest pain and suspected pulmonary embolism.

Figure 11-2*C* and *D* illustrates the pulmonary digital angiogram obtained in the same patients shown in Fig. 11-2*A* and *B* and demonstrates a saddle embolus.

This information can also be obtained with MRI (Chap. 6) and CT (Chap. 7), although these techniques are still being refined and improved and are not always available.[3–9]

Figure 11-3 is an electron beam CT (EBCT) scan in a similar patient with pulmonary embolism. Thrombus is seen as an elongated filling defect extending into the contrast-enhanced right and left main pulmonary arteries. This modality can also detect peripheral emboli, as shown in Fig. 11-3. The EBCT technique can be helpful for primary diagnosis and also for following patients undergoing treatment with anticoagulants; it is a welcome alternative to more invasive riskier angiography.[8] Computed tomography has the added advantage of providing a detailed display of lung parenchyma and vessels by altering the computer settings for CT window and level, as shown in Fig. 11-4 (see also Chap. 7).

The vast majority of emboli are thrombi and arise in the deep veins of the legs and pelvis. The most significant large emboli originate in the ileofemoral and popliteal venous system. However, air, amniotic fluid, bacterial vegetation, fat, parasites, and tumor as well as thrombus may embolize to the lungs. Fat embolism produces a clinical picture dominated by cerebral symptoms. The radiologic appearance resembles massive alveolar edema. Large emboli usually consist of thrombus, hydatid cysts, or occasionally tumor. When they lodge in the main pulmonary trunk and arteries, the presentation is one of collapse, dyspnea, tachycardia, and hypotension. Lobar embolism may present a similar clinical picture. Conversely, small emboli in peripheral vessels may be asymptomatic. Multiple recurrent emboli will result in chronic pulmonary hypertension; this may be due to thrombus, bilharzia, filaria, hydatid cyst, choriocarcinoma, or right atrial myxoma.[9] The incidence of pulmonary embolism is much greater than that usually reported.[2] The usual statistics quote an incidence of about 663,000 cases per year in America, of which 200,000 are fatal. Approximately 11 percent of patients with significant symptoms die within the first hour.

Infarction is not invariable with embolism, because the bronchial circulation supplies the lung. Infarction is most likely to occur in the presence of chronic pulmonary venous hypertension. If an infarct is small, it is often clinically silent; but when it involves half a segment or more, it may cause fever tachypnea, hemoptysis, and pleurisy with or without a pleural effusion.

Acute Pulmonary Embolism—Radiographic Findings

Lung ischemia or the Westermark sign, described in 1938, of abnormal radiolucency with few vessels, is almost never seen convincingly. The hilar arteries and pulmonary trunk are not dilated. When lobar or segmental arteries are embolized, the lower lobes are most often affected. Compensatory dilation of the large proximal pulmonary arteries may occur, but more dilation may involve the unaffected areas of the lung, resulting occasionally in pulmonary edema due to over perfusion. Diaphragmatic elevation may occur if an embolus lodges in a lower lobe. The artery containing the thrombus may appear enlarged and have an amputed appearance just proximal to the ischemic area. The heart is only rarely enlarged.[9] (See also Chap. 3.)

PULMONARY INFARCTION

Infarcts are a complication of pulmonary embolism (PE) and occur when collateral bronchial artery flow is inadequate. The lung is consolidated from effusion, with blood and fluid in the alveolar spaces. The infarct may develop immediately or be delayed for 5 days, but there is no delay between infarction and its appearances on the chest radiograph.

The radiological features of PE are the infarct infiltrate, pleural effusion, and diaphragmatic elevation. Infarcts are commonest in the lower zones and rare in the upper lobes. Infarcts are often reversible and may clear in a day or two. If not, the consolidation becomes more defined. Only the base of the infarct cone is actually infarcted, so a triangular infiltrate should not be expected. The infiltrate may have any shape from a linear band to a crescent or circle, depending on the projection and the location and size of the infarct. Very rarely, an infarct cavitates due to either necrosis or secondary infarction. The differential diagnosis includes trauma and lung contusion with hematoma.

Embolic Pulmonary Hypertension

Widespread occlusion of the vascular bed due to multiple recurrent emboli may cause pulmonary hypertension. Signs of chronicity include patchy vascular obliteration, pulmonary arterial calcification, infarct scars, and diaphragm elevation with pleural thickening. Tumor embolism causing pulmonary hypertension and parasites should not be forgotten. Angiography, radionuclide studies (Chap. 5), CT (Chap. 7), and MRI (Chap. 6) can all play a part in confirming or excluding the diagnosis of pulmonary embolism; however, the differential diagnosis can be broad.[9]

PULMONARY ARTERIOVENOUS MALFORMATIONS

The majority of pulmonary arteriovenous fistulas encountered by the cardiologist will be congenital. Acquired fistulas do occur in association with cirrhosis, schistosomiasis, and malignancy, notably metastatic thyroid carcinoma. The congenital form is progressive, with enlargement of the fistulas and sometimes development of new ones. Approximately 50 percent of patients have hereditary hemorrhagic telangiectasia (Osler-Weber-Rendu disease). [9–12] An example of this disease is illustrated in Fig. 11-5. These patients are not suitable candidates for surgery. The disease has a broad spectrum; often, there is only one large lesion, which presents as an oval or lobulated mass on the chest radiograph, usually in a lower lobe, and it may be found incidentally. Tubular structures arise from it and usually appear to course toward the hilum. Since the fistula is from a pulmonary artery to a pulmonary vein and is therefore a right-to-left shunt, the patient may present with symptoms of cyanosis and heart failure, dyspnea, or hemoptysis. Paradoxical embolism can cause a cerebral abscess or thrombosis, and this may bring the patient to the hospital. Most symptoms occur in the third or fourth decade.

The diagnosis can be made with CT, MRI, or digital subtraction arteriography (DSA); however, pulmonary arteriography is usually needed to define the feeding artery and identify the draining vein or veins to the left atrium. It should be remembered that selective angiography of both lungs must be obtained, since in 30 percent of cases multiple lesions are present, which are often not evident on chest roentgenography. Figure 11-6 demonstrates a large arteriovenous fistula with at least two draining veins. Figure 11-7 shows successful obliteration of the largest vein by intervention using catheter embolization with Gianturco coils.[13–15]

Stenosis and aneurysms of the pulmonary arteries may also occur. The majority are congenital disorders and are described in Chap. 3. Takayasu's arteritis can involve the pulmonary arteries.[16] Aneurysms of the pulmonary artery are also usually of congenital origin. Those caused by septic emboli usually associated with intravenous drug abuse represent a notable exception. Bacterial endocarditis of the tricuspid or pulmonary valves may also lead to mycotic aneurysms. Such aneurysms enlarge rapidly and are at risk of rupture.

Modern cross-sectional imaging obtained by MRI and CT—and probably, in the future, by digital ultrasound and nuclear medicine—involve the acquisition of a vast number of images. Automated boundary detection and three-dimensional displays are necessary to allow physicians to comprehend the anatomic and functional data more rapidly and to provide accurate quantitation. Some examples of how the pulmonary vessels can be segmented from overlying bone and soft tissues and then displayed on a TV monitor in any desired angle or cross-section are shown in Figs. 11-8 to 11-12.

The value of these newer techniques will be realized only when they are made accessible on standard work stations. The imaging data must be made available to the physician as soon as possible following the appropriate examination. This will become a reality as the complexity of microprocessors continues to increase while their cost diminishes. Many of the remarkable advances that have already appeared were due to close collaboration between physicists, computer scientists, and clinicians in medical centers and in industry. Outcome analysis studies are needed to demonstrate that this new technology is justified and that it improves patient diagnosis and care.

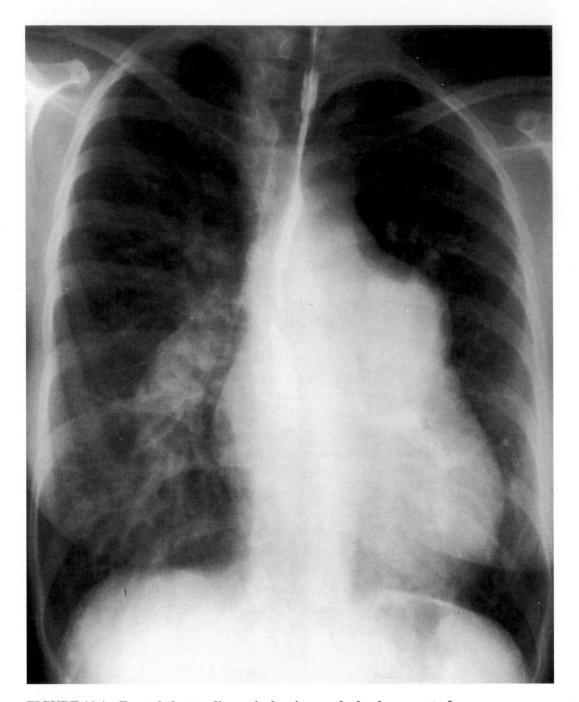

FIGURE 11-1 **Frontal chest radiograph showing marked enlargement of the pulmonary trunk and proximal hilar pulmonary arteries. The cardiac apex is elevated and the left cardiac border is indicative of right ventricular enlargement. The heart is moderately enlarged. These appearances are consistent with pulmonary arterial hypertension. The diaphragm and lung bases are clear, which denies chronic pulmonary embolism as the cause. A large left-to-right shunt was present at catheterization at the atrial level. (See also Chap. 3.)**

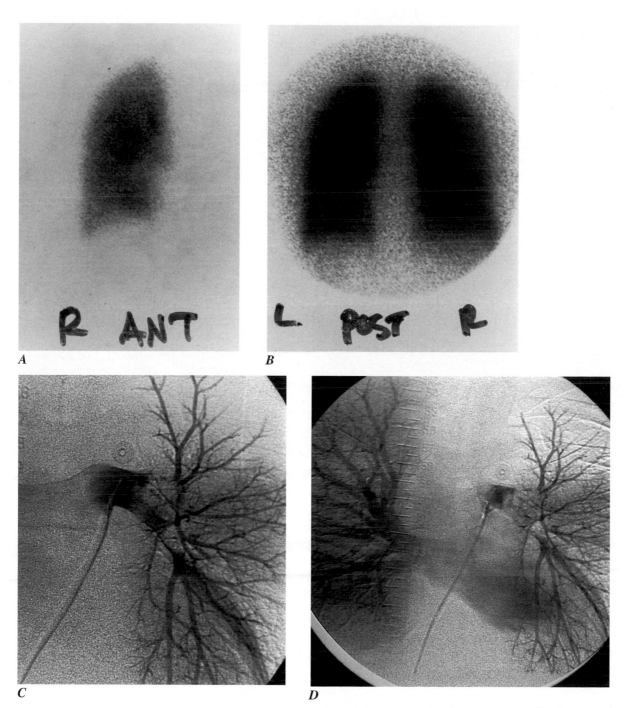

FIGURE 11-2   A ⁹⁹ᵐTc macroaggregated albumin (MAA) perfusion and ¹³³Xe ventilation scan performed in a 45-year-old man with deep vein thrombosis of the lower extremity and abrupt shortness of breath. *A.* This is the perfusion study *(anterior view)*, demonstrating nonperfusion of the left lung. *B.* The single-breath ventilation study shows normal, symmetrical distribution of xenon in both lungs. Findings of ventilation/ perfusion mismatch of this type are typical of a central pulmonary artery obstruction. *C.* A single frame from the arterial phase of a digital subtraction pulmonary arteriogram obtained in the same 45-year-old patient whose radionuclide ventilation/perfusion scans are illustrated in *A* and *B*. The catheter is positioned in the proximal left main pulmonary artery. The filling defect outlined by contrast medium represents a large saddle pulmonary embolus, which partially obstructs the proximal ascending and descending pulmonary artery branches and delays flow to the left lung. *D.* This is also the same study as illustrated in *C*, showing delayed flow through the left lung compared to the more normal rapid venous filling phase on the right side, where contrast can be seen opacifying the left atrium; arterial filling persists on the left.

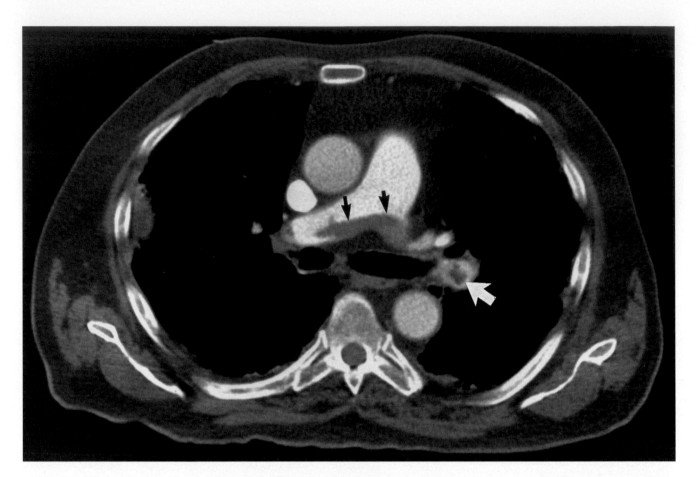

FIGURE 11-3   A 6-mm-thick section acquired in 0.2 s with an EBCT scanner through the chest, with intravenous contrast enhancement of the blood pool. Contrast is most dense at this time in the superior vena cava and the pulmonary arteries, where a large saddle pulmonary embolus produces the filling defect posteriorly (*black arrows*). There is also partial obstruction of the right main pulmonary artery as well as thrombus extension into the left main and left descending pulmonary arteries (*white arrow*). The rapid acquisition time of EBCT enables small emboli to be detected. (See also Chap. 7.)

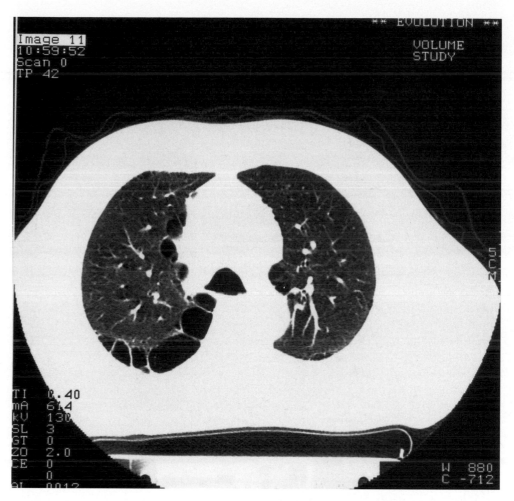

FIGURE 11-4   A 6-mm-thick EBCT scan through the chest obtained in 0.3 s, demonstrating the ability to examine lung parenchyma and pleura by appropriately adjusting the CT window and level. This information is obtained from the same acquisition as that used to image the heart and great vessels. This patient has severe bullous emphysema of the right lung, with much less involvement on the left side at this anatomic level. Volume scanning at multiple levels (40 in 13 s) provides not only a survey of the whole chest but also data for three-dimensional postprocessing and reconstruction.

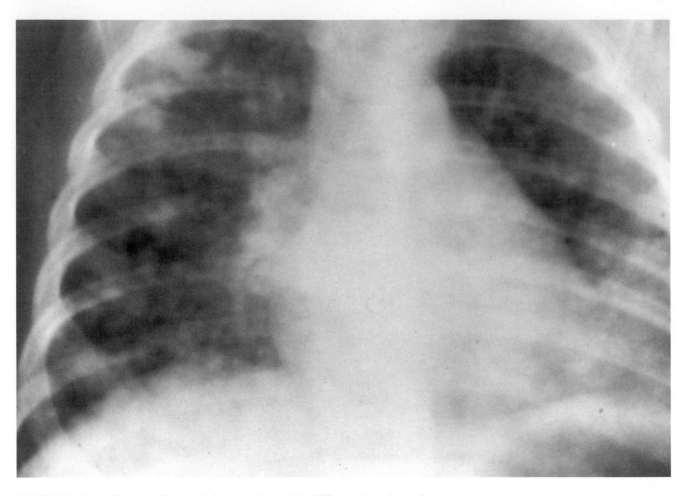

FIGURE 11-5   Chest radiograph in a patient with diffuse telangiectasia. The differential diagnosis includes heart failure, pulmonary edema, and extensive metastatic disease.

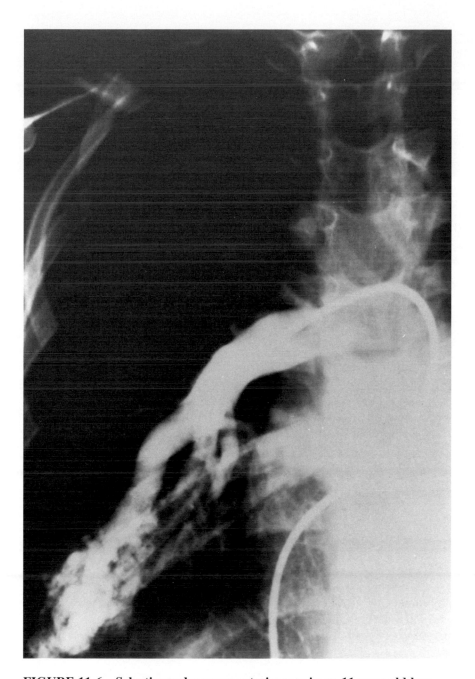

FIGURE 11-6 Selective pulmonary arteriogram in an 11-year-old boy with cyanosis and a right lower lobe nodular lesion on chest roentgenogram. The angiogram demonstrates a large arteriovenous malformation with at least two draining veins.

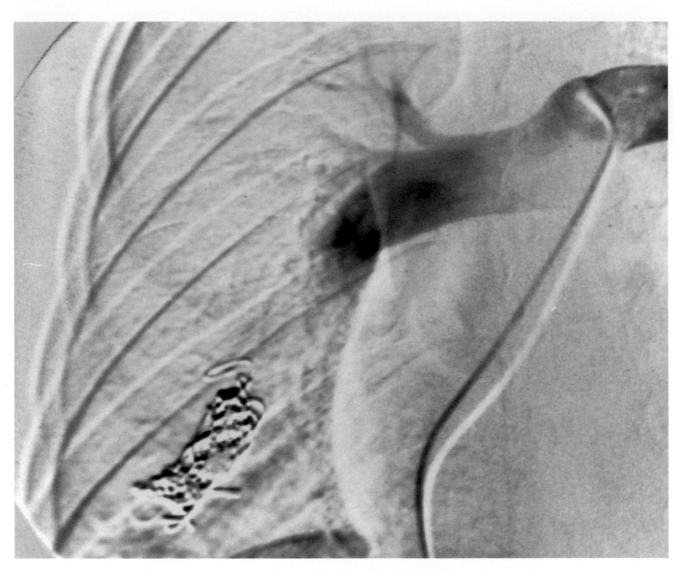

FIGURE 11-7   Same patient as in Fig. 11-6, illustrating the final angiogram obtained following embolization by interventional radiology using Gianturco coils of the largest draining vein. This shows near cessation of flow through the arteriovenous malformation, with a resultant 65 percent increase in arterial oxygen concentration.

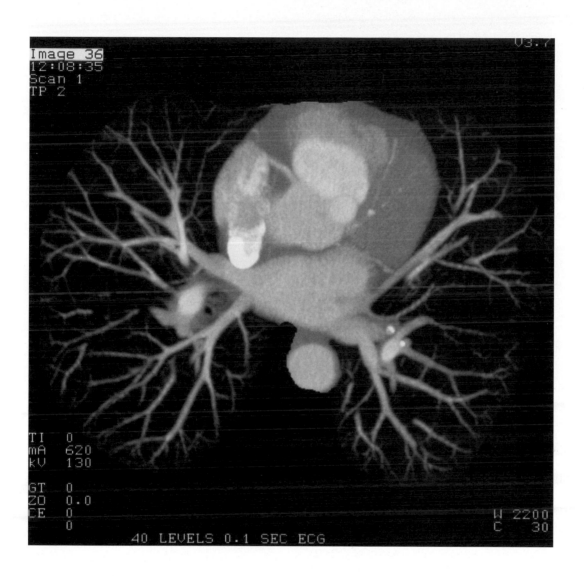

FIGURE 11-8   A maximum-intensity projection image of a 1.5-mm-thick EBCT scan acquired during the passage of an intravenously injected bolus of contrast agent with suspended respiration. The arterial and venous structures are enhanced. Note the excellent detail of the pulmonary venous system, including the pulmonary veins and the left atrium. Additional information concerning the aortic root and right coronary artery as well as calcification in branches of the left coronary artery should be noted. This three-dimensional volume image can be rotated in many planes and examined from many angles on a TV monitor. (Courtesy of Imatron Inc., San Francisco, and rendered by S. Napel, Ph.D., of Stanford University.)

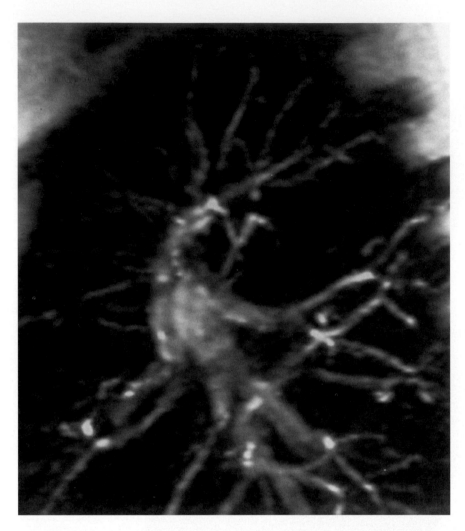

FIGURE 11-9 Maximum-intensity-projection MR image obtained with a prototype pulmonary phased-array coil in a sagittal plane, showing normal venous and arterial pulmonary vascular structures. The acquisition was cardiac-gated with variable delay via view recording and single breath-hold technique.

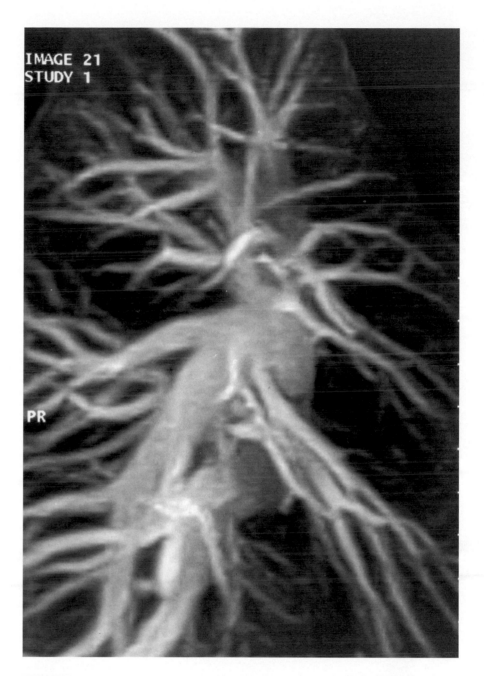

FIGURE 11-10 This MR image presented in a lateral projection was obtained on a 1.5-T (tesla) system in a healthy volunteer. The image acquisition time was approximately 15 min for each lung. The MRI technique used was a three-dimensional maximum projection rapid acquisition gradient echo (RAGE)-type sequence using a modified prepulse. The time to echo was 2.2 s. Third-and fourth-order vessels are sharply defined.

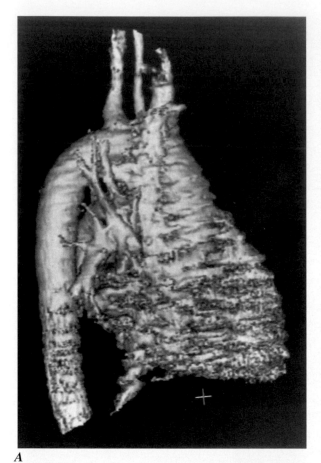

A

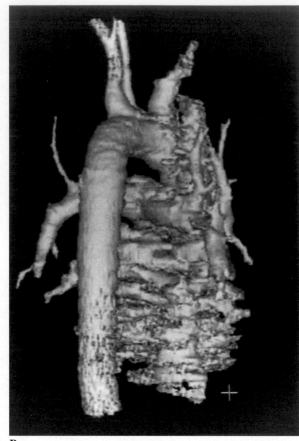

B

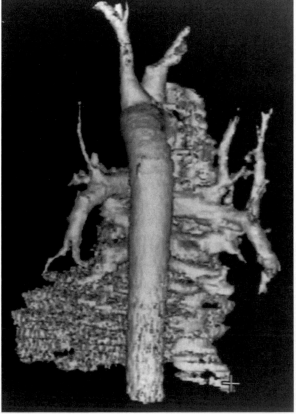

C

FIGURE 11-11 *A to C.* **These figures represent three different projections of a three-dimensional reconstruction obtained from continuous spiral CT volume scanning with a GE 9800 scanner through the chest during intravenous contrast enhancement. Contiguous 3-mm scans were obtained and the total volume CT data acquired were reconstructed at 1-mm intervals using a shaded surface display. The great vessels and aortic arch as well as the hilar and second-order pulmonary arteries are demonstrated. This type of segmented display can be combined with maximum-intensity images, which define the cardiac chambers and vessel lumens from the same image data set.**

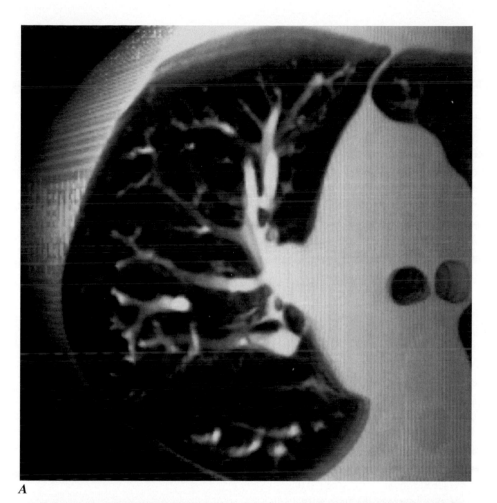

A

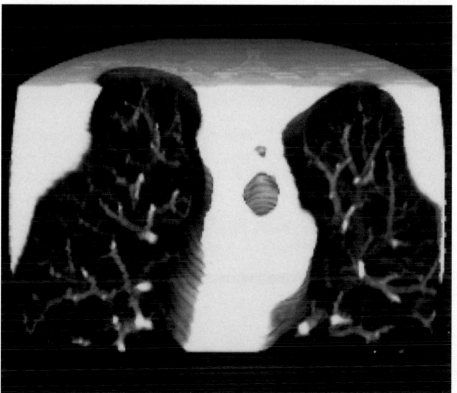

B

FIGURE 11-12   Volume visualization of lung structure from spiral CT scan parameters: 3-mm helical pitch, 1-mm slice reconstruction, 18-cm field of view (pixel size at 512 × 512 resolution = 0.35 mm), 95 slices. *A*. Right inferior oblique view, inclined 20° right from cephalo-caudal axis. *B*. Anterosuperior view, inclined 30° superior from AP axis with cutting plane normal to view direction. (Images rendered by Charles Pelizzari, Ph.D., Department of Radiation and Cellular Oncology, and Robert Grzeszczuk, Department of Radiology, University of Chicago.)

REFERENCES

1. Dash H, Lipton MJ, Chatterjee K, Parmley WW: Estimation of pulmonary artery wedge pressure from chest radiograph in patients with chronic congestive cardiomyopathy and ischemic cardiomyopathy. *Br Heart J* 1980; 44:322–329.

2. Dalen JE, Alpert JS: Natural history of pulmonary embolism. *Prog Cardiovasc Dis* 1975; 12:259–270.

3. DiCarlo LA, Schiller NB, Herfkens RJ, et al: Non-invasive detection of proximal pulmonary artery thrombosis by two dimensional echocardiography and computer tomography. *Am Heart J* 1982; 104:879–881.

4. Kareiakis DJ, Herfkens RJ, Brundage BH, et al: CT in chronic thromboembolic pulmonary hypertension. *Am Heart J* 1983; 106:1432–1436.

5. Gurney JW: No fooling around: Direct visualization of pulmonary embolism. *Radiology* 1993; 188:618–619.

6. Verschakelen JA, Vanwijck E, Bogaert J, Baert AL: Detection of unsuspected central pulmonary embolism with conventional contrast-enhanced CT. *Radiology* 1993; 188:847–850.

7. Teigen CL, Maus TP, Sheedy PF II, et al: Pulmonary embolism: Diagnosis with electron-beam CT. *Radiology* 1993; 188:839–845.

8. Stein PD, Hull RD, Saltzman HA, Pineo G: Strategy for diagnosis of patients with suspected acute pulmonary embolism. *Chest* 1993; 103:1553–1559.

9. Higgins DB, Lipton MJ: Pulmonary circulation. In: Grainger RG, Allison D (eds): *Diagnostic Radiology: An Anglo-American Textbook of Imaging,* Vol 1. London, Churchill Livingstone, 1986, pp 565–583.

10. Gomes MNR, Bernatz PE: Arteriovenous fistulas: A review and ten years experience at the Mayo Clinic. *Mayo Clinic Proc* 1970; 45:81–102.

11. Giampalmao A: The arteriovenous angiomatosis of the lung with hypoxemia. *Acta Med Scand* 1950; 139 (supp 248):1–67.

12. Godwin JD, Webb WR: Dynamic computed tomography in the evaluation of vascular lung lesions. *Radiology* 1981; 138:629–635.

13. White RI Jr: Embolotherapy with detachable balloons. In: Abrams HA (ed): *Interventional Techniques.* Philadelphia, Saunders, 1983; pp 2211–2222.

14. Castañeda-Zúñiga WR, Epstein M, Zollikofer C, et al: Embolization of multiple pulmonary artery fistulas. *Radiology* 1980; 134:309–310.

15. Jonsson K, Hellekant C, Olsson O, Holen O: Percutaneous transcatheter occlusion of pulmonary arteriovenous malformation. *Ann Radiol* 1980; 23:335–337.

16. Lupi H, Sanchez G, Horwitz S, Guttierrez E: Pulmonary artery involvement in Takayasu's arteritis. *Chest* 1975; 67:69–74.

CHAPTER 12

DIGITAL IMAGING OF THE HEART

Kenneth R. Hoffmann, Ph.D.

Shiuh-Yung Chen, Ph.D.

John D. Carroll, M.D.

Martin J. Lipton, M.D.

DURING the past 20 years, the revolution in the electronics and computer industries has made possible the development and application of a new technology known as digital imaging. *Digital imaging* is a general term applied to any image that has been in digital format at any stage between image acquisition and viewing. Images are stored as matrices of numbers (pixel values) in which each number corresponds to a picture element (pixel). The numbers range from 0 to 4095 currently, corresponding to 12 bits of information in the computer. These images can be displayed on video monitors, and the contrast in the digital image can be manipulated using the window and level functions. With digital imaging, quantitative analysis can be applied. Basic imaging techniques—such as edge enhancement, histogram analysis, image filtering, and boundary detection,[1,2] long used in other fields—are now being used in medicine.

With the digital data and sophisticated image processing methods, measurements of vessel sizes,[3–6] ventricular volumes,[7–9] and myocardial volumes can be performed. The three-dimensional anatomy of the heart, its chambers, and its blood supply can be flexibly displayed and studied using three-dimensional graphics. In addition, critical functional information can be estimated quantitatively. Analyses have been developed to quantitate myocardial motion,[10–13] perfusion,[14–17] and metabolism[18] and to present the data so as to facilitate appreciation of cardiac dynamics. The anatomic and functional data can then be integrated for even better understanding of disease states.[19] The ability to quantitate and visualize function and anatomy and combine them in a variety of ways is enhancing our understanding of disease in individual patients as well as in groups. These capabilities are further enhanced by digital storage and transfer technology—such as compact disks, tape archives, and networks—so that evaluation of images can be performed in the home or office. Digital imaging will continue to facilitate and improve our ability to assess patients and the way we care for them.

BASIC CONCEPTS IN DIGITAL IMAGING

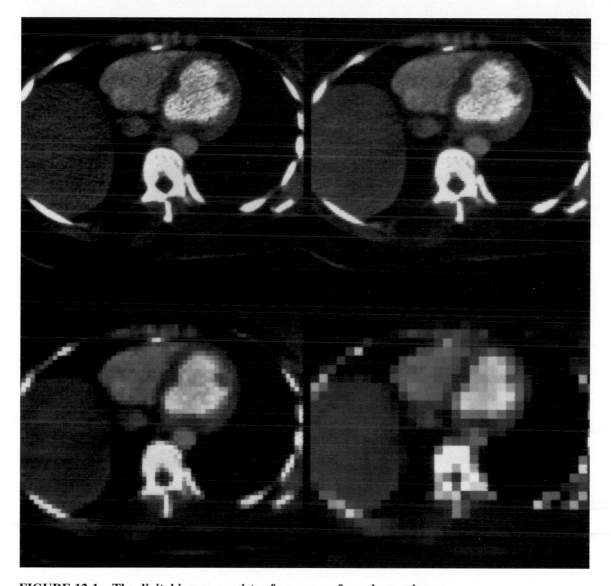

**FIGURE 12-1   The digital image consists of an array of numbers, where
each element in the array represents a physical characteristic of the image
in a finite region. The picture element or region represented by a number
is termed a *pixel* for two-dimensional and a *voxel* for three-dimensional (2D
and 3D) imaging. The size, and therefore the number, of pixels determines
the spatial resolution; for a given pixel size, more pixels are needed as the
image (or field of view) becomes larger. In order to illustrate the effect of
pixel size on the perceived visual information in an image, an electron beam
computed tomography (EBCT) image is presented with four different pixel
sizes: an original EBCT cardial image *(upper left)*, the original image with
the pixel size increased by 2 *(upper right)*, the original image with pixel size
increased by 4 *(lower left)*, and the original image with the pixel size
increased by 8 *(lower right)*. Note that as the pixel size increased, the
individual pixels become visible and edges of structures become more blocked.**

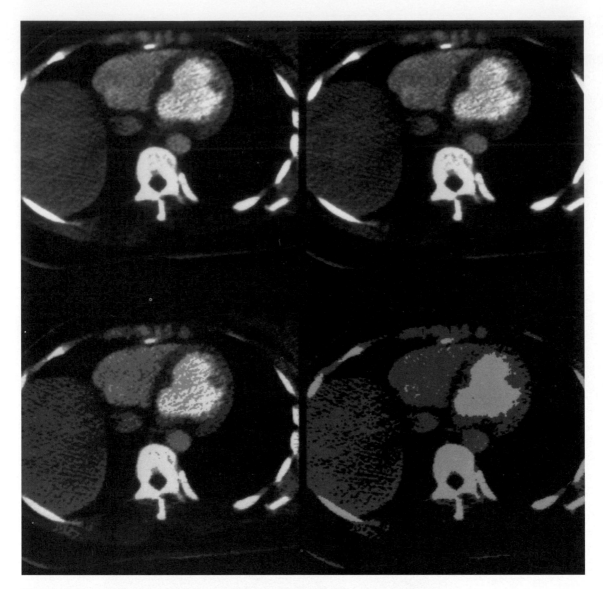

FIGURE 12-2   The physical characteristic represented by the number at
each position (pixel value) might be related to the x-ray attenuation coefficient (as in a computed tomography image), the transmitted x-ray intensity
(as in digital projection angiography), the proton density (as in magnetic
resonance imaging), the number of annihilations (as in positron emission
tomography), or the optical density of the film (as in digitized radiographs)
in the region represented by the pixel. Within a digital image, pixel values
are limited to a finite range termed the *pixel depth*, which is related to the
contrast resolution in the image. This depth is some power of 2, where a
power of 2 is 1 bit. Thus, if the pixel depth is 8 bits, the pixels can have any
value between 1 and 2^8, or 256 (actually between 0 and 255). To illustrate
the effect of pixel depth, the EBCT image shown in Fig. 12-1 (with 8 bits or
256 gray levels) is presented in which the pixel depth is varied from 6 bits
to 2 bits: the EBCT cardiac image with 64 gray levels (6 bits, *upper left*),
with 16 gray levels (4 bits, *upper right*), with 8 gray levels (3 bits, *lower left*),
and with 4 gray levels (2 bits, *lower right*). As the number of bits decreases,
contours appear in the image, and large regions of the image have a
common pixel value.

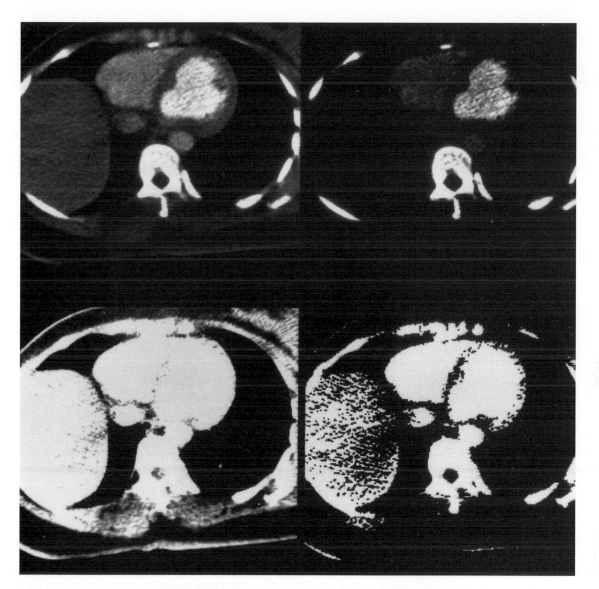

FIGURE 12-3   The mapping of the pixel values to the intensity displayed is determined by the window and level setting chosen in viewing an image. The window is the width of the range of pixel values chosen (the narrower the width, the higher the contrast in the image); the level is the central pixel value of this range. The effects of various window and level settings are illustrated here. *Upper left*: window and level setting to span the entire range of possible pixel values (window setting = 256, level = 128). All structures are visible, but contrast is relatively low. *Upper right*: window setting = 128, level = 192. Only those structures with high pixel values, corresponding to a high attenuation coefficient, such as the iodinated blood in the ventricle, are visible. *Lower left*: window setting = 128, level = 64. All structures with high pixel value are white, merging the different structures, but the contrast of the structures with lower pixel values has been increased. *Lower right*: a binary image, window = 1, level = 128. All structures with pixel values below the level are black and all above are white. This image is what the computer "sees" when thresholding operations (*below*) are performed.

BASIC ANALYSES IN DIGITAL IMAGING

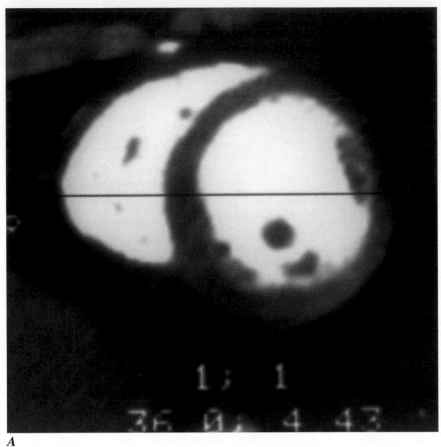

A

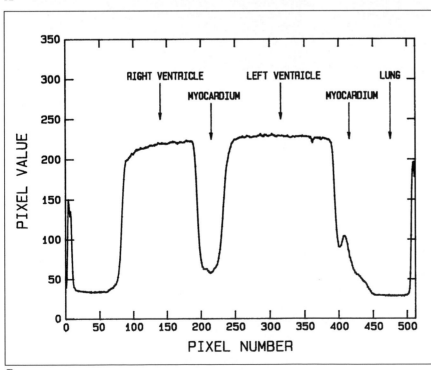

B

FIGURE 12-4   Image profiles.
A. An EBCT image acquired at near end diastole. The image is near the mitral valve and lies perpendicular to the long axis of the heart. *B.* Pixel values along a line indicated in *A.* This profile indicates that the pixel values tend to be high in the regions of the ventricles and low in the regions of the myocardium. This difference in pixel values between the two regions can be used to differentiate the pixels belonging to the ventricles from those corresponding to the myocardium. Image profiles can be a first step in the understanding and the analysis of an image. (From Hoffmann KR, Chen CT, Doi K: Automated region identification and its application to measuring cardiac function. *Am J Cardiac Imaging* 1991; 5:272–280. Reproduced with permission from the publisher and authors.)

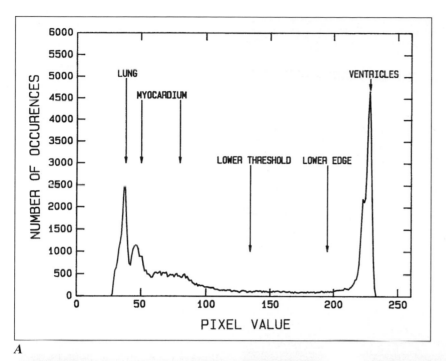

A

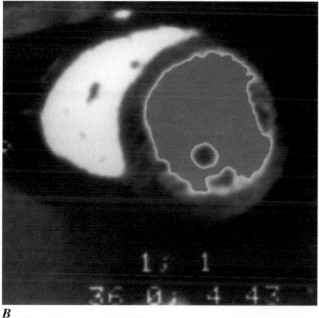

B

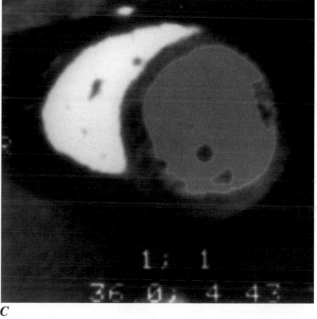

C

FIGURE 12-5 Histogram analysis. *A.* Histogram of pixel values of pixels in a region of the cardiac image shown in Fig. 12-4*A*. Accurate determination of the regions of the histogram—i.e., those pixel values that correspond to objects in the image—is essential to accurate identification of the pixels that belong to the object. Because other structures such as the right ventricle also have the same pixel values as the left ventricle, the additional criterion of connectivity is included in the analysis to determine the pixels that correspond only to the left ventricle. Only those pixels that are connected to the other pixel of the left ventricle and are above the threshold are identified, using region-growing,[1,2] as belonging to the left ventricle. With this technique, only those pixels that satisfy these criteria are included; thus, the papillary muscles are not included as part of the ventricles. *B.* Results of region growing with the pixel value at the "lower edge" used as the threshold value. Simply finding the edge of the region of the histogram is insufficient. *C.* Results of region growing with the pixel value of the "lower threshold" used as the threshold value. This halfway point between the pixel values of the myocardium and the ventricle yields better results. (From Hoffmann KR, Chen CT, Doi K: Automated region identification and its application to measuring cardiac function. *Am J Cardiac Imaging* 1991; 5:272–280. Reproduced with permission from the publisher and authors.)

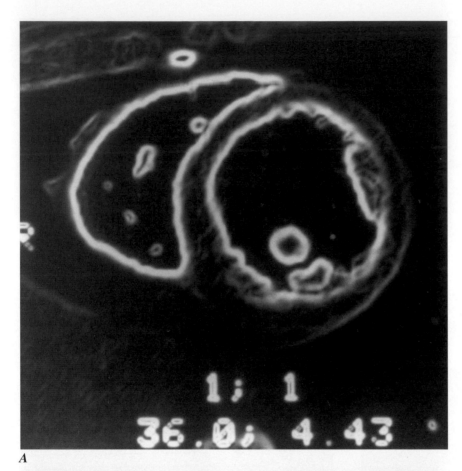

A

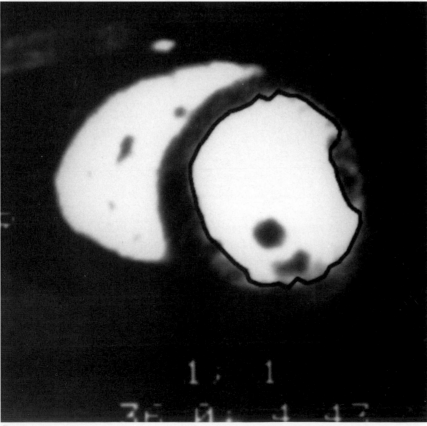

B

FIGURE 12-6 Edge enhancement and edge tracking. Edge-enhancing filters are usually based on derivatives; therefore they enhance regions with rapid spatial changes in pixel value, such as boundaries. For quantitative measurements, the determination of the boundaries of structures in the images is essential. *A*. The image in Fig. 12-4*A* after convolution with a 3-pixel × 3-pixel Sobel filter. The edges are clearly visible. When filters are applied to images, the edges can be shifted from their true position, and the shift can depend on the structures in the image itself. Thus, it is important to understand the effect of the applied filters on the edges of interest. *B*. The result of edge tracking of Fig. 12-6*A*. The boundary is tracked after an initial starting point is given by finding a series of contiguous pixels, with the maximum pixel value in the edge-enhanced image. The tracking of the boundary continues until a condition, such as closure, is met. Note that the papillary muscles have been included within the ventricle boundary, which will give an incorrectly high estimate of the ventricular area in this slice. (From Hoffmann KR, Chen CT, Doi K: Automated region identification and its application to measuring cardiac function. *Am J Cardiac Imaging* 1991; 5:272–280. Reproduced with permission from the publisher and authors.)

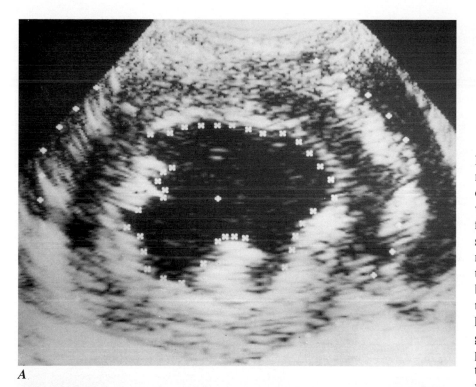

A

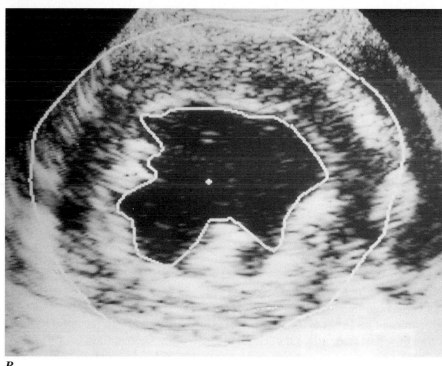

B

FIGURE 12-7 When the signal-to-noise ratio (SNR) is low, as in echocardiographic images, edges are not well defined and region-growing and filtering techniques fail. For these situations, additional a priori information must be incorporated, such as the continuity of the ventricular boundary and the noise properties of the image. Numerous techniques have been developed for echocardiographic images. In this image, we present the results of a technique that combines edge detection, ventricular continuity, and fuzzy reasoning techniques to estimate the ventricular boundary.[20,21] In fuzzy-reasoning techniques, features of the image (such as pixel value, local texture, or distance from the center) are extracted from image data. Each pixel is thereby represented by a point in the multidimensional feature space. Each pixel is then given a probability of membership in one or more types of regions in the feature space based on the pixel's location in the space. Boundaries are then determined based on the membership probabilities in the image. (From Hoffmann KR, Chen CT, Doi K: Automated region identification and its application to measuring cardiac function. *Am J Cardiac Imaging* 1991; 5:272–280. Reproduced with permission from the publisher and authors.)

VASCULAR ANALYSIS

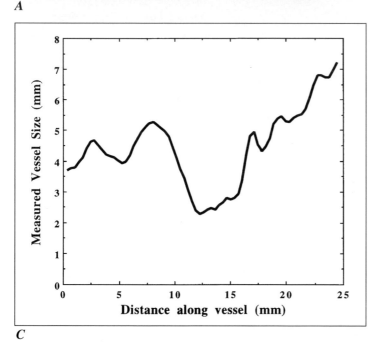

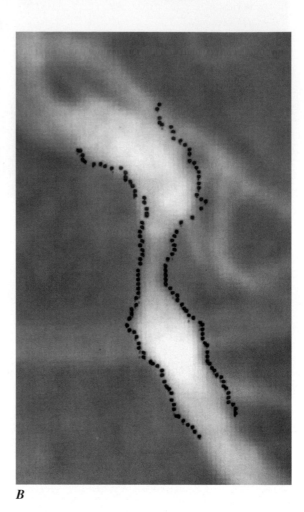

A

B

C

FIGURE 12-8 Vessel size measurement is one of the more frequently used analyses in cardiac imaging. Unfortunately, visual measurements of stenosis can be unreliable.[22] To improve the precision and accuracy of vessel size measurements, quantitative techniques have been developed.[3–6] *A.* Cardiac image with a stenosis in the left anterior descending (LAD) artery. *B.* The vessel edge along the length of the vessel. The result of analysis with the iterative deconvolution technique.[6] This technique takes the line-spread function of the imaging system into account and has been shown to have an accuracy and precision of 0.1 mm for vessels as small as 0.5 mm. The techniques available on clinical machines are based on vessel edges determined using first- and second-derivatives of the vessel profiles. With calibration, these techniques can yield reliable vessel sizes for vessels with diameters larger than the full width at half maximum (FWHM) of the resolution function of the imaging system. The resolution function relates the input to the II-TV system to the output. It can be measured using known pointlike and linelike objects and the images they produce.[23] The resolution function is usually shaped like a Gaussian function, and the width of this function at 50 percent of the maximum value is the FWHM. *C.* The vessel size is measured as a function of distance along the length of the vessel from which measurements of vessel morphology can be obtained. (Images courtesy of Yang Chen, M.S.)

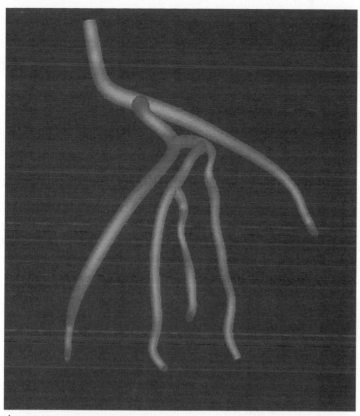

A

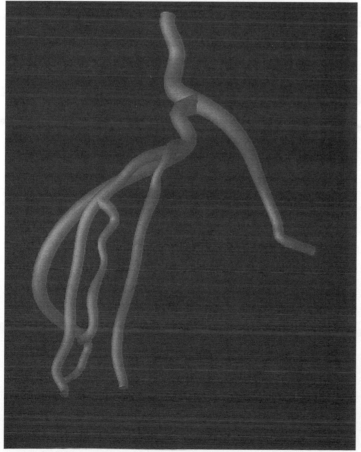
B

FIGURE 12-9   Three-dimensional coronary trees. Three-dimensional visualization or quantitation of the vascular tree can be obtained with stereoscopic imaging.[24] As images are acquired, the x-ray source alternates between two positions separated by approximately 2 to 6 cm. When the two images are viewed together, with each eye looking at a different one of the two stereoscopic images, the eye-brain system can perceive the 3D relationships between the vessels. When the stereoscopic images are digitized, the vessels can be tracked and the centerline position of the vessels in the images determined.[25] From these positions and the known stereoscopic imaging geometry, the 3D positions of the vessel centerlines can be determined.[26] The 3D positions and the measured vessel sizes can then be used for rendering the 3D vasculature at arbitrary projection angles. The right anterior oblique (RAO) (*A*) and 45° from RAO (*B*) projections of the left coronary tree are generated by the computer after determination of the 3D positions by means of vessel tracking and correlation of the vessels in the tree and knowledge of the imaging geometry. In the second projection, the several vessels overlap, which can hinder diagnosis. With the 3D rendered tree, projections can be identified with minimal obscuring of the vessels of interest, and the gantry can be positioned for that acquisition geometry. Techniques have also been developed to determine 3D vascular positions from biplane views, from which 3D renderings can also be generated. In addition, methods have been developed to determine the "triple-orthogonal axis," i.e., the axis that is perpendicular to the vessel centerline in the two views.[27] (*See color Plate 41A and B.*)

VENTRICULAR ANALYSIS

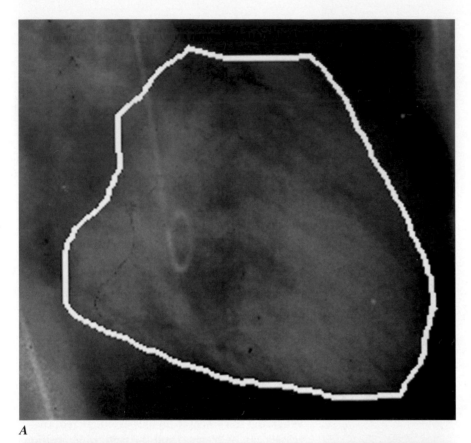

A

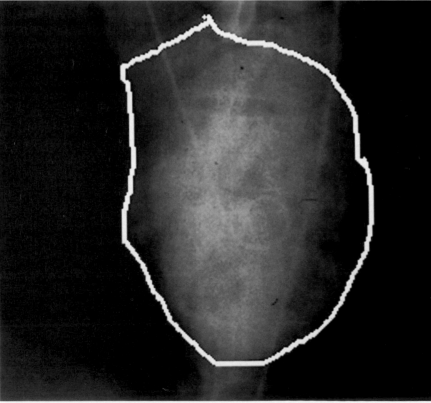

B

FIGURE 12-10 Quantitative ventricular measurements from biplane ventriculography. Ventriculography is often used to assess heart function. Images are acquired as contrast material is injected into the ventricle either in a single-plane or biplane mode. From these images, motion can be appreciated qualitatively, or digital techniques can be applied to quantitate the motion of the ventricle. Quantitation of the motion requires first the detection of the ventricular boundaries either manually or automatically.[28] The right anterior oblique (*A*) and left anterior oblique (LAO) (*B*) views of the opacified ventricle, with the boundaries drawn using commercially available software are depicted. With the boundaries in a single projection, slicewise circular models or elliptical models of the ventricle (for single-plane or biplane acquisitions, respectively) can be employed to calculate the ventricular volume (see Fig. 12-11*C*). The stroke volume is then calculated as the volumetric differences at diastole and systole.

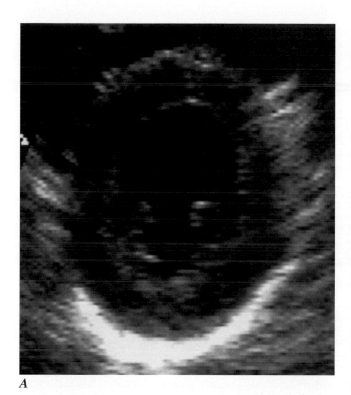

A

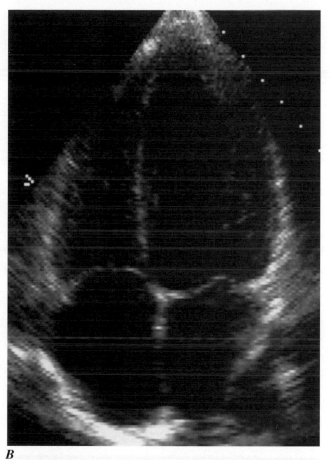

B

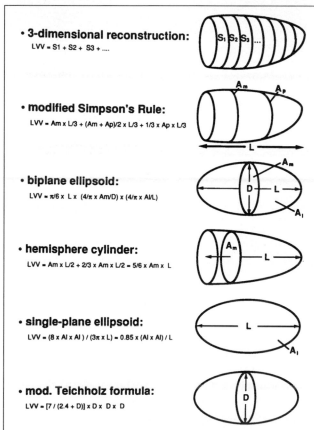

C

FIGURE 12-11 Ventricular volume measurements based on echocardiographic imaging. Echocardiography is a tomographic technique in which cross-sectional images of the heart are obtained. Ventricular volumes are frequently measured in echocardiography by acquiring cross sections of the heart at one or more orientations, such as the short (*A*) and long (*B*) axis images of the heart. With these cross sections, models are used for calculating ventricular volumes. *C*. The algorithm and formula for geometric models for determination of left ventricular (LV) volumes. Al = cross-sectional area of the LV cavity in the horizontal long-axis planes; Am = cross-sectional area of the LV cavity in the selected short-axis planes, approximately 1 cm below the leaflets of the mitral valve; Ap = cross-sectional area of the LV cavity in the selected short-axis plane, approximately at the base of the papillary muscles; D = diameter of the LV cavity, approximately 1 cm below the leaflets of the mitral valve in the selected short-axis plane; L = longest length of the LV cavity in the horizontal long-axis plane; LVV = LV volumes. (From Dulce MC, Mostbeck CH, Friese KK, et al: Quantification of the left ventricular volumes and function with cine MR imaging: Comparison of geometric models with three-dimensional data. *Radiology* 1993; 188:371–376. Reproduced with permission from the publisher and authors.)

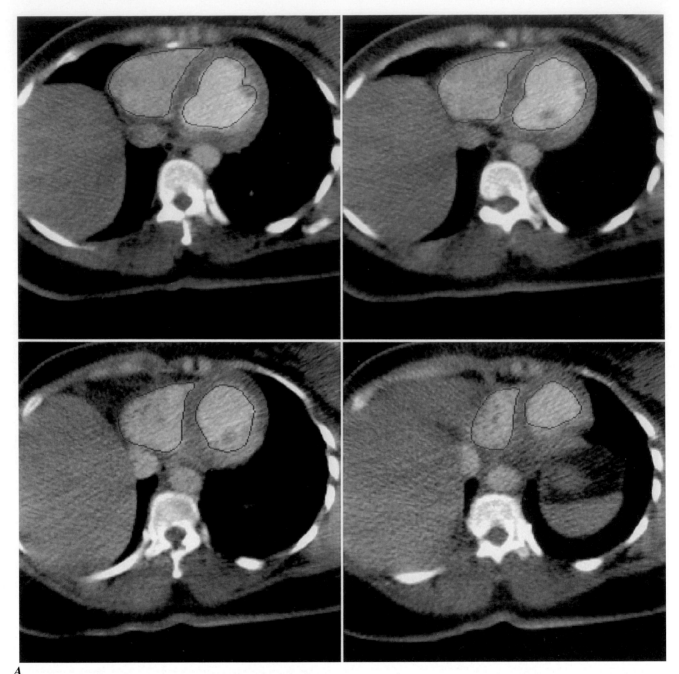

A

FIGURE 12-12 **Three-dimensional extraction and rendering of the ventricular surface. When cross-sectional images of the heart are obtained, the various levels of the heart can be inspected visually. Because CT and MRI are digital modalities, quantitative techniques can be applied. In particular, the ventricular regions can be identified using boundary-detection techniques. *A*. Individual contours (*red*) extracted semiautomatically from EBCT using an adaptive segmentation algorithm.[29,30] These contours can be stacked (*B*) and interpolated (*C*) or the surface can be shaded (*D*) to give a 3D perspective of the ventricular and aortic surfaces. *E*. When the boundaries of the epicardium are also obtained, volume-rendering techniques can be employed to render the cardiac structures for visualization. From such data, ventricular or myocardial volumes can be calculated by summing the areas of the individual regions and multiplying by the slice thickness (Simpson's rule). (From Chen SY, Carroll JD, Chen CT, et al: Three-dimensional ventricle reconstruction from serial cross sections. *Proc SPIE* 1993; 1905:93–99. Reproduced with permission from the publisher and authors.) (*See color Plate 42A–E.*)**

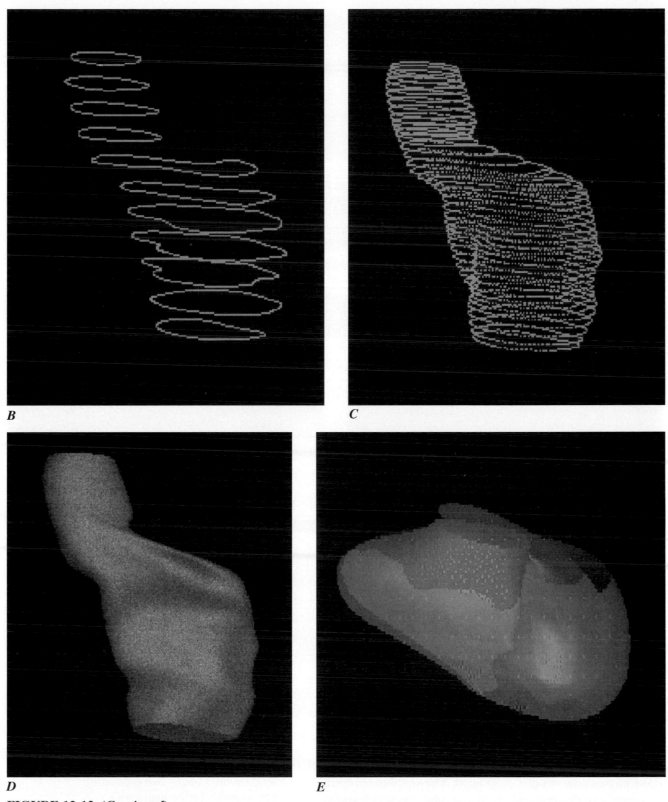

B

C

D

E

FIGURE 12-12 *(Continued)*

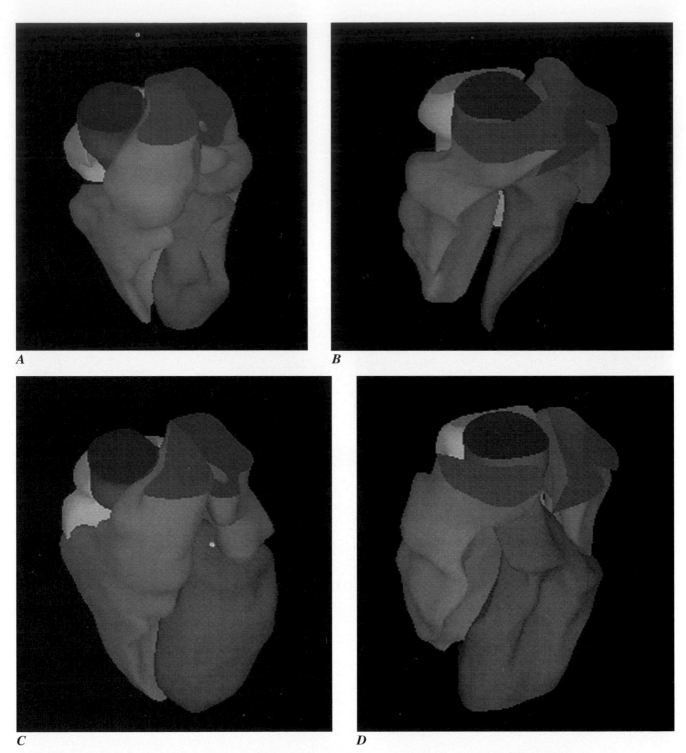

A

B

C

D

FIGURE 12-13　Ventricular motion from EBCT. Cardiac images are usually obtained at various phases of the cardiac cycle. Thus, the ventricular or myocardial surfaces can be rendered for each of these phases and volumes calculated. The standard procedure is to analyze the images corresponding to systole and diastole and to calculate the ejection fraction or visualize ventricular or heart wall motion. The ventricles can be rendered from EBCT images obtained at end-diastole and end-systole. Illustrated are a normal heart at end-diastole (*A*) and end-systole (*B*), and a heart with dilated cardiomyopathy at end-diastole (*C*) and end-systole (*D*). With the 3D-rendered surfaces, the difference in the volume of the left ventricle of the two hearts at end-diastole is readily apparent. By comparing the changes between end-diastole and end-systole for the two hearts, the reduction of motion (or change of volume) for the heart with dilated cardiomyopathy is also apparent. (*See color Plate 43A–D.*)

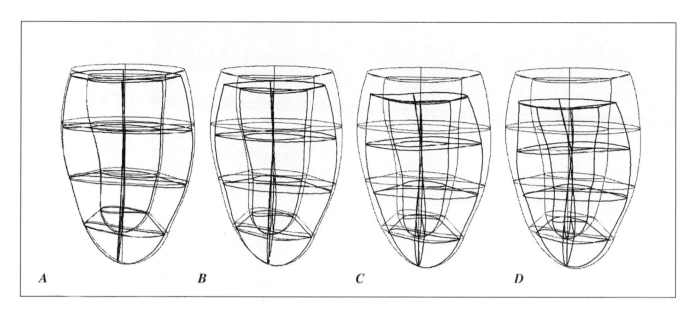

A   B   C   D

FIGURE 12-14   Ventricular motion from MRI. With EBCT, individual points in the myocardium cannot be tracked directly. Thus, local motion of the heart muscle cannot be determined. However, using spatial modulation of magnetization (SPAMM),[31] individual points in the myocardium can be tracked as a function of time and can provide useful kinematics and motion data. From these data, myocardial stress and strain can be calculated.[32] While out-of-plane motion cannot be directly tracked with this technique, methods are being developed to estimate this component of the motion.[33] Because of the multidimensional nature of the data, spatial and temporal, wire frame displays facilitate interpretation. In this figure, the deformation fits for five time points during the cardiac cycle are shown. To facilitate visualization of the change in the myocardial shape during the cycle, the mycardial boundaries and connecting points at time point 1 are shown in each figure (A–D) by a series of connected broken lines. The myocardial boundaries and connecting points at time points 2–5 are shown by a series of connected solid lines in A–D, respectively. The viewpoint is slightly elevated and in front of the septum. Using such renderings and by viewing them for a number of time points in the cardiac cycle, features, such as the anisotropy of the contraction of the heart, can be appreciated. (From Young AA, Axel L: Three-dimensional motion and deformation of the heart wall: Estimation with spatial modulation of magnetization—A model-based approach. *Radiology* 1992; 185:241–247. Reproduced with permission from the publisher and the authors.)

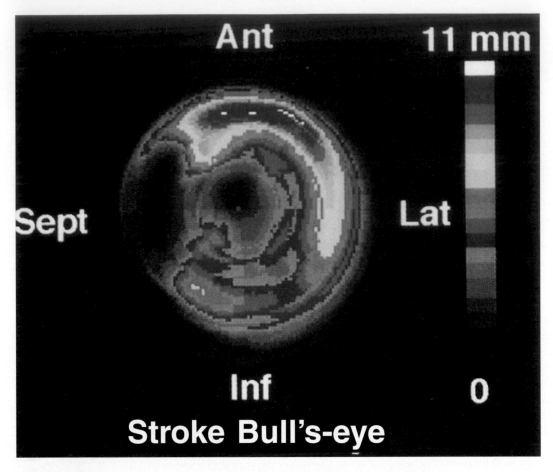

FIGURE 12-15 Ventricular motion from PET. Methods have also been developed for measurement of wall motion from PET data. An ECG/seven-slice PET series was obtained using ^{15}O-carbon monoxide; the slice spacing was 14.2 mm, and the transaxial spatial resolution was 8.5 mm. By calculating the difference between the end-systolic data and end-diastolic data, "stroke" images were obtained. These data were then displayed using a polar bull's-eye display.[34,35] The results presented in this figure indicate that the patient had poor wall motion centered at the apex (center of the bull's-eye) and in the septal region, with good motion in the basal and lateral regions. Although PET studies do not have the spatial resolution of EBCT or MRI, PET can provide metabolic information (see Fig. 12-17) currently unavailable with the other modalities. (From Miller TR, Wallis JW, Landy BR, et al: Measurement of global and regional left ventricular function by cardiac PET. *J Nucl Med* 1994; 35:999–1005. Reproduced with permission from the publisher and authors.) (*See color Plate 44*. See also Chap. 8.)

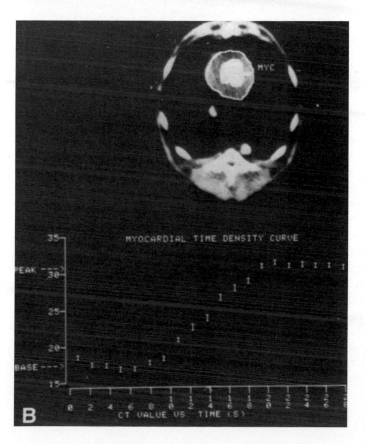

MYOCARDIAL PERFUSION

FIGURE 12-16 Determination of myocardial perfusion. In addition to motion, perfusion of the cardiac muscle or regions of it is a useful indicator of cardiac function (e.g., late arrival times indicate possible stenoses in the feeder vessels, and long washout times indicate poor perfusion of the muscle). With the regions identified in the images acquired during the phases of the heart cycle temporal variations in CT number can be measured and plotted as time-density curves. *A*. Ventricular time-density curve. *B*. Myocardial time-density curve. These data can then be analyzed for each of the regions of the heart to calculate the temporal progression of perfusion of the heart muscle for evaluation of ischemia. (From Wolfkiel CJ, Ferguson JL, Chomka EV, et al: Measurement of myocardial blood flow by ultrafast computed tomography. *Circulation* 1987; 76:1262–1273. Reproduced with permission from the publisher and authors.)

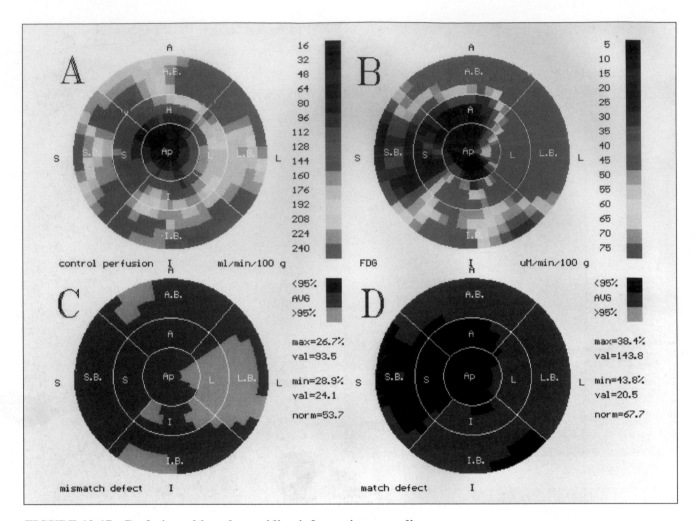

FIGURE 12-17 Perfusion, although providing information regarding ischemia, may not reflect the functional health of a region of the heart muscle. Studies with radio-isotope labeled [18]FDG (fluorodeoxyglucose) can provide information on glucose consumption and thereby metabolic function. Parametric polar maps of myocardial perfusion (*A*) and glucose consumption (*B*). The color scales pertinent to the maps are displayed to the right. In the bottom panel at left (*C*), the mismatch map is displayed as the ratio of *B* and *A*. In the map, the regions exceeding the 95 percent confidence interval are displayed in light green (increased [18]FDG uptake related to perfusion), the remainder in blue. At right, in the bottom panel (*D*), the match map is displayed. This is obtained by multiplying *A* and *B* and normalizing for mean flow. The match defect is the region below the 95 percent confidence interval (concomitant low perfusion and [18]FDG uptake) and displayed in black, the remainder in blue. In the right portion of *C* and *D*, the percentages of the myocardium that lie within, below, and above the 95 percent confidence interval are indicated along with their values. This example is from a patient with extensive myocardial infarction in the anteroseptal region and ischemia in the posterolateral and inferior regions. (From Blanksma PK, Willemsen ATM, Meeder JG, et al: Quantitative myocardial mapping of perfusion and metabolism using parametric polar map displays in cardiac PET. *J Nucl Med* 1995; 36:153–158. Reproduced with permission from the publisher and authors.) (*See color Plate 45.*)

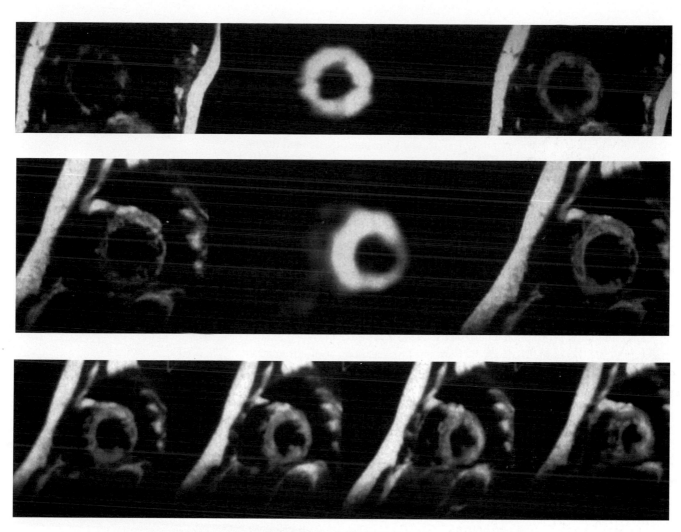

FIGURE 12-18   The different modalities often present complementary data, which must be integrated in the cardiologist's mind. Computational methods have been developed to facilitate this image integration when digital data are available. To integrate data, they are first registered (i.e., the corresponding regions in the two image sets must be made to overlap accurately). Registration can be performed with the individual planes of data. However, the different acquisitions are usually not obtained with the exact same imaging geometry; in addition, out-of-plane motion of the heart may further frustrate registration and thereby comparison of the image data. Thus, registration of the 3D data sets is required. Faber and colleagues[19] have developed techniques for registration of 3D single photon emission computed tomography (SPECT) and MR image sets of the heart. After registration, the information from the two modalities is combined by using the MRI to indicate anatomy as a gray scale image and the SPECT information as a color wash. The results are shown here. *Top*: One section of cardiac MR image is on the left, the corresponding section from the registered SPECT image is in the middle, and the fused image combining the MR and SPECT images is on the right. Note the uniformity of perfusion. These images are from a healthy subject. *Middle*: Registration and fusion of images from a subject with coronary artery disease. The MR image is on the left, the stress perfusion SPECT image is in the middle, and the fused image is on the right. Note the perfusion abnormality in the lateral wall, corresponding to an infarction. *Bottom*: Multiple frames of the rest study from the first subject. Fused short axis sections from end diastole (*left*) to end systole (*right*). (From Faber TL, McColl RW, Opperman RM, et al: Spatial and temporal registration of cardiac SPECT and MR images: Methods and evaluation. *Radiology* 1991; 179:857–861. Reproduced with permission from the publisher and authors.) (*See color Plate 46*.)

REFERENCES

1. Pratt WK: *Digital Image Processing*. New York, Wiley, 1978.
2. Castleman KR: *Digital Image Processing*. Englewood Cliffs, NJ, Prentice-Hall, 1979.
3. Brown BG, Bolson E, Frimer M, Dodge HT: Quantitative coronary arteriography: Estimation of dimensions, hemodynamic resistance, and atheroma mass of coronary artery lesions using the anteriogram and digital computation. *Circulation* 1977; 55:229–337.
4. Haase J, DiMario C, Slager CJ, et al: In-vivo validation of on-line and off-line geometric coronary measurements using insertion of stenosis phantoms in porcine coronary arteries. *Cathet Cardiovasc Diagn* 1982; 27:16–27.
5. Kruger RA: Estimation of the diameter of and iodine concentration within blood vessels using digital radiography devices. *Med Phys* 1981; 8:652–658.
6. Fujita H, Doi K, Fencil LE: Image feature analysis and computer-aided diagnosis in digital radiography: 2. Computerized determination of vessel sizes in digital subtraction angiography. *Med Phys* 1987; 14:549–556.
7. Lipton MJ, Hayashi TT, Body D, Carlsson E: Measurement of left ventricular cast volume by computed tomography. *Radiology* 1978; 127:419–424.
8. Reiter SJ, Rumberger JA, Feiring AJ, et al: Precision of measurements of right and left ventricular volume by cine computed tomography. *Circulation* 1986; 74:890–900.
9. Dodge HT, Sandler H, Ballew DW, Lord JD Jr: The use of biplane angiocardiography for the measurement of left ventricular volume in man. *Am Heart J* 1960; 60:762–778.
10. Zerhouni EA, Parish DM, Rogers WF, et al: Human heart: Tagging with MR imaging—A method for noninvasive assessment of myocardial motion. *Radiology* 1988; 169:59–63.
11. Pelc NJ, Herfkens RJ, Pelc LR, et al: Three-dimensional motion analysis by means of phase-contrast cine MRI. *Radiology* 1991; 181P:218.
12. Dulce MC, Mostbeck GH, Friese KK, et al: Quantification of the left ventricular volumes and function with cine MR imaging: Comparison of geometric models with three-dimensional data. *Radiology* 1993; 188:371–376.
13. Axel L, Goncalves RC, Bloomgarden D: Regional heart wall motion: Two-dimensional analysis and functional imaging with MR imaging. *Radiology* 1992; 183:745–750.
14. Dumay ACM, Minderhoud H, Gerbrands JJ, et al: Three-dimensional reconstruction of myocardial contrast perfusion from biplane cine-angiograms by means of linear programming techniques. *Int J Cardiol Imaging* 1988; 3:141–152.
15. Gould RG: Perfusion quantitation by ultrafast computed tomography. *Invest Radiol* 1992; 27:S18–S21.
16. Pope DL, Parker DL, Clayton PD, Gustafson DE: Left ventricular border determination using a dynamic search algorithm. *Radiology* 1985; 155:513–518.
17. Wolfkiel CJ, Ferguson JL, Chomka EV, et al: Measurement of myocardial blood flow by ultrafast computed tomography. *Circulation* 1987; 76:1262–1273.

18. Blanksma PK, Willemsen ATM, Meeder JG, et al: Quantitative myocardial mapping of perfusion and metabolism using parametric polar map displays in cardiac PET. *J Nucl Med* 1995; 36:153–158.

19. Faber TL, McColl RW, Opperman RM, et al: Spatial and temporal registration of cardiac SPECT and MR images: Methods and evaluation. *Radiology* 1991; 179:857–861.

20. Chu CH, Delp EJ, Buda AJ: Detecting left ventricular endocardial and epicardial boundaries by digital two-dimensional echocardiography. *IEEE Trans Med Imaging* 1988; 7:81–90.

21. Feng J, Lin WC, Chen CT: Automatic left ventricular boundary detection in digital two-dimensional echocardiography using fuzzy reasoning techniques. *Proceedings of the SPIE Conference on Biomedical Image Processing*. 1990; 1245:19–105.

22. Zir LM, Miller SW, Dinsmore RE, et al: Interobserver variability in coronary angiography. *Circulation* 1976; 53:627–632.

23. Metz CE, Doi K: Transfer function analysis of radiographic imaging systems. *Phys Med Biol* 1979; 24:1079–1106.

24. Doi K, Patronas NJ, Duda EE, et al: X-ray imaging of the vessels to the brain by use of magnification stereoscopic technique. In: Carney AL, Anderson EM (eds): *Advances in Neurology*. New York, Raven Press, 1981; pp. 175–189.

25. Hoffmann KR, Doi K, Chen SH, Chan HP: Automated tracking and computer reproduction of vessels in DSA images. *Invest Radiol* 1990; 25:1069–1075.

26. Hoffmann KR, Doi K, Chan HP, Takamiya M: Three-dimensional reproduction of coronary vascular trees using the double-square-box method of tracking. *Proc SPIE* 1988; 914:375–378.

27. Wollschlaeger H, Zeiher AM, Lee P, et al: Computed triple orthogonal projections for optimal radiological imaging with biplane isocentric multidirectional x-ray systems. *Proc Comp Cardiol* 1987; 185–188.

28. Slager CJ, Hooghoudt TEH, Serruys PW, et al: Automated quantification of left ventricular angiograms. In: Short MD et al (eds): *Physical Techniques in Cardiological Imaging*. Bristol, England, Hilger, 1982; pp. 163–172.

29. Chen SY, Lin WC, Chen CT: Split-and-merge image segmentation based on localized feature histograms and statistical inference. *CVGIP: Graphical Methods Image Processing* 1991; 53:457–475.

30. Chen SY, Carroll JD, Chen CT, et al: Three-dimensional ventricle reconstruction from serial cross sections. *Proc SPIE* 1993; 195:93–99.

31. Axel L, Goncalves R, Bloomgarden D: Regional heart wall motion: Two dimensional analysis and functional imaging with MR imaging. *Radiology* 1992; 183:745–750.

32. Young AA, Axel L: Three-dimensional motion and deformation of the heart wall: Estimation with spatial modulation of magnetization—A model-based approach. *Radiology* 1992; 185:241–247.

33. Rogers WJ, Shapiro EP, Weiss JL, et al: Quantification of and correction for left ventricular systolic long axis shortening by magnetic resonance tissue tagging and slice isolation. *Circulation* 1991; 84:721–731.

34. Garcia EV, VanTrain K, Haddahi J: Quantification of rotational thallium-201 myocardial tomography. *J Nucl Med* 1985; 26:17–26.

35. Miller TR, Starren JB, Brothe RB: Three-dimensional display of positron emission tomography of the heart. *J Nucl Med* 1988; 29:530–537.

36. Miller TR, Wallis JW, Landy BR, et al: Measurement of global and regional left ventricular function by cardiac PET. *J Nucl Med* 1994; 35:999–1005.

CHAPTER 13

CORONARY ANGIOSCOPY

James S. Forrester, M.D.

Robert J. Siegel, M.D.

Frank Litvack, M.D.

Neal L. Eigler, M.D.

F OR interventional cardiologists and vascular surgeons, angioscopy provides unique information that is different from and complementary to that from both intravascular ultrasound and angiography. The interventional cardiologist can determine the etiology of unstable coronary chest pain syndromes, assess the trauma created by angioplasty, determine the appropriateness of stent placement, and evaluate the completeness of thrombolysis. Vascular surgeons can inspect anastomoses and determine the completeness of valvotomy and thrombectomy. Although angioscopy probably will not come into routine use in catheterization laboratories because decisions rarely depend on such information, it continues to have great value in clinical coronary research. In contrast, angioscopy is widely used by peripheral vascular surgeons for intraoperative decision making.

ANGIOSCOPIC TECHNOLOGY

Angioscopic fiberoptic instruments are composed of an inner core that conveys light and a surrounding cladding that traps the light within the inner core.[1,2] When the ratio between the refractive indices of the core and cladding material is appropriately chosen, light is completely reflected within the core, resulting in the transmission of light around bends with minimal loss of intensity. Individual fibers are assembled into a bundle such that each fiber forms one pixel of the intravascular image. A lens is attached to the distal end of the bundle to focus the output.

To steer the angioscope through tortuous vessels and center the lens in the vessel during imaging, monorail systems and balloons are used.[3] The balloon obstructs antegrade blood flow, allowing more prolonged imaging during flushing of blood from the imaging site. With these technologic advances, percutaneous intracoronary angioscopy can be performed with relative ease in the catheterization laboratory.[4,5]

ANALYSIS OF ANGIOSCOPIC IMAGES

Angioscopic images are classified using color, mass, and the surface characteristics of the vessel.[6–8] The normal vessel surface is smooth, white, and without masses (Figs. 13-1 and 13-2). Stable atheromas are white or yellow masses with a smooth surface (Figs. 13-3 and 13-4). Sites of intimal disruption have a torn surface without thrombus (Figs. 13-5 through 13-8). Thrombus appears as a red or white mass that partially or completely obstructs the lumen (Figs. 13-9 and 13-10; see also Table 13-1).

Angioscopy and angiography are complementary. Angioscopy is far superior for detecting localized damage (e.g., intimal tears, thrombosis) to the vessel surface; angiography is best for defining the magnitude of coronary luminal obstruction throughout the length of a vessel.[9–12] The differences between angioscopic and angiographic detection of thrombus are clearly related to the size of the lesion. Whereas angiography detects 100 percent of large angioscopic thrombi, it detects only 30 percent of small ones. Thus, the unique value of angioscopy is its superiority for detecting small- to medium-sized intracoronary thrombi and intimal disruptions that are undetectable by angiography. (See Table 13-2.)

Angioscopy has played a central role in defining the pathogenesis of acute ischemic syndromes. Whereas patients with stable angina have stable atheromas (Fig. 13-3), those with unstable angina typically have disrupted atheromas (Fig. 13-6) or partially occlusive thrombi.[13,14] Patients with acute myocardial infarction have totally occlusive thrombi[15] (Fig. 13-10). After infarction, the thrombus frequently disappears at 1 to 6 weeks, leaving a plaque that gradually returns to a stable appearance. Among patients with unstable angina, 71 percent have gray-white thrombi, whereas virtually all of the

TABLE 13-1
Classification of Native Lesions in Coronary Arteries

	Normal	Stable Atheroma	Disrupted	Thrombus
Surface	Smooth	Smooth	Torn	Smooth
Color	White	White or yellow	White or yellow[a]	Red
Mass	None	Obstructs lumen	Usually	Obstructs or occludes

[a]Some disrupted surfaces have subintimal hemorrhage.

TABLE 13-2

Limitations of Angioscopy and Angiography

Angioscopy	Angiography
Length of vessel examined is limited	Major damage is often undetectable
Quantitative measurements are impractical	Underestimates complex lesion morphology
Interpretation is subjective	Does not detect small thrombi
Difficult to perform in tortuous vessels	Does not identify plaque composition

patients with acute infarction had red thrombi.[16] This angioscopic observation suggests that the thrombi in unstable angina are older and more platelet-rich.

ANGIOSCOPY DURING CORONARY INTERVENTIONS

In the catheterization laboratory, the interventional cardiologist deals with acute closure due to arterial dissection and/or thrombosis (Fig. 13-8). Angioplasty damages the blood vessel surface in ways that are largely undetectable by angiography.[4] Since some of this damage (e.g., undetected partial thrombosis) may be correctable, angioscopy could provide a means for reducing the rate of both acute complications and late restenosis. Angioscopy also has been used to evaluate the effect of new interventional devices, including excimer and holmium YAG lasers and extraction atherectomy.[5,17–19] These studies reveal that the magnitude of procedure-induced injury is comparable to that created by balloon angioplasty. Flaps, fractures, and abundant tissue remnants are common. (See also Chap. 9.)

Angioscopy has also been used during and after the placement of coronary stents. Investigators have reported that angioscopy influenced their clinical management in 30 to 50 percent of their cases.[20–23] The great majority of these cases involved detection of unsuspected thrombus or withholding of thrombolytic therapy in patients with suspected thrombus. Serial angioscopy reveals absence of a neointimal layer at 8 to 18 days and its uniform presence at 65 to 142 days.[24] Although it now seems likely that routine stent placement will not require both intravascular ultrasound and angioscopy, angioscopy may find a role among the choices of interventional devices in some clinical subsets (e.g., vein graft stenosis) or when stent placement is difficult.

ANGIOSCOPY DURING CARDIAC AND VASCULAR SURGERY

Angioscopy has been used sparingly during coronary vascular surgery and extensively in peripheral vascular surgery. The value of angioscopy during cardiac surgery remains undefined. On the one hand, unexpected pathologic abnormalities can be detected, albeit in low prevalence. On the other, the added time and minimal risk associated with intraoperative angioscopy suggest that it is unlikely to be used routinely. In contrast, angioscopy has clear value in peripheral vascular surgery. Most authors report changes in intraoperative management based on angioscopic findings in about 25 percent of cases.[25–28] Follow-up studies suggest that angioscopic evaluation may significantly alter long-term outcomes. By the use of life-table analysis, the patency rate for patients in whom angioscopy was used was 62 percent at 1 year, compared to 44 percent in patients in whom it was not.[29] Because angioscopy alters both intraoperative decisions and probably also long-term outcomes, it probably will have an expanding role in peripheral vascular surgery.

In summary, flexible, steerable angioscopes with diameters suitable for coronary use provide unique information about the surface of coronary vessels. Although interpretation of images is subjective, angioscopic image analysis is reasonably accurate and reproducible when compared to histopathologic data. Angioscopy consistently detects clinically important intimal disruption and partially occlusive thrombosis that is undetectable by angiography. Images before and after atherectomy as well as balloon and laser angioplasty indicate that angioplasty causes severe trauma that is not detected by angiography. These data provide insight into the mechanisms responsible for angioplasty-induced acute closure and restenosis. Finally, although the value of angioscopy continues to stem from its ability to clarify the pathogenesis of a broad spectrum of vascular syndromes, it has direct relevance to clinical decision making in selected clinical subsets.

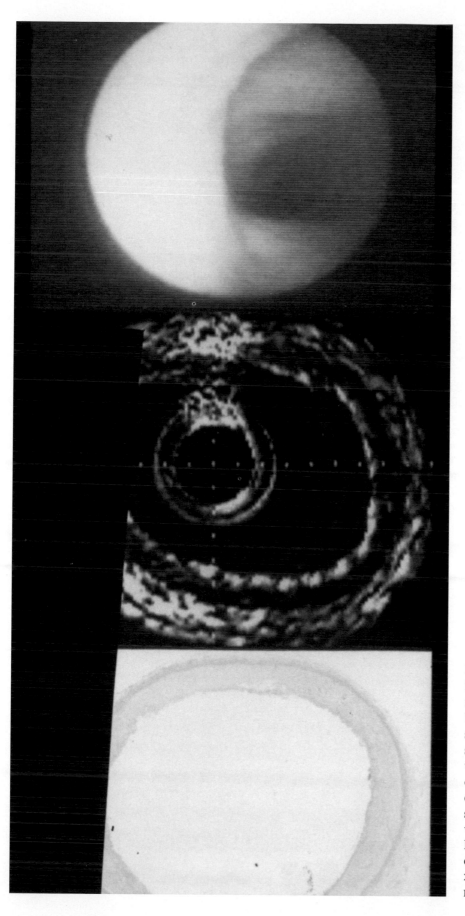

FIGURE 13-1   Angioscopic, intravascular ultrasound, and microscopic images of the normal blood vessel surface. The angioscopic image shows a white, smooth, flat surface. The intravascular ultrasound image reveals circular vessel with normal echodensity, smooth luminal surface, and normal thickness with a "three-ringed" appearance. Microscopy (hematoxylin and eosin stain, original magnification × 2) demonstrates a normal muscular artery.

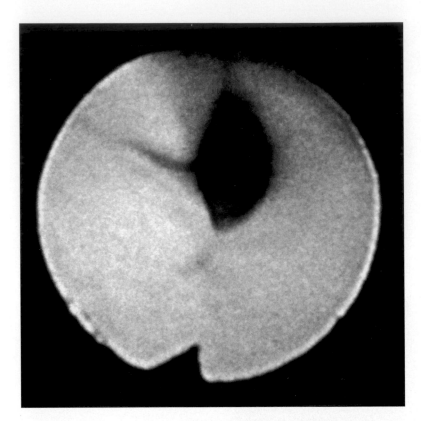

FIGURE 13-2 An 84-year-old woman underwent a femoral popliteal bypass with a composite graft comprising a reverse saphenous vein and a cephalic vein. This is an image of a typical normal blood vessel surface as seen by angioscopy. There are two vessel segments: the distal anastomosis and the outflow tract. Both vessels are white, smooth, and flat.

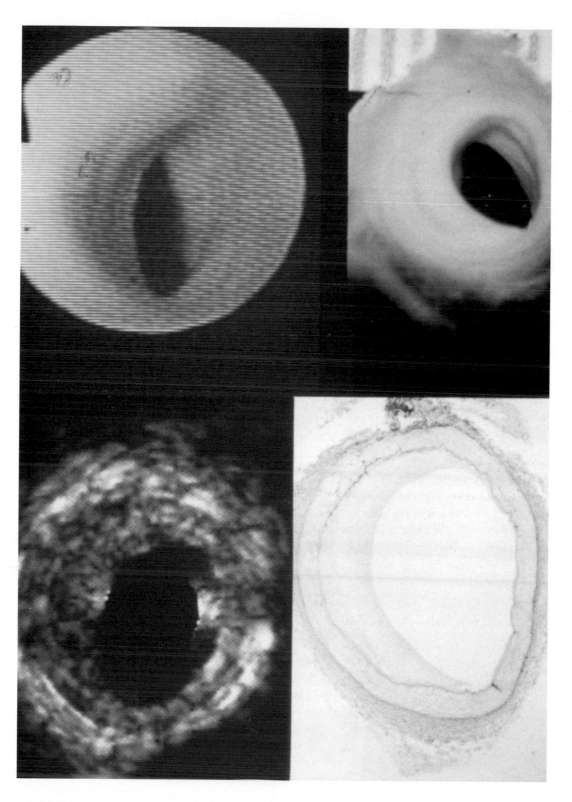

FIGURE 13-3   A stable atheroma. The angioscopic image shows a yellow mass with a smooth surface; the lumen is elliptical. The intravascular ultrasound image reveals increased wall thickness from 3 to 9 o'clock and a smooth luminal surface. Gross pathology and histology (hematoxylin and eosin stain, original magnification × 2) demonstrate an eccentric fibrous plaque in the area of increased wall thickness.

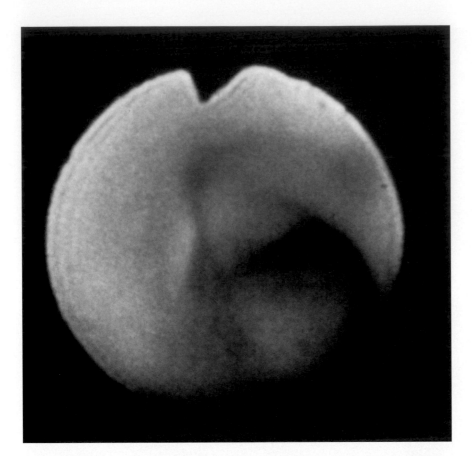

FIGURE 13-4   A stable atheroma in vivo as seen by angioscopy. A 68-year-old man presented with stable angina. He had multivessel disease by angiography, was unresponsive to medical therapy over a 12-h period, and was sent to bypass surgery. This lesion in the proximal left anterior descending coronary artery is smooth and yellow; it partially occludes the coronary lumen.

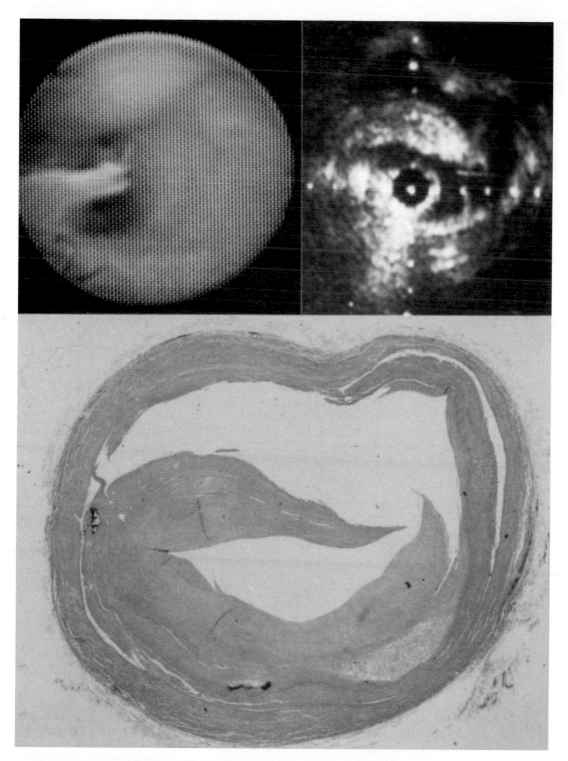

**FIGURE 13-5   A typical intimal disruption. The angioscopic and
ultrasound images demonstrate separation of plaque from the arterial wall.
These findings are confirmed by microscopy (hematoxylin and eosin stain,
original magnification × 2).**

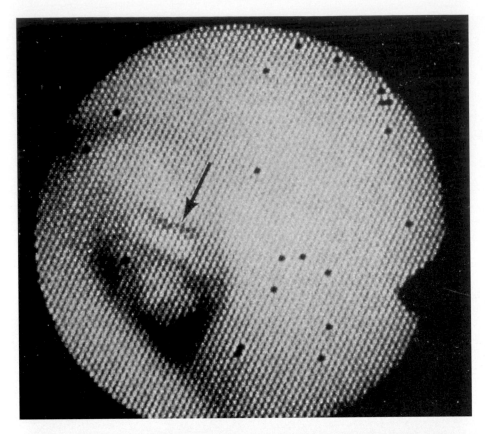

FIGURE 13-6 This image is from a 72-year-old man with unstable angina who was unresponsive to medical therapy, which included aspirin, a beta blocker, and a calcium antagonist. Angiography revealed no thrombi or intimal disruption. Angioscopy, however, revealed a disrupted atheroma in the left anterior descending coronary artery. This disruption was undetectable in multiple angiographic views. (*See color Plate 47.*)

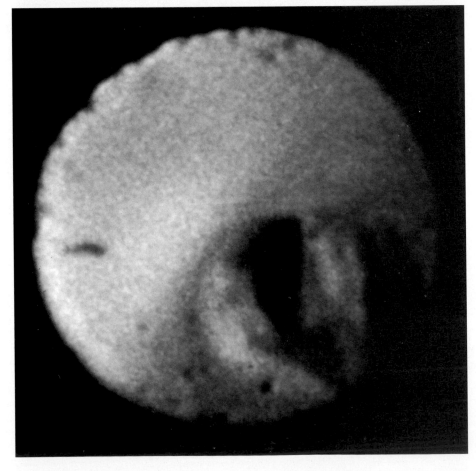

FIGURE 13-7 A 74-year-old diabetic woman underwent an in situ femoral-popliteal bypass. This is an angioscopic image of a partially disrupted venous valve after initial valvotomy. (*See color Plate 48.*)

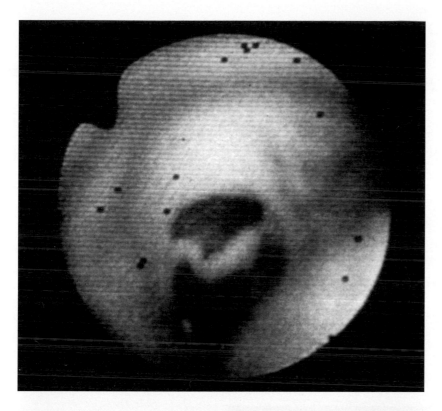

FIGURE 13-8 This image is from a 52-year-old man with severe stable angina who had acute closure during balloon angioplasty. Angiography revealed a long spiral dissection. By angioscopy, there is severe intimal change caused by the balloon angioplasty. The image shows the double lumen created by the dissection as well as subintimal hemorrhage. (*See color Plate 49.*)

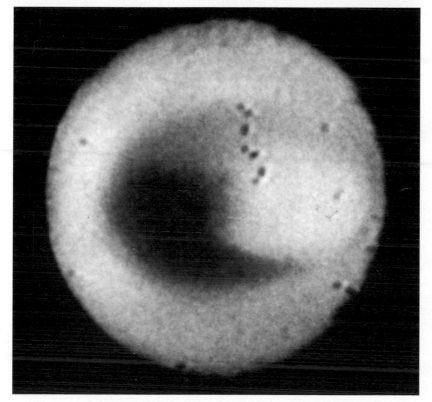

FIGURE 13-9 This image is from the left anterior coronary artery of a 68-year-old woman with acute unstable angina pectoris at rest that was unresponsive to medical therapy. There is a crescent-shaped, fresh, partially occlusive coronary thrombosis. The surface of the clot undulated during routine flushing to clear blood from the imaging field. Coronary thrombi are typically adherent and do not dislodge during flushing. (*See color Plate 50.*)

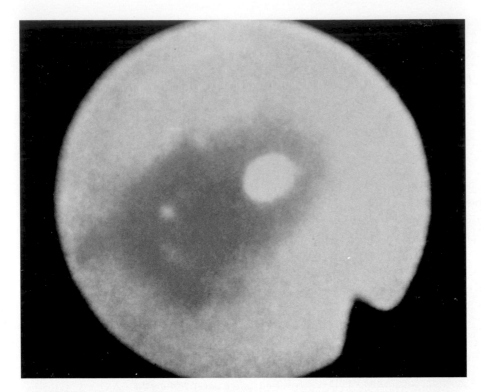

FIGURE 13-10   A 70-year-old woman with known coronary artery disease presented with unrelenting chest pain of 4 h duration. Acute myocardial infarction was documented by electrocardiography and enzymes. Angioscopy revealed a completely occlusive coronary thrombosis in the left anterior descending coronary artery. The angioscope is very close to the thrombus. The vessel walls are outside the field of view. The central white spot is the angioscope's imaging light reflected back off the glistening thrombus. (*See color Plate 51.*)

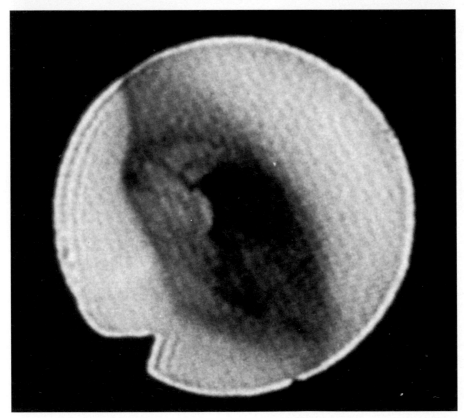

FIGURE 13-11   A 56-year-old man was studied by angioscopy 2 weeks after transmural myocardial infarction. The image reveals an atheroma with residual disruption but without thrombosis. The patient had not been treated with a thrombolytic agent. Thus, this is an example of spontaneous endogenous thrombolysis after presumed coronary occlusion. (*See color Plate 52.*)

REFERENCES

1. Katzir A: Optical fibers in medicine. *Sci Am* 1989; 120–125.
2. Auth D: Physical principles and limitations of fiberoptic angioscopy. In: Moore WS, Ahn SS (eds): *Endovascular Surgery*. Philadelphia, Saunders, 1989, pp. 31–38.
3. Franzen D, Hopp HW, Korsten J, Hilger HH: A prospective study on percutaneous coronary angioscopy with different guiding techniques in patients with coronary heart disease. *Eur Heart J* 1992; 13:655–660.
4. den Heijer P, van Dijk RB, Hillege HL, Pentinga ML: Serial angioscopic and angiographic observations during the first hour after successful coronary angioplasty: A preamble to a multicenter trial addressing angioscopic markers for restenosis. *Am Heart J* 1994; 128:656–663.
5. Larrazet FS, Dupouy PJ, Rande JL, Hirosaka A: Angioscopy after laser and balloon coronary angioplasty. *J Am Coll Cardiol* 1994; 23:1321–1326.
6. Siegel RJ, Ariani M, Fishbein MC, et al: Histopathologic validation of angioscopy and intravascular ultrasound. *Circulation* 1991; 84:109–117.
7. den Heijer P, Foley DP, Hillege HL, Lablanche JM: The d'Ermonville classification of observations at coronary angioscopy—Evaluation of intra- and inter-observer agreement. European Working Group on Coronary Angioscopy. *Eur Heart J* 1994; 15:815–822.
8. Schwartz A, Burrig KF, Aulich A: Usefulness of angioscopy in stenotic processes of the carotid—A comparison with morphological findings. *Endoscopy* 1988; 20:107–110.
9. Van Stiegman G, Perace W, Bartle, E, et al: Flexible angioscopy seems faster and more specific than arteriography. *Arch Surg* 1987; 122:279–283.
10. Johnson C, Hansen D, Vracko R, Ritchie J: Angioscopy—more sensitive for identifying thrombus, distal emboli, and subintimal dissection. *J Am Coll Cardiol* 1989; 13:146A.
11. den Heijer P, Foley DR, Escaned J, Hillege HL: Angioscopic versus angiographic detection of intimal dissection and intracoronary thrombus. *J Am Coll Cardiol* 1994; 24:649–654.
12. Mizuno K, Yanagida T, Shibuya T, Arakawa K: The effectiveness of coronary angioscopy in detecting intraluminal pathologic changes. *Jpn Circ J* 1992; 56:586–591.
13. Sherman CT, Litvack F, Grundfest W, et al: Demonstration of thrombus and complex atheroma by in-vivo angioscopy in patients with unstable angina pectoris. *N Engl J Med* 1986; 315:913–919.
14. Forrester J, Litvack F, Grundfest W, et al: Symposium: Intravascular imaging and flow: Cardiac angioscopy in acute ischemic syndromes. *Am J Cardiac Imaging* 1988; 2:178–184.
15. Mizuno K, Miyamoto A, Satomura K, et al: Angioscopic coronary macromorphology in patients with acute coronary disorders. *Lancet* 1991; 337:809–812.
16. Mizuno K, Satomura K, Miyamoto A, et al: Angioscopic evaluation of coronary-artery thrombi in acute coronary syndromes. *N Engl J Med* 1992; 326:287–291.
17. Nakamura F, Kvasnicka J, Uchida Y, Geschwind HJ: Percutaneous angioscopic evaluation of luminal changes induced by excimer laser angioplasty. *Am Heart J* 1992; 124:1467–1472.

18. Ito A, Miyazaki S, Nonogi H, et al: Angioscopic and intravascular ultrasound imagings before and after percutaneous holmium-YAG laser coronary angioplasty. *Am Heart J* 1993; 125:556–558.

19. Annex BH, Sketch MII Jr, Stack RS, Phillips HR: Transluminal extraction coronary atherectomy. *Cardiol Clin* 1994; 12:611–622.

20. Teirstein PS, Schatz RA, Wong SC, Rocha-Singh KJ: Coronary stenting with angioscopic guidance. *Am J Cardiol* 1995; 75:344–347.

21. Strumpf RK, Heuser RR, Eagan JT Jr: Angioscopy: A valuable tool in the deployment and evaluation of intracoronary stents. *Am Heart J* 1993; 126:1204–1210.

22. den Heijer P, van Dijk RB, Twisk SP, Lie K: Early stent occlusion is not always caused by thrombosis. *Cathet Cardiovasc Diagn* 1993; 29:136–140.

23. Resar JR, Brinker J: Early coronary artery stent restenosis: Utility of percutaneous coronary angioscopy. *Cathet Cardiovasc Diagn* 1992; 27:276–279.

24. Ueda Y, Nanto S, Komamura K, Kodama K: Neointimal coverage of stents in human coronary arteries observed by angioscopy. *J Am Coll Cardiol* 1994; 23:341–346.

25. Bessou JP, Melki J, Bouchart F, Mouton-Schleifer D, et al: Intraoperative coronary angioscopy—Technique and results: A study of 38 patients. *J Card Surg* 1993; 8:483–487.

26. White GH, Siegel SB, Colman PD, et al: Intraoperative coronary angioscopy: Development of practical techniques. *Angiology* 1990; 41:793–800.

27. Grundfest W, Litvack F, Glick D, et al: Intraoperative decisions based on angioscopy in peripheral vascular surgery. *Circulation* 1988; 78:113–117.

28. Dietrich EB, Yoffe B, Kiessling JJ, et al: Angioscopy in endovascular surgery: Recent technical advances to enhance intervention selection and failure analysis. *Angiology* 1992; 43:1–10.

29. Trubel W, Magoometschnigg H, al-Hachich Y, Staudacher M: Intraoperative control following femorodistal revascularization: Angioscopy is superior to angiography. *Thorac Cardiovasc Surg* 1994; 42:199–207.

INDEX